AF790828

Portraits of Human Monsters in the Renaissance

Monsters, Prodigies, and Demons:
Medieval and Early Modern Constructions of Alterity

SERIES EDITORS

Kathleen Perry Long
Cornell University

Luke Morgan
Monash University, Australia

SERIES ADVISORY BOARD

Elizabeth B. Bearden
University of Wisconsin

Maria Fabricius Hansen
University of Copenhagen

Jeffrey Jerome Cohen
George Washington University

Virginia A. Krause
Brown University

Surekha Davies
Western Connecticut State University

Jennifer Spinks
University of Melbourne

Richard H. Godden
Louisiana State University

Debra Higgs Strickland
University of Glasgow

Wes Williams
University of Oxford

See our website for further information on this series and its publications.

Medieval Institute Publications is a program of
The Medieval Institute, College of Arts and Sciences

WESTERN MICHIGAN UNIVERSITY

Portraits of Human Monsters in the Renaissance

Dwarves, Hirsutes, and Castrati as Idealized Anatomical Anomalies

Touba Ghadessi

Monsters, Prodigies, and Demons:
Medieval and Early Modern Constructions of Alterity

MEDIEVAL INSTITUTE PUBLICATIONS
Western Michigan University
Kalamazoo

Copyright © 2018 by the Board of Trustees of Western Michigan University

Publication is made possible in part by a gift from Elizabeth and Todd Warnock to the Department of Art History at Northwestern University.

Library of Congress Cataloguing-in-Publication Data are available from the Library of Congress.

ISBN 978-1-580442-75-6
e-ISBN 978-1-580442-76-3

All rights reserved. Without limiting the rights under copyright reserved above, no part of this book may be reproduced, stored in, or introduced into a retrieval system, or transmitted, in any form, or by any means (electronic, mechanical, photocopying, recording or otherwise) without the written permission of both the copyright owner and the author of the book.

Contents

List of Plates

List of Illustrations

Acknowledgements

THE PLEASURE OF ACKNOWLEDGING THE many institutions and people who made this book a reality is one I am delighted to welcome. This book would simply not have been written without their financial, intellectual, and personal support. I found extraordinary help wherever I conducted archival research. Specifically, I would like to thank the staff at the Archivio di Stato di Firenze; the Istituto e Museo della Storia della Scienza in the Palazzo Castellani in Florence; the Biblioteca Nazionale Centrale di Firenze; the Opificio delle Pietre Dure e Laboratori di Restauro in Florence; the Biblioteca Angelica in Rome; the Biblioteca Universitaria di Bologna; the Département des manuscrits anciens du site Richelieu de la Bibliothèque nationale de France; the Bibliothèque Interuniversitaire de Médecine de Paris; the Institut d'Histoire de la Médecine et de la Santé de Genève; the Musée des Beaux-Arts du Château de Blois; the Prints and Drawings Department and the European Paintings Department at the Metropolitan Museum of Art in New York; and the Pierpont Morgan Library in New York.

My home institution, Wheaton College in Massachusetts, contributed to my research in the form of grants from the Provost's Office and I thank Linda Eisenmann and Renée White for them. Many of my colleagues have been a part of this book in one form or another. Tripp Evans has a brilliant plume and I was the fortunate beneficiary of his generous reading. Leah Niederstadt, Daniel Becker, Kate Boylan, and Jessica Kuszaj hunted tirelessly for obscure images. James Mancall repeatedly made the impossible possible. My, then, research student Logan Hinderliter tracked countless references with much patience. We are now intellectual partners at the Rhode Island Council for the Humanities where I have the enviable position of regularly being in conversations with fascinating people who are changing the world. The Providence reading group—Fran de Alba, Yuen-Gen Liang, James Mulholland, Rolf Nelson, and Gail Sahar—provided me with stimulating discussions and friendship, as did Josh Stenger.

As a graduate student thinking about the ideas that, eventually, formed the core of this book, I was privileged to benefit from the incredible academic environment of Northwestern University. The Art History department helped shape the thoughts that led to this book and, in the end, supported its publication through a generous gift from Elizabeth and Todd Warnock brought to my attention by Jesús Escobar, to whom I am thankful. There, not only did I study with formidable professors—Claudia Swan, Hollis

Clayson, and David van Zanten's knowledge and generosity are unmatched—but my peers also were and still are the most amazing cheerleaders: Leah Boston, Laura Bruck Renzelman, Jessica Keating, Meredith TeGrotenhuis Shimizu, Janeen Traen Turk, Leslie Ureña, and Meghan Wilson Pennisi. My advisor, Lyle Massey, offered her unwavering confidence in the project's potential. She provided me with indispensable guidance and incisive suggestions, while fostering scholarly originality. I admire both her intellectual and personal integrity and I am still learning invaluable lessons from her inspiring choices. From my undergraduate days and until this very moment, I am immensely grateful to Jacqueline Musacchio, whose flawless scholarship, dedicated teaching, and strong mentorship have motivated my career choices for twenty years. I am proud and honored to have been her student and I am humbled by her friendship.

Throughout the years, I have had the great blessing of encountering scholars who have gone above and beyond academic largesse. They have vastly improved this book by reading drafts, sharing unpublished research and documents, offering inestimable insights, and simply discussing ideas and encouraging me when the project seemed impossible to complete. I owe a debt of gratitude to: Sheila Barker, Molly Bourne, Andrea Carlino, Surekha Davies, Chet van Duzer, Marco Fiorilla, Lisa Goldenberg, Guido Guerzoni, Fredrika Jacobs, Caroline zum Kolk, Diane Kunzelmann, Rafael Mandressi, Lia Markey, Régis Michel, Caroline Murphy, Katharine Park, Deanna Shemek, and Evelyn Welch. Particularly, I would like to thank Ed Goldberg's detailed reading of my manuscript when it was far from being a book. I would also like to recognize Sefy Hendler's continued intellectual generosity—his academic work is as gracious as his persona.

And I have made my colleagues very envious by working with Erika Gaffney. She is thoughtful, sharp, and most of all incredibly patient. This book is in your hands because of her.

While writing can be a very solipsistic endeavor, it can only be so because of the many people who, indirectly but indispensably, allow it to happen. Thanking all of these individuals adequately would require a separate volume added to this book. But I do have to single out one person—my person. John Richard has been my indefatigable champion and my rock. Every day, I wonder what marvelous twist of fate brought our lives together. His love, his strength, and his infinite kindness are my most precious gifts.

I have to end my acknowledgments by mentioning someone who has shaped my intellectual path in more ways than I can count. My father taught me that knowledge, courage, and integrity are inseparable in a respectful society. He turned words into actions and, until his last breath, fought to save his beloved country from ignorance and darkness. As the world continues to use difference as a weapon toward divisiveness, this book calls for another approach, one that assesses the queries made to understand difference, even maladroitly. I think my father would have enjoyed this book's historical narrative and would have contrasted it with the dangerous and self-serving political discourse that fearful autocratic leaders endorse. I miss his counsel.

Introduction

> "This may be the curse of the human race," responded Mogor. "Not that we are so different from one another, but that we are so alike."[1]

IN 1560, PIERRE BOAISTUAU (1517–1566) wrote that monsters were a source of pleasure, horror, and admiration.[2] But what and who were monsters? The use of the term in the sixteenth and the seventeenth centuries allowed for many different "others" to fall under its umbrella: from imaginary marine creatures, to fabricated hybrid beings, to created terrifying and destructive species, and to human beings who simply diverged from ideal norms. The present study concerns itself with the latter set—while it considers the philosophical and intellectual parameters that abstracted otherness into monsters, it mainly examines human beings who were different from expected societal standards in their appearance. In doing so, I hope to call attention to the heterogeneity that the Renaissance category of "monster" encompassed, without the pretension of an impossible exhaustive coverage of all things monstrous in the Renaissance. The pointed lens and the chosen case studies of this book are intentionally limited, as they allow for richer and more precise intellectual investigations. Because this book is grounded in historical language, the term monster is used to describe these human beings, in accordance with sixteenth-century rhetoric, practice, and etymological history. In the Renaissance, monsters were phenomena that fell outside the normal course of nature and they were often associated with signs of divine wrath or omens. They were also beings intended to be shown (*mostrare*). While respecting the historical use of the word monster, this book is far from a teratological treatise—I intend to underline the diversity of human qualities found in the differences that made these beings monstrous. This diversity is as wide as the reasons that determined why certain otherness fell outside a typical normative Renaissance discourse.

The difficulty of writing a book that addresses cases and thoughts grounded in intellectual discourses devised centuries ago is manifold. Beyond the usually challenging—but invigorating—work all historians face in deciphering documents based on distinct time-dependent semantics, this book also confronts the delicate task of addressing subjects that demand sensitive and sensible rhetorical approaches. It is with great delight that I have noted a strong increase in considering "otherness" in medieval and early modern studies.[3] These considerations have taken many forms and are analyzed through various disciplines, often grouped under the denomination of disability studies. At its core, this book aligns itself with central tenets guiding inquiries into disability-oriented approaches, namely in the questioning of what constitutes a normal body.[4] Yet, this book also intentionally respects the historical modes of thoughts used to assess, understand, and describe the individuals that it studies—hence the use of adjectives such as monstrous, anomalous, and abnormal. While these terms may create unease in a twenty-first-century reader, they are purposed words that carry an early modern mediated reasoning. Perhaps a welcome compromise could be the use of "extraordinary bodies" to qualify the bodies of individuals whose physical features did not conform to the visible norm determined by a dominant cultural group.[5] However, it is important to note that the sixteenth-century bodies of dwarves, hirsutes, and castrati were first and foremost anatomically anomalous bodies before they became extra-ordinary sites of intellectual inquiries, delight, wonder, and horror. I will, thus, ask for the reader's participation in acknowledging the thoughtful historical choices made in regard to the physical descriptions of the—indeed—extraordinary bodies studied in this book. The alternating of words should not deter from what early modern sensibilities understood as monstrous and what such categorizations implied.

The individuals at the center of this book occupied several intellectual dimensions. As subjects of study, they were categorized scientifically into relevant categories, often monstrous ones. As such, they were also seen as divine signs and theological omens, as curiosities of nature, and as pathological anomalies and attention was paid to documenting the specific anatomical features that made these people into objects of wonder. Additionally, they were seen as comical implements and were associated with entertaining traditions. Finally, they were emblems of courtly life and cultural markers of the social sphere in which they lived. They became conventional symbols of the court milieu. These aspects overlapped with each other and it is in their portraits that we see these components in fruitful conversations.

Images of humans who fell outside normative aesthetic standards—such as dwarves or hirsutes—offer a fertile and new way to approach debates in Renaissance portraiture. And yet, the canonical scholarship on Renaissance portraiture does not provide an adequate model for interpreting these works. Most investigations on Renaissance portraiture have followed the frame provided by sixteenth-century theorists regarding the superiority of *ritrarre* versus *imitare*—or literal record versus artistic imitation. Consequently, most scholarship has focused on the prominence of the individual through his or her idealized visual projection and the meanings behind such visual documentations. The few attempts at alternate readings that propose to redirect the centrality of idealization over mimesis have not directly explored the tension between the two to see its application in portraits of individuals whose physical appearance and social station defied easy categorizations.

Based on Jacob Burckhardt's (1818–1897) assertion that the Renaissance gave rise to notions of individuality, scholarship on Renaissance portraiture has focused on how the outward appearance of the sitter is connected visually to his or her character.[6] Building on Burckhardt while also following sixteenth-century theoretical writings about artistic practice, modern scholars have emphasized the importance of idealization over likeness; mimesis has thus been regarded as a lesser component of Renaissance portraiture. However, portraits of physically different individuals allow us to play with this balance: in these representations, mimesis and idealization worked hand in hand to highlight the accurate details of the sitter's physical differences and to make a statement regarding the subject's social station. Posing a challenge to more conventional theories of portraiture applied to typical court dwellers, these paintings require an approach that underscores the importance of discourses tied to anatomy, natural scientific studies, and collecting practices. Because physical abnormality was the source of these individuals' employment, identity and general interest during the sixteenth and early seventeenth centuries, it is also the focus of their portraits. On the one hand, by clothing this deformity in the trappings of court portraiture, the sitters are given more dignity and humanity than in other forms of representation. On the other hand, their anatomical anomalies are explored and used to justify their status as marvels and curiosities in courtly settings.

The painted portraits examined in this book adopt conventions of traditional courtly representations, while exploring the physical variations of the sitters empirically and metaphorically. In addition to unveiling pertinent social and cultural details, depictions such as Agnolo Bronzino's (1503–1572) *Morgante* (ca. 1547) (Plate 1), Lavinia Fontana's (1552–1614) portrait of *Antoinette Gonsalvus* (1595) (Plate 2), or Andrea Sacchi's (1599–1661) 1640 portrait of *Marc'Antonio Pasqualini* (Plate 3) also question the boundaries of Renaissance portraiture as a painterly tradition. They problematize the usually unchallenged triangular relation (patron–artist–subject) dictating the production of a portrait; they re-examine the theoretical principles guiding artistic emphases on representation; and they make anatomical anomalies legible through terms borrowed from scientific explorations. Precisely because each of these cases diverge from each other in terms of their otherness, they demonstrate that there is diversity in difference and that the homogeneous approach scholarship has adopted in discussing portraiture's theories are too restrictive.

All of the human subjects presented in this book have known identities. It is in fact part of this project to determine how their identities were established through their physical differences and their subsequent integration within a highly regulated social milieu. This active participation was then visually expressed in their portraits, either through open iconography or through more concealed subtext. Far from only emphasizing the derisive aspects of the subjects, the portraits at the center of this book contribute to solidifying the character of the sitters and thus to inscribe these works as true articulations of traditional Renaissance portraiture.

Display and wonder were essential elements for both the natural/scientific collection and the classical art collection; the experience felt by a visitor in either type of collection would have called upon his or her sense of wonder, whether it was wonder arisen from curiosity, in the case of a scientific/natural collection, or wonder based on the emotion evoked by a work of art.[7] The effect of a collection was as important to the owner as it was to the visitor, as it was meant to serve as "a marvel, which gave pleasure and pride to its owner and induced pleasure and awe in the privileged visitor."[8] Collecting individuals, who, by virtue of their physical difference were seen as actual marvels, or collecting representations of them, thus capitalized on the same kind of response from the viewer. The portraits of these beings, therefore, stood at the crossroads between living and breathing "curiosities," scientific illustrations found in treatises on the monstrous and the wondrous, and traditional collections of art and antiquities.[9]

These portraits, however, were neither traditional portraits, nor scientific illustrations, nor mere *mirabilia*. For instance, the idealization, and at times allegorization, that was present in portraits of dwarves, hirsutes, or castrati distinguished them from scientific records that solely focused on cataloguing physical traits. While comparable in subject matter to many visual documents that were produced in the context of collecting evidence of the bizarre, portraits of physically intriguing individuals integrated an aspect that was absent from these visual records: a tension between idealization and likeness specific to Renaissance portraiture, as well as an emphasis on the sitter's character, in spite—or perhaps because—of his or her physical divergences.[10] The pictorial representations that are the focus of this book are "portraits," with all this word entails. The unusual bodies that were presented to a courtly audience became acceptable precisely because these paintings alluded to the already known vocabulary of traditional portraiture.

It has been common in the scholarship on Renaissance portraiture to group these representations with objects collected in *Wunderkammern*, and this classification with other curiosities is not completely misconstrued. Indeed, treatises such as Ulisse Aldrovandi's (1522–1605), Ambroise Paré's (1510–1590), or Fortunio Liceti's (1577–1657) presented hairy individuals under the denomination of monsters.[11] Dwarves were seen as objects of wonder, in fact, in some inventories, dwarves, hirsutes, or deformed individuals were categorized as natural curiosities. European courts

> most often considered natural wonders as examples of God's ingenuity; less frequently they described them as cases of 'nature errings.' A great many animal, botanical, and geological specimens were regarded as marvels, but normally the term was applied when the object was unusually large or small, extremely rare, exotic, abnormally or grotesquely shaped, or spectacularly beautiful. [...] No less fascinating to the European mind were the human prodigies: dwarfs, freaks, and other human anomalies often became the subject of art and poetry and were discussed at length in natural histories. Although sometimes viewed as nature's 'mistakes,' they were most often regarded, like geniuses, as God's marvelous work and the products of his divine wisdom.[12]

It may thus seem appropriate to add portraits of dwarves and the likes as a supplementary category to the already existing scholarship on curiosities. Yet the intentional pictorial language employed in these portraits—the compositions, references, and formal elements—are those used in canonical court portraiture, in spite of the *Wunderkammer*-quality of its subject. Portraits of physically different individuals were not mere extensions of curiosity collections, but they existed as a combination of two worlds: they incorporated visual court conventions to a cabinet of curiosity.

In addition to their *Wunder*-like qualities, most portraits of non-normative individuals contained anatomical subtexts. The Renaissance development of anatomical knowledge was at its peak in the middle of the sixteenth century with the publication of Andreas Vesalius's *De humani corporis fabrica* in 1543 and its emphasis on a normative body.[13] Following the drive for a regulated body, portraits of physically abnormal beings attempted to normalize anomalies through the use of courtly standard representational topoi; however, they complicated this language by presenting the viewer with visual testimonies of observations akin to anatomical inquiries.[14] Falling between the search for general rules in science and the need to deal with actual anomalies, portraits of these different beings were the sites of a conflation between the two. The visual language adopted in these portraits allowed the "irregular" to become familiar and effectively tamed the anatomically unusual.

The first chapter of this book addresses the importance of natural sciences in understanding monsters and how this discourse seeped into collecting practices. These collecting practices, in turn, were often the result of a court system that regulated behavior and appearance strictly. It is in these courtly environments that we found most of the records for the human subjects at the core of this book, which is why the second chapter of this book analyses their centrality. Additionally, this chapter also addresses the theoretical debates framing artistic productions in the early modern period. Together, courtly behaviors and art theoretical discourses on representations allow for subjects such as human monsters to find their way in portraits, with the dwarf Morgante as a first case study. Chapter 3, therefore, examines dwarves, their position in small Italian courts, and their subsequent visual portrayals. What chapter 3 offers as a discursive structure is applied to hirsutes, who become the focus of chapter 4. From mythological understandings, to medical analyses, this chapter uses the Gonsalvus family as a paradigm to discuss juridical personhood and shifting politics made legible through portraits. Finally, this book concludes with a chapter on castrati. The figure of the castrato may seem at odds with those of dwarves and hirsutes—they are not analogous because the castrato's physical difference is created, rather than genetic, and its visibility is not as obvious (if visible at all) as the non-normative bodies of dwarves and hirsutes. But, while the castrato's physical difference was celebrated when he became successful, similar theoretical parameters dictated the understanding, categorization, and visualization of his portrayal: he was physically out of the natural norm, he was groomed by a court setting to which he belonged, and his legacy and juridical personhood was tied to his anatomical difference. Additionally, he, too, shook the rigid boundaries that normative bodies categorized—gender norms were challenged by his body, made audible for all and visible through portraits and caricatures.

Portraits of sitters with intriguing physical diversity stand as paradigmatic examples of shifts occurring in early modern scientific debates, as well as in intellectual discourses defining the theoretical place for other disciplines to come to build a richer context for the images, as it is the most productive way to understand not only the nature of monstrousness in early modern thought, but also the contribution of this visual material to the historiographic debates on portraiture. Studies on collecting practices in the early modern period are also deployed here to establish the strong connections existing between possessing objects that generated wonder and the collector's self-presentation. Additionally, this book analyzes inquiries into human anatomy. These investigations allowed for an examination of the body as an object that could possibly be displayed and possessed. Ultimately, these ideas solidified within an art historical framework and early modern scientific investigations help guide my considerations of artistic debates, as well as political and social situations. Because of such examinations, the knowledge of a dwarf's independent juridical personhood balances his comical aspect. Similarly, the glory of a castrato gives way to the knowledge of his possible impotence and unsettled legal status, and the image of a hairy savage girl shifts progressively to that of a civilized girl.

Whereas these portraits have been explored individually, there has not been a cohesive narrative to help frame them adequately in early modern terms. Scholars *have* addressed monsters—widely—in visual representations in art historical studies, but without failing, they justify these images as indices of courtly wit and humor, or as vague references to collections of curiosities. Also, even though historians of science have provided great resources for the study of collecting practices, teratology, and anatomy in the early modern period, their scholarship has yet to be fully included into studies on portraiture. Therefore, portraits of anatomically different beings have evaded methodical examinations since they have been seen as either scientific illustrations only, or as marginal and isolated artistic endeavors. This book proposes to situate these portraits at the center of early modern artistic considerations, rather than in the borders of canonical productions. It is precisely in these portraits that visual theoretical debates, peppered with scientific impulse and social oscillations, become palpable. And it is only by understanding early modern scientific inquiries into the practice of collecting and human anatomy that the different layers underlining these portraits can come together. By allying the premises that dictate typical Renaissance portraits with the varied discourses that inform the visualization of monsters, we see a concentric area appearing, that of courtly portraits of monstrous human beings. It is this juncture, this coincidental area that highlights essential characteristics for both "normative" portraits and monstrous ones. However, in order to disentangle both discourses, we need to examine the multiple fields that inform such representations: from natural philosophy, to court determinations, and finally, to the specific anatomical characteristics that established the social places held by the individuals discussed here. It is therefore why this book starts with examining early modern scientific thoughts, then moves to discussing court settings and collecting practices associated with them, to finally arrive at three case studies. From the dwarf Morgante, to the hirsute Antoinette Gonsalvus, and finally to the castrato Marc'Antonio Pasqualini, all three subjects exemplify the ways in which monsters—as visible others—defined normative social grounds and established exceptions needed to reinforce conventions. Dwarves were miniature foils to the perfect courtly body; hirsutes stood as savage foils to civilized courtly behavior; and castrati were problematic gender foils to uniform courtly masculinity. It is through monsters' overt signs of difference that constructed perfection could be made legible. It is through the portraits of these sitters that perfect courtly subjects found reassurance. However, this book also problematizes a linear discourse on difference: as the complex layers of meanings in these portraits are revealed, it is the sitters' similarities to universal human qualities that eventually become apparent, and not their more overt asperities.[15]

Notes

[1] Salman Rushdie, *The Enchantress of Florence* (New York: Random House, 2009), 135.

[2] Pierre Boaistuau, *Histoires prodigieuses* (Paris: Robert le Mangnier, edition of 1566 from the original publication of 1560), preface following the dedication: "Monseigneur, entre toutes les choses qui se peuvent contempler soubs la concavité des cieux, il ne se voit rien qui plus efeuille l'esprit humain, qui ravisse plus les sens, qui plus espouvente, qui engendre plus grande admiration ou terreur aux creatures, que les monstres [...].

[3] Though one can certainly lament the lack of diversity represented in those heralding some of these studies.

[4] In this regard, Jonathan Hsy has explored many avenues and has provided scholars with original and necessary intellectual paths. See, for instance, "Disability," in *The Cambridge Companion to the Body in Literature*, ed. David Hillman and Ulrika Maude (Cambridge: Cambridge University Press, 2015), 24–40 and 27 in particular.

[5] Rosemarie Garland Thomson provides a strong theoretical model for the intellectual nomenclature attached to physical disability. See *Extraordinary Bodies: Figuring Physical Disability in American Culture and Literature* (New York: Columbia University Press, 1997).

[6] Jacob Burckhardt, *The Civilisation of the Renaissance in Italy*, trans. S.G.C. Middlemore (London: George Allen & Unwin, 1921).

[7] Lorraine Daston and Katharine Park, *Wonders and the Order of Nature 1150–1750* (New York: Zone Books, 1998), 22.

[8] Martin Kemp, "'Wrought by No Artist's Hand': The Natural, the Artificial, the Exotic, and the Scientific in Some Artifacts from the Renaissance," in *Reframing the Renaissance: Visual Culture in Europe and Latin America 1450–1650*, ed. Claire Farago (New Haven and London: Yale University Press, 1995), 185.

[9] Julius von Schlosser, "Italienische Kuriositätenkammern," in *Dir Kunst- und Wunderkammern der Spätrenaissance* (Leipzig: Klinkhardt & Biermann, 1908).

[10] Such documents were often engravings representing the actual collection onto which a dwarf might have been added. See Ferrante Imperato, *Dell'historia naturale* (1672); Benedetto Ceruti and Andrea Chiocco, *Musaeum Francisci Calceolari Iunioris Veronensis* (1662); Lorenzo Legati, *Museo Cospiano annesso a quello del famoso Ulisse Aldrovandi e donato alla sua patria dall'illustrissimo Signor Ferdinando Cospi* (1677); and Ulisse Aldrovandi's illustrations in *Monstrorum historia* (1642).

[11] Ulisse Aldrovandi, *Monstrorum historia* in *Opera Omnia* (Bologna: Manolesiana, Feronii, Thebaldinum, 1638–1681); Ambroise Paré, *Vingt cinquième livre traitant des monstres et prodiges* (Paris: G. Buon, 1585); and Fortunio Liceti, *De monstrorum caussis, natura, et differentiis, libri duo* (Padua: Frambotti, 1634).

[12] This classification is taken from Joy Kenseth, *The Age of the Marvelous* (Hanover: Hood Museum of Art, Dartmouth, 1991), 33. Also, Tobia Aldini, naturalist and prefect of the Farnese gardens, includes humans among the other marvels of the cardinal's court. Tobia Aldini, *Exactissima descriptio rariorum quarandarum plantarum quae continentur Romae in Horto Farnesiano* (Rome: Typis Iacobi Mascardi, 1625), 10, as cited in Roberto Zapperi, "Arrigo le Velu, Pietro le Fou, Amon le Nain et autres bêtes: Autour d'un tableau d'Agostino Carrache," *Annales: Économies – Sociétés – Civilisations* 40, no. 2 (March–April 1985): 310 and 324, footnote 11.

[13] J.B. deC. M. Saunders and Charles D. O'Malley, *The Illustrations from the Works of Andreas Vesalius of Brussels* (New York: Dover Publications, 1950).

[14] In fact, artistic interest in anatomy was more than a mere parallel. For works on artists' burgeoning interest in anatomy in the Renaissance, see Andrea Carlino, *Books of the Body: Anatomical Ritual and Renaissance Learning* (Chicago and London: University of Chicago Press, 1999); Andrea Carlino, *Paper Bodies: A Catalogue of Anatomical Fugitive Sheets 1538–1687* (London: Wellcome Institute for the History of Medicine, 1999); Mimi Cazort et al., eds., *The Ingenious Machine of Nature: Four Centuries of Art and Anatomy* (Ottawa: National Gallery of Canada, 1996); Julie V. Hansen and Suzanne Porter, *The Physician's Art: Representations of Art and Medicine* (Durham: Duke University Medical Center Library and Duke University Museum of Art, 1999); Martin Kemp and Marina Wallace, *Spectacular Bodies: The Art and Science of the Human Body from Leonardo to Now* (Los Angeles: University of California Press, 2000); and Bernard Schultz, *Art and Anatomy in Renaissance Italy* (Ann Arbor: UMI Research Press, 1985).

[15] Fredrika H. Jacobs uses the term "asperity" to define the unequal qualities that form an anatomically non-normative subject—a choice that is both intellectually apposite and innovative. See *The Living Image in Renaissance Art* (Cambridge: Cambridge University Press, 2005), 146.

Chapter 1

Difference as an Inquiry

THE IMPORTANCE OF ANATOMICALLY UNUSUAL individuals in the early modern scientific discourse parallels their positions in various Renaissance courts. Scientific treatises and incipient discussions on anatomical differences informed ideas about monstrousness, images of sitters who were considered to be monstrous, and the reality of individuals deemed monstrous. This is precisely why this chapter examines monsters as systematic objects of inquiry subject to the early modern scientific gaze. Just as medical anomalies framed the nature of normative bodies for early modern philosophers and scientists, so too portraits of dwarves, hirsutes, and castrati reveal for the historian of art the true nature of normative constructions in Renaissance portraiture. Ultimately, these sources turned the fascination with monsters into an established science; anatomical treatises, dialogues emanating from natural philosophy, and medical approaches allowed for the visualization of monsters to occur. These discussions informed not only the relationship between the physically different sitters and their patrons/owners, but also the subsequent portraits that emerged from such interactions.

The acquisition of knowledge about the normative human body acquired through dissections was circulated through the production of images at a time when the ascendency of perspective had newly secured the truthfulness, verisimilitude, and objectivity of visual representation. What emerged, then, was a nexus in which science and art combined to effectively transmute physiognomy into veracity—a move that facilitated the application of anatomical knowledge and the staging of public dissections to the study of *visibly* non-normative bodies.[1] Superimposing the scientific authority upon which human dissection depended onto the study of anomalous beings meant that their representations expanded beyond mere curiosity; in fact, these pursuits became tantamount to discovering the "truth" about monsters, monstrousness, and monstrosity, and by extension the truth about human nature.[2]

This development derived from the primacy of the visual sense. Textual descriptions of monsters emphasized graphic traits for the reader, and in tandem with visual representations, these studies became both titillating and instructive. Indeed, as scientific interest in monsters' anatomy lent representations of monsters an element of documentary authenticity, these representations stood in as visual dissections—not only of monsters, but also of monstrousness itself. Thus the subjects' wondrousness and deformities were rendered accessible to multiple viewers, who felt comforted via their sense of sight that they were presented with accurate and true knowledge.

Monsters only gradually became systematic objects of inquiry. One of the most important characteristics of the early modern discourse on monsters is the multiplicity of sources that touch upon the subject. The diversity of visual representations and textual descriptions that invoke monsters ensured that their study was proportionally complex and multifaceted. Prior to this period, various authors and publishers typically reproduced mythical images of monsters and only slightly rewrote accounts found in ancient texts. Increasingly, however, a great number of new images and texts dealing with recently-discovered monsters began to appear, thus whetting popular interest in the monstrous.[3] One of the most widely recognized and discussed early modern monsters was the famed Papal Ass, discussed notably by Martin Luther and Philipp Melanchthon. The Papal Ass (Fig. 1.1) was found on the banks of the Tiber river (Rome) in 1495; twenty-eight years later, both Luther and Melanchthon wrote an apocalyptic and anti-papal pamphlet that interpreted the details of the visual appearance of this monster as portentous signs. From the head of the ass symbolizing the divinely condemned pope, to the foot of the creature representing the corrupted servants of the church, each part of the monster—and even his death, which spoke to the end of papacy—built on theological, secular, and political beliefs, and therefore appealed to a large audience.[4] These accounts serve as a testimony to the changing understanding of the relation between Man and divine forces, channeled through the power of the natural world. They also provide information regarding the place of the marvelous, the curious, and the scientific in the early modern conception of the world.

The question of monsters engaged several fields of knowledge in the sixteenth century: medical traditions from ancient, medieval, and contemporaneous early modern sources; theological disputes ranging from early Christian era to the Middle Ages; mythological writings from ancient authors and their fantastic adaptations in the Middle Ages; and finally, popular culture informed by selected samples of medical, theological, and mythological themes. As medical inquiries grew stronger during the sixteenth and seventeenth centuries—fueled by first-hand anatomical observations—the second, third, and fourth components that defined the monstrous grew weaker in published works.[5] The causes of monstrousness were not understood solely as the results of the opposition between devilish and divine forces, or only as the product of sympathetic magic during pregnancy. Methodical explanations were increasingly applied to shed light on the origins of physical difference. Ultimately, in the nineteenth century, Isidore Geoffroy Saint-Hilaire (1805–1861) established teratology as an acknowledged science.[6]

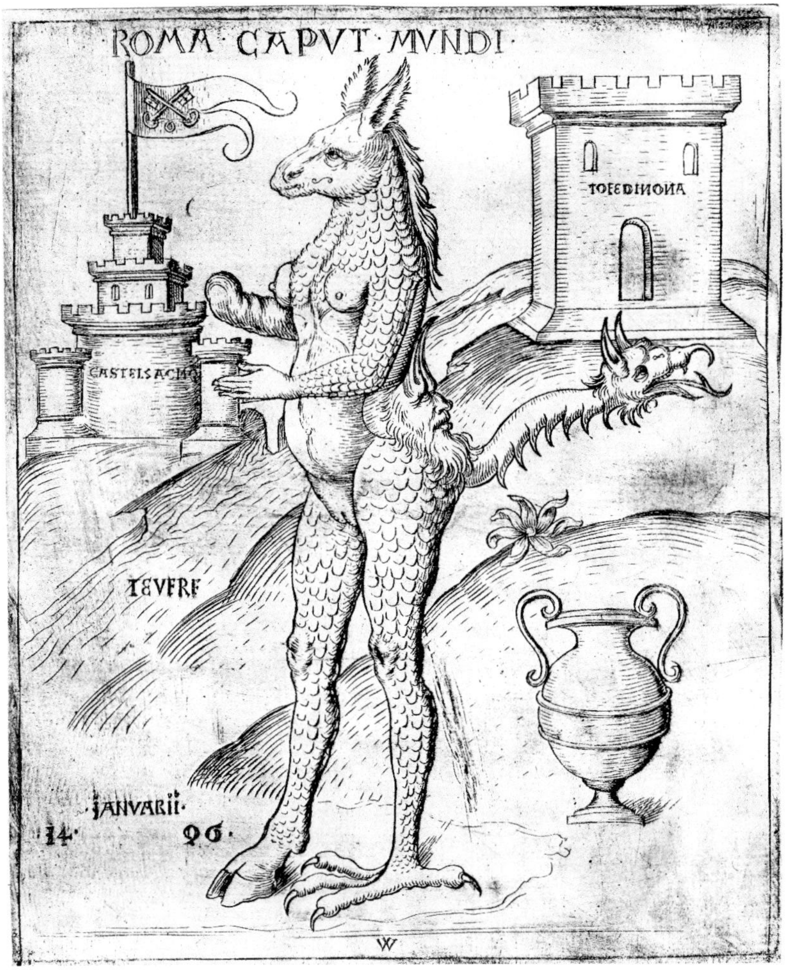

Figure 1.1. Lucas Cranach the Elder, *The Papal Ass of Rome*, from Melanchthon and Luther *Deuttung der zwo grewlichen Figuren*, 1523, © The Trustees of The British Museum, London

Even though interest in the marvelous, rare, curious, and inexplicable had never waned, rational scientific accounts added a new component to this pursuit. Indeed, the vacillation between popular imagination and systematic, medicalized explanations actively structured the public's attention toward and the experts' scrutiny of monsters from the early modern period forward. For instance, the story of the monster of Ravenna (Fig. 1.2) in the early sixteenth century touched the imagination of many people, from Florence to Munich and beyond. The monster's description is found in the diary of Luca Landucci, an apothecary from Florence who wrote in 1512:

> We heard that a monster had been born at Ravenna, of which a drawing was sent here; it had a horn on its head, straight up like a sword, and instead of arms it had two wings like a bat's, and at the height of the breasts it had a *fio* [Y-shaped mark] on one side and a cross on the other, and lower down at the waist, two serpents, and it was a hermaphrodite, and on the right knee it had an eye, and its left foot was like an eagle's. I saw it painted, and anyone who wished could see this painting in Florence.[7]

Because days later the city of Ravenna fell to a coalition of papal, Spanish, and French troops, the birth of this monster was widely interpreted as a bad omen. This monster became instantly well-known, thanks to *avvisi*, broadsheet, and pamphlets that circulated widely and at a fast pace.[8] Combining religious fears with popular convictions and political thoughts, the monster of Ravenna became a perfect site for all these notions to coexist. Different understandings of monsters were in fact not in competition, but rather complemented each other. As Lorraine Daston and Katharine Park have argued, it would be misguided to assume a teleological schema that charts an evolution of monstrous categories according to the distinct time periods. For instance it would be misleading to claim that medieval audiences regarded the monster solely as a sign of theological superstition, or that those of the early modern period understood the monster only as a source of delight and pleasure. Nor is it accurate to claim that, suddenly, in the late sixteenth and seventeenth centuries, the monster became an object of medical and scientific inquiry. Rather, these epistemologies tended to overlap—often in socially or culturally expedient ways. This is particularly evident in early modern reconfigurations, where the monster begins to comprise an alternate body of knowledge that served, in part, to strengthen anatomical standards such as those put forth by Andreas Vesalius (1514–1564). The normalizing discourse that framed anatomical inquiries—especially in the wake of Vesalius's *Fabrica* (1543)—turned the slightest deviation into an object of inquiry. Such deviations provided the exceptions needed to reinforce the structure of a new canon—departures from the norm that served strategically to delineate the boundaries of the very norms beyond which they were doomed to remain.

The methodical examination of monsters' visible anomalies revealed a constructive intellectual system that affected the reality of individuals at court who were seen as monsters, the collective imaginary tied to monsters, and their subsequent visual translations. The images and texts that resulted from the study of monsters provided a model of anatomical knowledge that became a valid alternative to the normative ideals promoted by anatomists like Vesalius, who upheld the idea that truth lay in practice-based processes and their textual and visible translations. The ways in which monstrous bodies were explored echoed these practices, and thus reinforced the epistemological maquette proposed by early modern dissections of normalized human bodies.

The early modern development of anatomical knowledge reached its peak in the middle of the sixteenth century. In 1543, Vesalius published the first edition of his landmark *De Humani Corporis Fabrica* (Fig. 1.3)—a work that combined artistic originality with

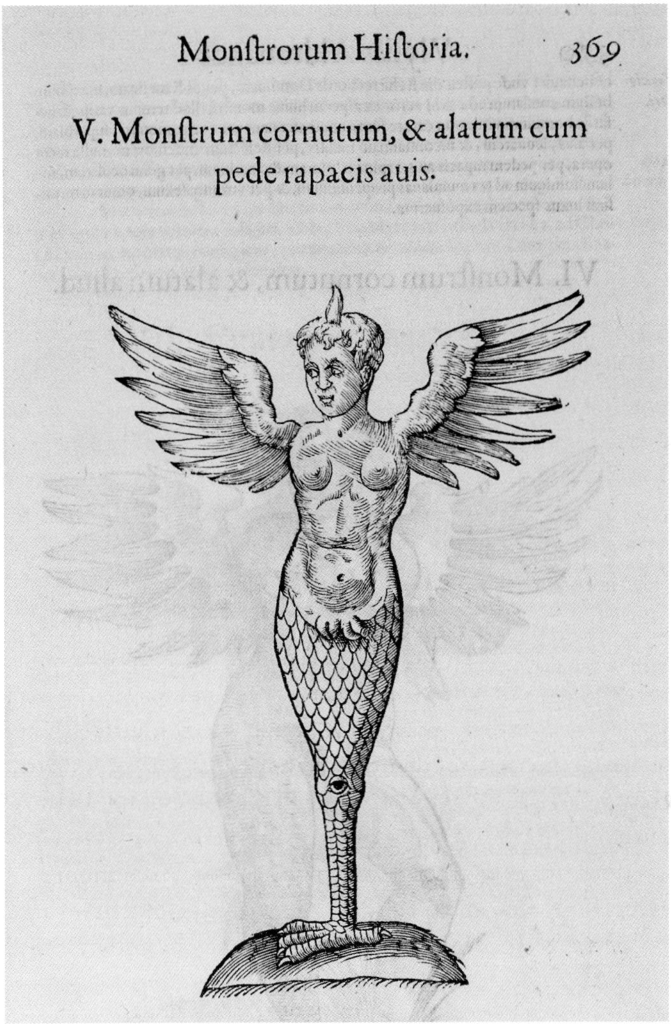
Monſtrorum Hiſtoria. 369
V. Monſtrum cornutum, & alatum cum pede rapacis auis.

Figure 1.2. Ulisse Aldrovandi, the monster of Ravenna, page 369, *De monstrorum historia*, 1642, Wheaton College Permanent Collection, Newell Bequest Fund, Norton, Massachusetts

radical anatomical inquiries. A compendium, entitled the *Epitome* appeared in tandem with the *Fabrica* and was meant to give an introduction and topographical approach to the novice in medicine.[9] Vesalius emphasized direct observation, eliminated the divisions of roles between the anatomist, the barber surgeon, and the pointer, made this practice part of the curriculum of academic teaching, and finally challenged the hegemony of the Galenic tradition.[10] A student of Gunterius Andernacus (1505–1574) and Jacobus Sylvius (1478–1555) in Paris in 1533, Vesalius performed dissections that broke with tradition: he eradicated the varied channels that stood between the student of anatomy

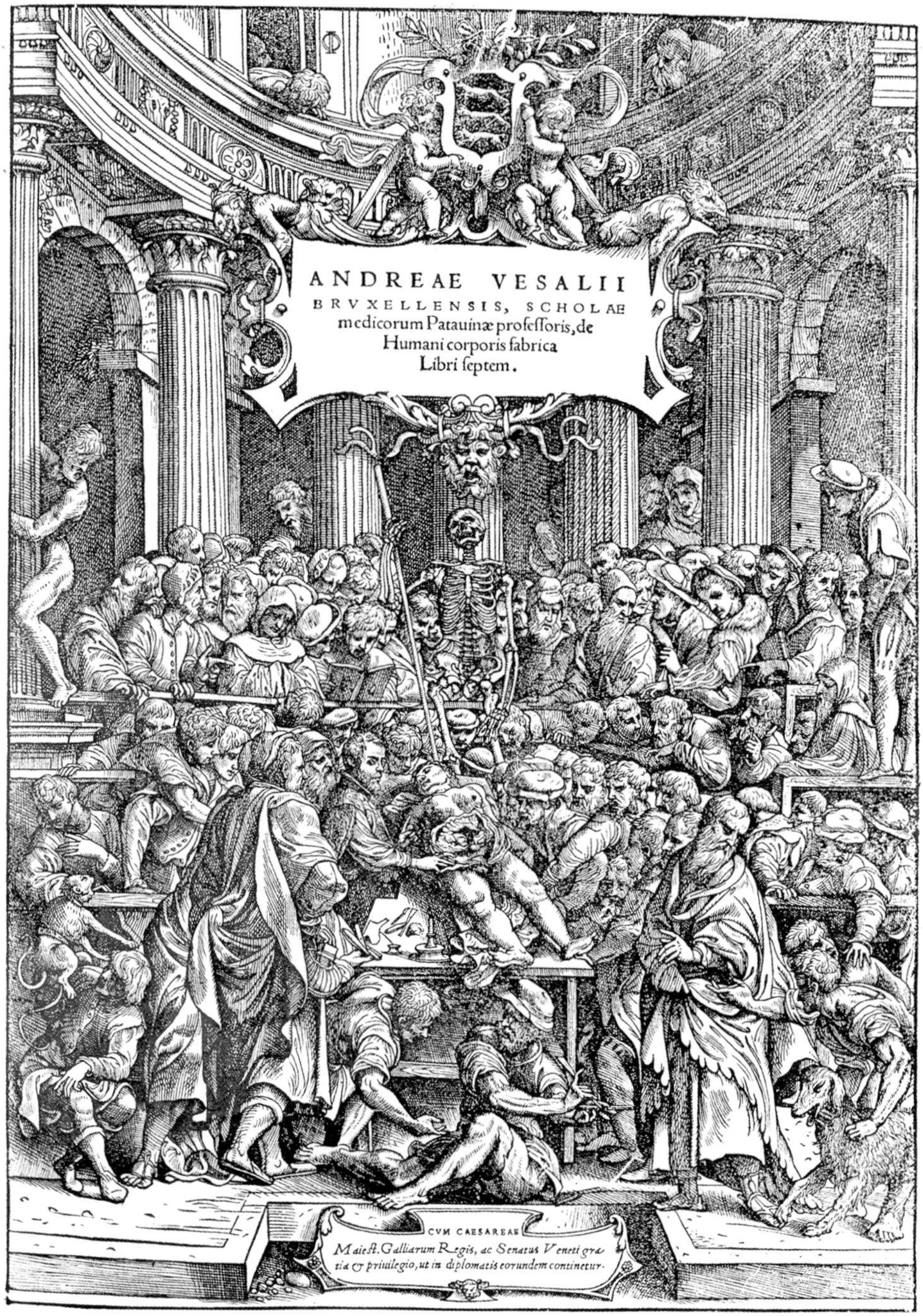

Figure 1.3. Jan van Kalkar, title page of Andreas Vesalius *De humani corporis fabrica*, 1543. HIP/Art Resource, New York

and the immediate knowledge the dissected body offered. This method allowed him to appreciate the numerous errors made by Galen of Pergamum (130–200) and to challenge the textual basis of medieval medicine.[11] The *Fabrica* therefore not only changed the ways science and anatomy were taught and learned, but it also provided a strong paradigm for anatomical illustrations that would last approximately two hundred years.[12]

However great the significance of this publication for subsequent inquiries about the human body, anatomical treatises had existed prior to the publication of the *Fabrica*. The first writings on human anatomy were part of the *Corpus hippocratum* that circulated in Greece around 400 BCE.[13] About a hundred years later, and for approximately two centuries during the Hellenistic period, the first recorded human dissections allowed the "black box" of knowledge to be opened and reveal its secrets.[14] Yet in spite of this early foray into an empirical experience of the human body, it is the imprint of Galen that influenced the transmission of anatomical knowledge from Antiquity to the Renaissance. Prior to becoming the physician of the emperor Marcus Aurelius (121–180), Galen worked in a gladiator school and treated severe wounds that served as his "windows into the human body."[15] Although he grounded his inquiries concerning the human body in Aristotelian teleological philosophy and empirical methods of investigation, Galen never actually practiced a human dissection.[16] As a result, his descriptions of human anatomy were often inaccurate and the mistakes found in his *On the Usefulness of the Parts of the Human Body* (ca. 175) became unquestioned truth repeated by later authors. From the fourth-century Alexandrian physician Magnus of Nisibis to the thirteenth-century Bolognese Mondino de Liuzzi, most physicians and anatomists persisted in their use of the Galenic canon and thus perpetuated some of his incorrect assessments along with his methodological approaches.

Human dissections were officially reintroduced into Western teaching practice at the end of the thirteenth century in Bologna.[17] Yet the logical confrontation of the visual knowledge of the body with the erroneous Galenic textual tradition did not occur until Vesalius addressed this in his *Fabrica*.[18] A proponent of Galenic principles—at least in theory—Vesalius followed the advice set by the anatomist from Pergamum, that experience trumps hypothesis. For instance, via the practice of human dissections, Vesalius clearly established that the sternum had three segments and not the seven Galen had proposed.[19] The title page of the 1543 *Fabrica* is a woodcut showing a crowded public dissection in which Vesalius demonstrates anatomy directly on a body, thus speaking to his insistence on the empirical acquisition of knowledge. Much has been written on this woodcut print, but one of the most interesting and salient discussions is that of Katharine Park who points to the importance of the female corpse being dissected by Vesalius.[20] By choosing to center his title page on the body of a hanged *female* criminal executed in Padua, Vesalius achieved several goals: he enhanced his reputation with a curious male audience; made a strong *memento mori* statement visibly linking birth to death (from the womb to the skeleton); undeniably asserted his superiority over Galen in matters of female anatomy; and dissociated the viewer from the subject being dissected by emphasizing the gendered distance—rather than the identification—between (male) viewer and (female) corpse.[21] In the *Fabrica*, Vesalius proposed a new way to anatomize and made clear from the outset that this treatise and his inquiries were distinct from those of his predecessors.[22] Notably, in spite of his insistence on an empirical examination and understanding of individual bodies, Vesalius still believed in the principle of an idealized normative body.[23] The Vesalian thrust toward a normative ideal—followed for centuries by various anatomists and physicians—purposefully did not take the physically deformed into account.[24] This was not the case, however, for everyone working within the Vesalian paradigm.

Concomitant with intellectual and scientific developments pertaining to an ideal human body, attention to anatomical irregularities grew from a marginal interest to a defined science. In fact, awareness of physical irregularity was fed by the normative ideals upheld by Vesalius and adopted by his followers. By promoting his regulated standards of anatomy, ironically Vesalius had recreated the intellectual system that shaped the transmission of Galenic textual knowledge in the first place.[25] The Vesalian body became the new standard "body of knowledge," and departures from its strict norms fueled interest in anatomical deviations by creating a parallel scientific pursuit that used the same heuristic tools.

Gradually, during the early modern period, popular and theological beliefs were perused under a medical lens and audiences started to study monsters in a rigorous and systematic scientific manner. Early modern scientific communities emphasized empirical examination and natural philosophers employed it to explain both normative and unusual natural phenomena. Anatomical inconsistency and its visual symptoms fell under this pragmatic scrutiny.[26] It made sense for intellectual strategies that controlled the understanding of ordinary bodies to find resonance in the investigation of extraordinary physical attributes. And thus a few attempts at cataloguing extraordinary humans, animals, organic matters, and fantastic beings were made throughout the sixteenth century. The first systematized and published attempt appears to have been the 1503 treatise on signs and wonders—*De signis portentis, atque prodigiis*—by a Freiburg scholar and genealogist to the Holy Roman Emperor Maximilian, Jakob Mennel (ca. 1460–1525). In 1560 Pierre Boaistuau (ca. 1520–1566) published his *Histoires prodigieuses*, in which he presented various stories gathered from ancient authors, devised from imaginary biblical occurrences, and featuring fantastic animals, and combined them with descriptions of congenital diseases.[27] Even though Boaistuau's organizational scheme came close to an actual classification, he made no direct attempt to define categories of abnormal beings. He provided detailed descriptions and an elaboration on the ideas of the bizarre and the imaginary, but did not demonstrate a scientific causality for the existence of unusual beings. In addition, the title, preface, dedication, and the entirety of the text were in French, rather than Latin, despite the fact that Boaistuau clearly meant to target an elite audience. The book is dedicated to a scientific novice, the noble lord Jean Rieux, Seigneur d'Assérac and the preface left no doubt as to the courtly pretensions of the text and illustrations through which Boaistuau intended to flatter his patron:

> My Lord, among all things that may be seen under the skies, nothing touches the human spirit more, nothing pleases the senses more, nothing horrifies more, nothing generates more admiration or terror to creatures than the monsters, prodigies and abominations in which we see the errors of nature or only assumed, reversed, mutilated and shortened, but (in addition) we discover most often a secret judgment and scourge of God's wrath, through the object of things that are presented, which make us feel the violence of his justice , which is so bitter that we have to look inside ourselves and hit our consciousness with a hammer, peel away at our own vices, be appalled by our wrong-doings, particularly when we read in sacred and secular stories that sometimes the elements were heralds, trumpets, ministers and executors of God's justice.[28]

Shortly after the publication of *Les histoires prodigieuses*, Ambroise Paré (1510–1590) wrote and edited several editions of *Des monstres et prodiges*, first published in 1573.[29] Paré chose to write in the vernacular French and was aware of the stigma this decision had on a scientific text. Yet, in the preface, he insisted that his decision to write in French was a conscious one, meant to enrich the practice of medicine by adding to it the knowledge of rare things such as monsters.[30] In addition, unlike Boaistuau, whom he cited as a provider of some of his case studies, Paré provided a definition of monsters and distinguished the various terms he used:

> Monsters are things that appear outside of the course of nature (and are most often signs of some misfortune to come) such as a child who is born with one arm only, another with two heads, and other limbs that are out of the ordinary. Prodigies are things that happen against nature, such as a woman giving birth to a snake, or to a dog, or to anything that goes against nature. [...] The mutilated are the blind, one-eyed people, hunchbacks, lame people, or people having six fingers or toes, or less than five fingers or toes, or fingers and toes joined together, or arms that are too short, or noses that are set too deep like those with crooked noses, or lips that are big and reversed [...] or anything that goes against nature.[31]

Paré's work fell within a trend that spoke to the growing interest in marvelous and prodigious things. Indeed, the increase of published works dealing with medical cases in the sixteenth century signaled the rising interest of laymen and men of sciences for published accounts of various natural wonders, including monsters.[32] His many illustrations deal with different monsters, whose medical validity varied from conjoined

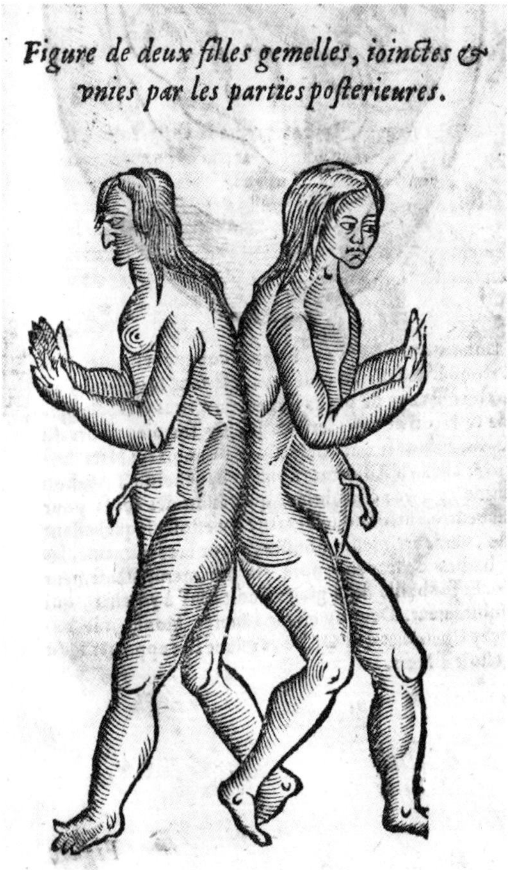
Figure de deux filles gemelles, ioinctes & vnies par les parties posterieures.

Figure 1.4. Ambroise Paré, illustration for conjoined twins, page 647, *Les Oeuvres d'Ambroise Paré, conseiller et premier chirurgien du roy. Douziesme Edition, Chez Jean Gregoire*, 1664, Bayerische Staatsbibliothek, Munich

twins (Fig. 1.4) to individuals with shortened limbs (Fig. 1.5), and finally to imaginary hybrid creations such as a half-man, half-piglet creature with no noteworthy explanation beyond the plain, matter of fact description of the two components that form his hybridism (Fig. 1.6). The conjoined twins on the left of the page are described as the "figure of *a* [italics mine] child having two heads, two arms, and four legs."[33] Interestingly, the twins are described as a single human being who is monstrous because of the duplicity of his heads and legs. Yet on the same page, the other set of conjoined twins are described as two human beings, only they have a single head that they share.[34] More unusual is the anonymous boy with shortened limbs whose monstrosity is, according to Paré, due to the lack of semen.[35] The anonymity of the boy is, however, compromised by the atypical hat he is wearing—the only clothes on an otherwise naked body. This item of clothing cancels his generic position as a mere case study and invites viewers to speculate about the possible identity of this boy—through a sartorial index—while becoming witnesses to the scientific truth presented by Paré. Through the preface and the rest of the volume, the reader is presented with case studies accompanied by illustrations, therefore guaranteeing that the work dealt with visually verifiable knowledge. Paré's training as a barber-surgeon, his experience with battlefield surgery, and his position as the official surgeon to several kings of France certainly determined his medical view of the body and its possible variances. His knowledge was one that was mostly experiential and garnered *in situ* rather than extracted from treatises and academic settings. Because of his reputation, many counted on his expertise and he encountered numerous patients and cases that, statistically, would have provided him with direct access to diseases that visibly manifested

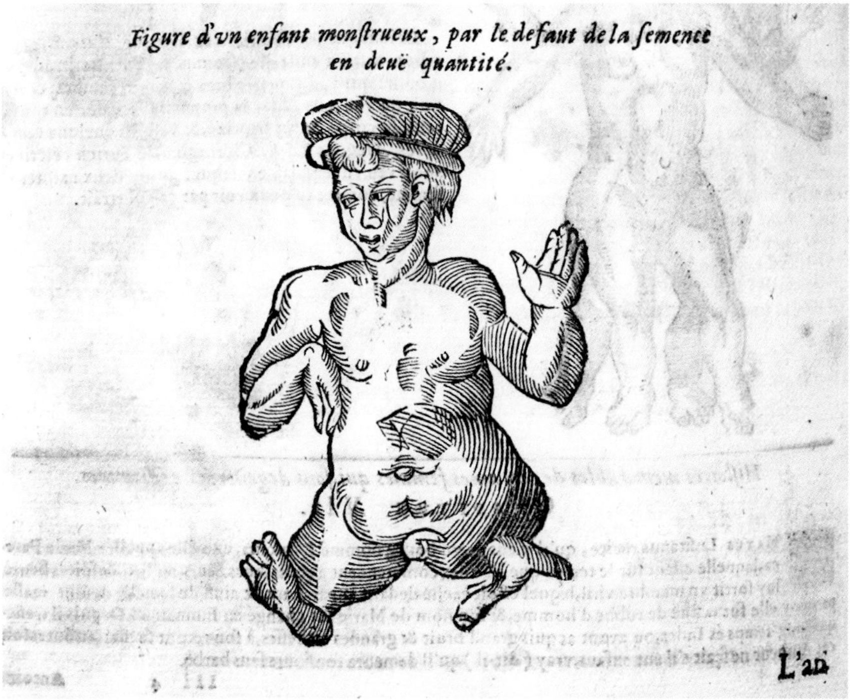

Figure 1.5. Ambroise Paré, illustration for a man lacking a limb, page 656, *Les Oeuvres d'Ambroise Paré, conseiller et premier chirurgien du roy. Douziesme Edition, Chez Jean Gregoire*, 1664, Bayerische Staatsbibliothek, Munich

themselves through monstrous symptoms. Furthermore, after Henri II's fatal tournament accident in 1559, Paré met Vesalius, who came to Paris in the hope of healing the dying king.[36] Undoubtedly this meeting led to the practice-based methods of the famous anatomist to influence the royal surgeon. Paré may not have directly applied Vesalius's techniques to his own inquiries, but, as a medical practitioner aware of the radical shift led by the author of the *Fabrica*, he certainly processed them as he was gathering material for his investigation on the nature, indications, and causes of monstrousness. While *Des monstres et prodiges* is not considered a strict medical assessment of the pathologies that led to anatomical deformities, it was a step toward medicalizing the discourse on monsters and using them as an alternate body of anatomical knowledge.

Here again, the term monster refers to individuals whose bodies deviated from the standard aesthetic norm promoted both by newly published anatomical treatises and courtly ideal set publicly. This history shows that systematic methods of inquiry used to understand monsters as phenomena outside the normal course of nature co-existed with the theological understanding of monsters as signs of divine wrath or omens.[37] For instance, Paré's medical assertions did not shatter his belief that monsters were a divine

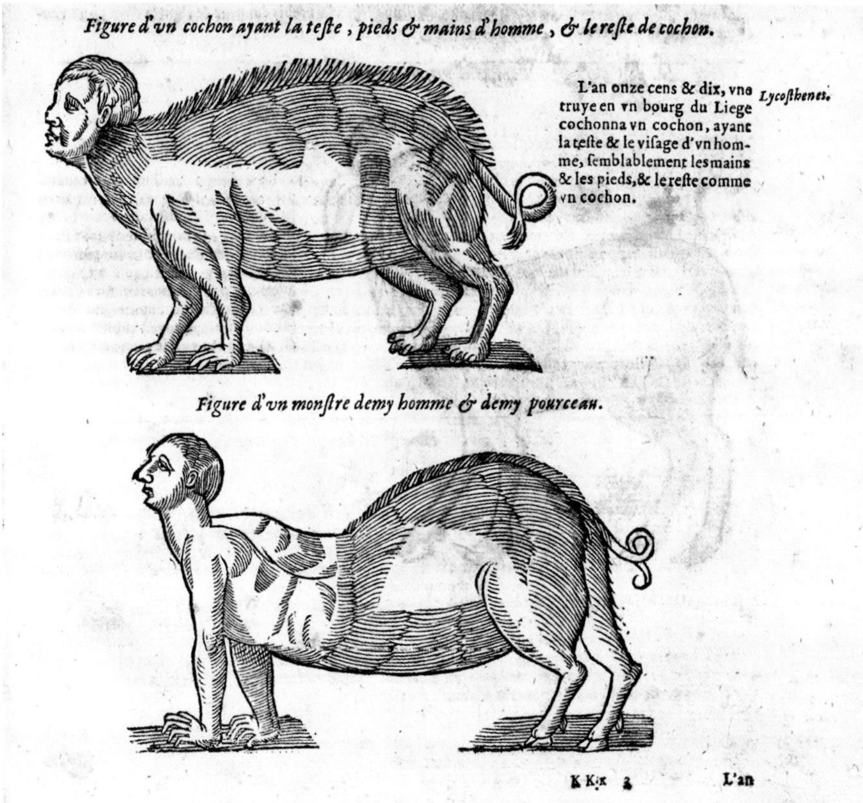

Figure 1.6. Ambroise Paré, illustration for a half-man, half-pig monster, page 665, *Les Oeuvres d'Ambroise Paré, conseiller et premier chirurgien du roy. Douziesme Edition, Chez Jean Gregoire*, 1664, Bayerische Staatsbibliothek, Munich

mark placed on nature or might represent what happened to those who faced God's wrath.[38] To support both these assertions, Paré recast the etymological origins of the term "monster" to support the assumptions that monsters were sacred signs to be shown. The origin of the word "monster" is found in the Latin *mostrare*, to show.[39] Paré himself discussed the monster as "a being that one shows."[40] One of the most famous instances described by Paré was that of conjoined twin sisters born in Verona in 1475. These sisters "were carried through several cities in Italy" by their poor parents who thus earned a significant amount of money thanks to the "people who were very eager to see this new spectacle of nature."[41] The essence of the monster as a creature "meant to be shown" was here presented as beneficial, since the conjoined twin sisters became a visible index of God's play with nature that relieved the family from financial distress. In addition to its ties to the verb *mostrare*, the noun *mostro* has also been related to the word *monere*, to warn.[42] Hence Paré, Boaistuau, and Conrad Lycosthenes (1518–1561), among others, included the notion of warning in their definitions of monsters. In the same vein, most authors in the sixteenth century saw monsters as a sign of *remonstrance* from God, but one that was neither simplistic nor invariable.

One of the first early modern authors to provide a more strictly conceived scientific treatise on monsters was Fortunio Liceti (1577–1657), who published *De monstrorum natura* ... in 1616. Liceti, a physician from Padua, expressed his disbelief in monsters as portentous heavenly signs and insisted on their importance as living beings who expressed certain truths of nature through their unusual physical appearance.[43] In doing so, Liceti privileged the sense of sight as a means to acquire true knowledge, since it was the outer appearance of these individuals that justified the scientific investigation of their bodies. Liceti saw monsters as beings whose deformities elicited the most wonder and admiration; he was thus not surprised that audiences were so intrigued by them and sought to understand their origins.[44] Liceti abandoned the idea of the monster as an ominous divine sign, justifying its existence not as a mistake made by nature, but as an expression of difference necessary in the face of adverse conditions. His work demonstrates that monsters in the seventeenth century began to be seen as valid variations of nature, indispensable contrasts to the normative body described by Vesalius. The approach adopted by Liceti exemplifies the inchoate constructions of monsters as authoritative epistemological alternatives. The categories assigned to nature are taken up much later by Michel Foucault, who explained early modern scientific difference in *The Order of Things* (1966). In this project, Foucault explored monsters not as simple errors of nature, but rather as Liceti-inspired constructed ideals. According to this conceptual model, monsters became required deviations. These deviations would in turn allow nature to preserve its continuum by allowing difference to exist not in *opposition*, but in *parallel* to its own course:

> The monster ensures in time, and for our theoretical knowledge, a continuity that, for our everyday experience, floods, volcanoes, and subsiding continents confuse space. [...] On the basis of the power of the continuum held by nature, the monster ensures the emergence of difference. This difference is still without law and without any well-defined structure; the monster is the root-stock specification, but it is only a sub-species itself in the stubbornly slow stream of history. [...] Thus, against the background of the continuum, the monster provides an account, as though in caricature, of the genesis of differences.[45]

A teleological approach is not the goal of this discussion, but it is worthy to note the strong theoretical parallel found in, arguably, one of the most influential assessments of philosophies regarding the early modern mind and Liceti's intellectual enterprise on monsters. Liceti's adherence to an Aristotelian view of nature, as well as the defined categories he gave his reader, provided his audience with a physician's gaze upon the—now—explainable anomalies of nature.[46]

Increasingly, the tension between the idea of monsters as medical objects of inquiry and that of monsters as theological warnings became more palpable. Although its resolution—if resolution there needed to be—did not imply mutual exclusivity, the position taken by anatomists and scientists for the stronger authority of methodical examination often settled the conflict—once again echoing the rationalization of knowledge, truth, and direct observation championed by Vesalius. Realdo Colombo (1510–1559) explored the anatomical anomalies of otherwise normative human beings in Book Fifteen of *De re anatomica*, published posthumously in 1559.[47] Colombo took over Vesalius's position as the chair of anatomy at the University of Padua; his medically-guided approach to the study of monsters is therefore no surprise, since he was teaching anatomy and immersed in medical treatises during his explorations of anomalous bodies.[48] Unlike Paré or Boaistuau, Colombo never mentioned monsters as portentous signs; he did not attack those who had treated them as such, but he purposefully omitted any reference to their prophetic dimension. Colombo's treatise, by virtue of its deliberate exclusion, was one of the few and first teratological treatises to deal with monsters as pathological anomalies *only*. Though I here agree with Andrea Carlino's claim that Colombo's pathological presentation of monsters represents a shift, placing monsters in the realm of medicine, I also believe that the opposition between medicine and the wonderful was not as clear-cut as Carlino may suggest. Therefore, I use the adverb "only" intentionally.[49] The dissections that Colombo performed—particularly that of a hermaphrodite—and discussed in his Book Fifteen made his series of illustrated case studies valid bodies of knowledge by making him, and by proxy his readers, witnesses to the truth found in anatomizing monstrous bodies.[50]

In spite of the numerous avenues opened by treatises on monsters on the medical, theological, and philosophical fronts, an exact and universal name for the science of studying monsters did not appear until the nineteenth century. Following in the footsteps of his father, who was a renowned zoologist, Isidore Geoffroy Saint-Hilaire (1805–1861) wrote a treatise on monsters in 1832, entitled *Traité de tératologie*.[51] From the onset of his book, Saint-Hilaire positioned "teratology" as a distinct and separate science from physiology and other related sciences. He confirmed the validity of studying monsters, not only as a branch of pathology or philosophical anatomy, but as an independently justifiable inquiry.[52] Saint-Hilaire denounced previous authors who purported to study monsters while constantly attaching them to different branches of zoology or embryology. Saint-Hilaire's work built upon centuries of inquiries; nevertheless, he validated the study of monsters as a uniquely scientific endeavor by not only attributing an exclusive technical term to the study of monsters, but also by renouncing any kind of supernatural claim pertaining to the formation or presence of physically deformed individuals.

Though Saint-Hilaire was aware of the major leap he was proposing, he was nonetheless certain about the legitimacy of his claim.[53] He finalized the numerous attempts made before him by proposing an exhaustive study of teratology based on his ultimate goal: to understand the modification of the normal order.[54] It is noteworthy to point out that Saint-Hilaire's effort to remove theological and supernatural components attached to the study of monsters was not entirely successful in its legacy. Even though "teratology" became an accepted word denoting the scientific study of monsters, some authors did take liberties with the term. They used it and were aware of its origins, yet they re-introduced some of the factors Saint-Hilaire had eradicated. Exemplifying this trend is Cesare Taruffi (1821–1902), professor of anatomical pathology in the medical school of Bologna. Between 1881 and 1886, Taruffi wrote and published his *Storia della teratologia* in four volumes. Taruffi was a medical doctor, but he did not completely part with theological or mythical discussions about monsters in his treatise. This is explicitly stated in the first volume of his treatise where Taruffi mentions a few theological vectors that drive the understanding of monsters, particularly their formation and their relation to nature; he also remarks on the mythical origins of monsters by elaborating on Ermafroditus.[55] Ultimately, Saint-Hilaire's scientific study was the result of numerous intellectual confluences, many of which were born of the original wonder felt in the presence of monsters or in front of their representations.[56] This wondrous feeling was explored and exploited during the early modern period, as exemplified in collections of curiosities amassed by princely, regal, and scientific collectors alike.

In the sixteenth and seventeenth centuries, new attitudes and modes of inquiry toward nature were the reason for, and the result of, the development of new collecting practices.[57] Natural/scientific collections reflected and paralleled, for the most part, the inquiries taking place in the development of early modern scientific thought.[58] They established a link between the person who possessed the collectible object, and the scientific ideas this object represented. Likewise, the antiquities and paintings in other collections spoke to the intellectual taste and knowledge of the collector. Display and wonder were essential elements for both the natural/scientific collection and the classical art collection; the experience felt by a visitor in response to either type of object would have called upon his or her sense of wonder, whether it was wonder inspired by curiosity, as in the case of a scientific/natural collection, or wonder based on the emotion evoked by a work of art.[59] The effect of a collection was as important to the owner as it was to the visitor, because it was meant to serve as "a marvel, which gave pleasure and pride to its owner and induced pleasure and awe in the privileged visitor."[60]

The anatomical experience and the revealing of the true knowledge of the body during dissection was prolonged and refined by the subsequent process of the collection.[61] Further, anatomical collections and collections of curiosities often carried the stamp of truth beyond the theater because of their association with the visual experience of dissection. The objects thus collected and displayed held both the validation of scientific practice and the wonder associated with the spectacle of dissection. Early Italian collections were not meant to call only upon the senses of the viewers and to elicit undifferentiated emotional responses. Papal collections, for instance, were meant to maintain a specific heritage and assert the validity of the Catholic faith throughout the Christian world. In the same vein, the study of Christian Antiquarianism served to trace the roots of Christian belief and practice. As genealogy emerged as a recognized study—linked to a large literature on antiquities and nobility—collections of antiquities affirmed the prominence of one family while legitimizing such things as claims of lineage through the possession of antique sculptures, bronzes, gems, and cameos.[62]

Collecting as an activity, however, transcended its status as a princely or noble pursuit and during the sixteenth and seventeenth centuries became favored by scholars and medical men alike. It is in fact the latter group who elaborated new categories that shaped Renaissance collections by intensifying their wondrous, curious, and scientific characteristics.[63] As for what things (or live beings) best invoked wonder in a collection, several factors were considered. For the collection to be wondrous as a whole, number, variety, and organization were essential. For single elements to belong to such a collection, they had to be particularly beautiful, rare, exotic, or possess occult powers.[64] Monstrous beings, who were seen as marvels, fit the requirements necessary to belong to a collection of curiosity—and portraits of these beings stood at the crossroads between living and inanimate "curiosities." These images were considered quasi-scientific illustrations of the physically deformed and were found in collections such as Ulisse Aldrovandi's (1522–1605), one of the most eminent figures in Bologna. Over the course of more than fifty years, the naturalist Aldrovandi gathered a personal collection of over twenty thousand paintings, objects, plants, and prints housed in a public studio as well as a private museum in his home.[65] In 1595, Aldrovandi described his collection in these words:

> Today in my microcosm, you can see more than 18,000 different things, among which 7,000 plants in fifteen volumes, dried and pasted, 3,000 of which I had painted as if alive. The rest—animals terrestrial, aerial and aquatic, and other subterranean things such as earths, petrified sap, stones, marbles, rocks, and metals—amount to as many pieces again. I have paintings made of a further 5,000 natural objects—such as plants, various sorts of animals, and stones—some of which have been made into woodcuts. These can be seen in fourteen cupboards, which I call the Pinacotheca.[66]

Establishing specific *tabulae* to organize his entire collection, Aldrovandi emphasized the different links between nature and knowledge in his writings as much as in the physical organization of his collection.[67] In addition, in accordance with an Aristotelian system of thought, Aldrovandi stressed the importance of direct observation in order to better grasp the relationship between natural philosophy, medical knowledge, and sensory experience.[68] Aldrovandi's interest in anatomical and pathological rarities comes as no surprise, since monstrous individuals allowed curious scientists to apply at once their medical, natural, and sensory knowledge. Aldrovandi did not include woodcuts representing human monsters or hybrid monsters in a specific order in his posthumously published *Monstrorum Historia* (1642); rather, the mixture of images seems quite arbitrary

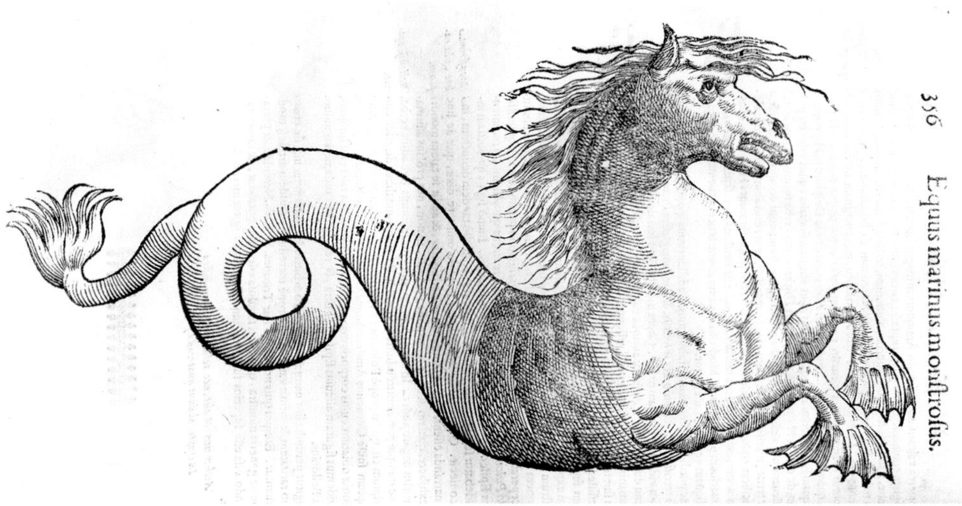

Figure 1.7. Ulisse Aldrovandi, a marine monster, page 356, *De monstrorum historia*, 1642, Wheaton College Permanent Collection, Newell Bequest Fund, Norton, Massachusetts

and possibly related to the enormous number of illustrations Aldrovandi commissioned during his lifetime.[69] But the amalgamation of imaginary and real historical monsters could also, in fact, serve to give legitimacy to the former. For instance, a marine monster (Fig. 1.7) precedes the imaginary half-dog, half-human conjoined twins (Fig. 1.8) and is directly followed by the monster of Ravenna (Fig. 1.2). Similarly, dwarves appear at the beginning of the *Historia* (Fig. 1.9), as well as much later in the book (Fig. 1.10).

In addition to Aldrovandi's *Monstrorum Historia*, some inventories categorized dwarves, hirsutes, or deformed individuals as natural curiosities—a testament to the fact that these individuals were in fact seen as collectible objects.[70] The third chapter of this book includes several examples of Medici inventories, thus providing additional substantiation for the categorization of dwarves as collectible objects. Similarly, the fourth chapter notes the presence of hirsutes in listings that underline their liminal positions.

On a different but comparable level, the acquisition of textual sources relating to monsters formed another dimension of this collecting activity. The scientific authority of such texts was not meant to weigh against that of printed images, since their goal, though not necessarily their audience, was different.[71] These texts, *sans* visual image, depended on the instinctive response of the reader in the same way collections of curiosities did. Such textual sources spanned from casual descriptions given to a French soldier by his cousin, to an assortment of scientific letters addressed to the Dauphin of France.[72] In both cases, lengthy descriptions of monstrous births, filled with many graphic details recalled the visual techniques employed in collections of curiosities, treatises on monsters, and

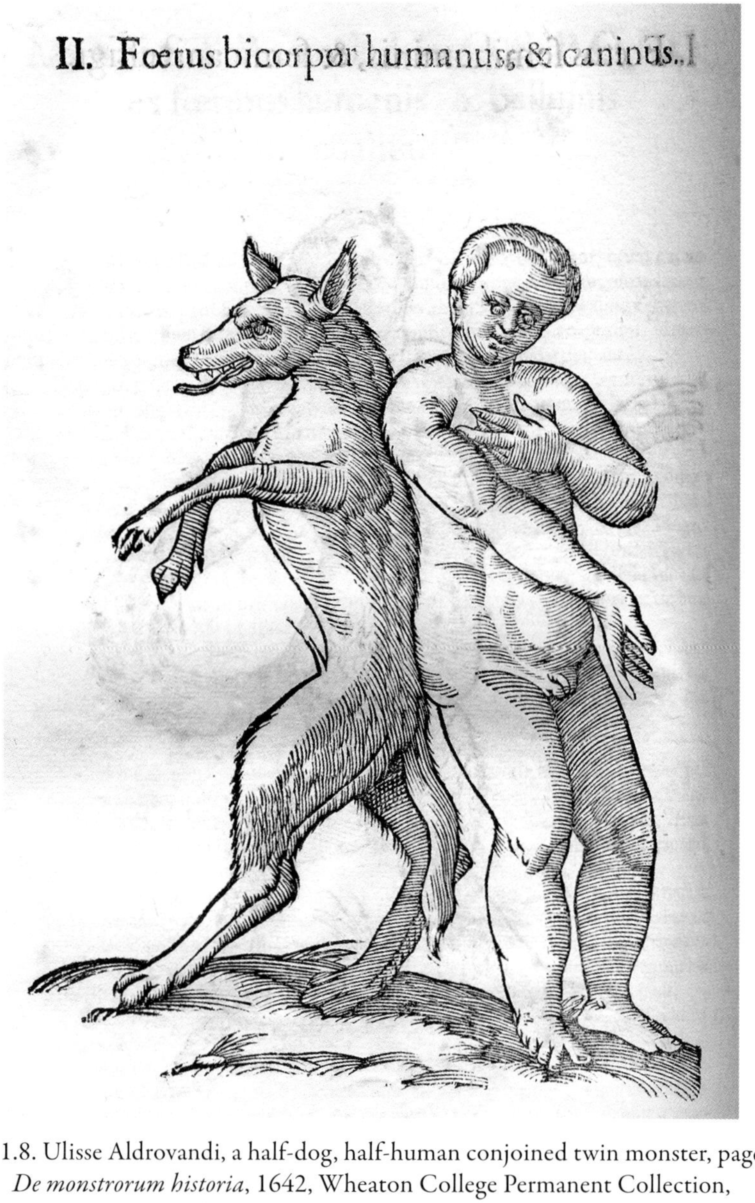

Figure 1.8. Ulisse Aldrovandi, a half-dog, half-human conjoined twin monster, page 366, *De monstrorum historia*, 1642, Wheaton College Permanent Collection, Newell Bequest Fund, Norton, Massachusetts

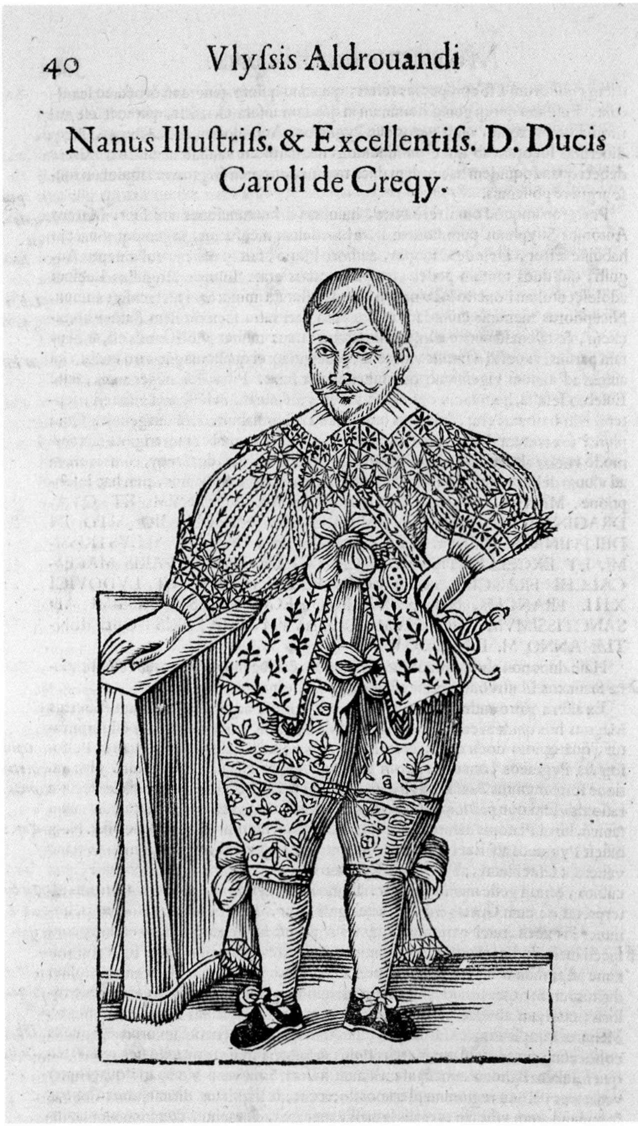

Figure 1.9. Ulisse Aldrovandi, the dwarf of Charles de Créquy, page 40, *De monstrorum historia*, 1642, Wheaton College Permanent Collection, Newell Bequest Fund, Norton, Massachusetts

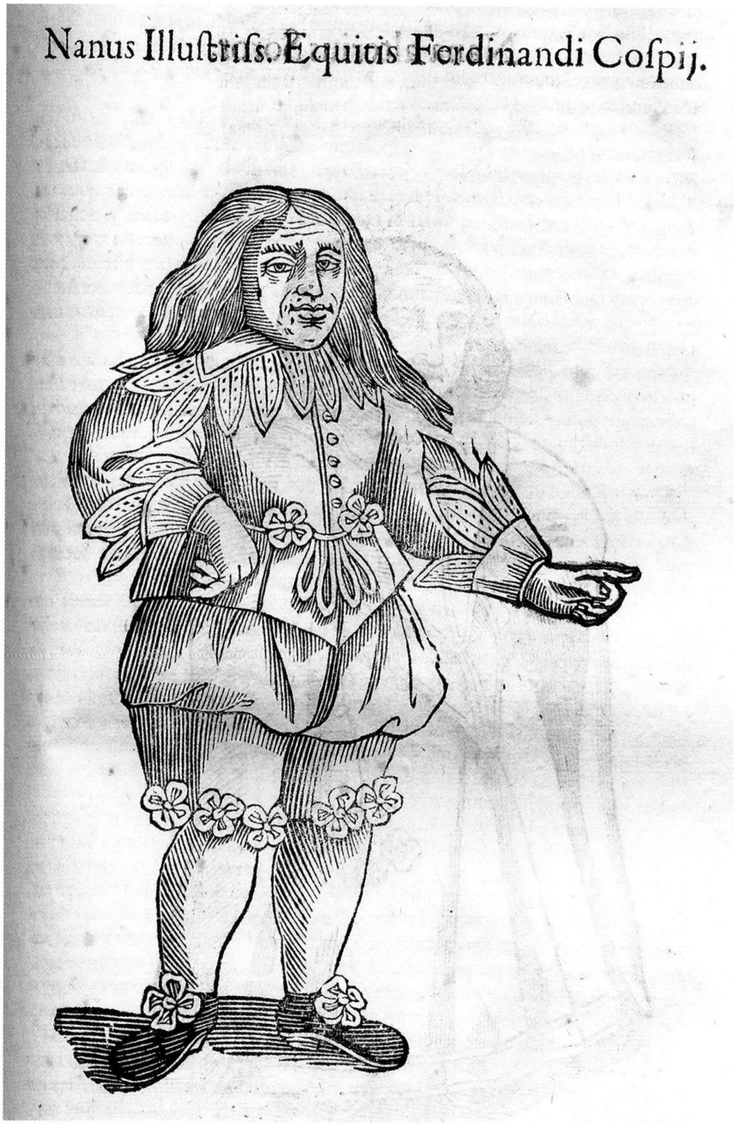

Figure 1.10. Ulisse Aldrovandi, the male dwarf of Ferdinando Cospi, page 603, *De monstrorum historia*, 1642, Wheaton College Permanent Collection, Newell Bequest Fund, Norton, Massachusetts

anatomical dissections. In addition to meticulous visual accounts, both letters gave locale, time references, and proper names when possible, so as to assert the veracity of the story being related. For instance, in a letter dated to 1649, the author mentions the city where the monster was born ("Mark"), how far this city was from Calais ("deux lieues"), the name of the father of the mother ("Quelin Soufré"), the date of her marriage and the origin of her husband ("mariée apres Pasques à un jeune Lorain"), the date when her contractions started and the day when they ended ("19 Fevrier" and "23 Fevrier"), and, finally, the name of the surgeon who helped the delivery ("Servais Cardon").[73] These extraneous details, repeated in several letters found in this collection, assured the reader of the validity of the event while enabling him/her to retrace the account, should s/he wish to do so.[74] Whereas the authorship and the true recipients of these "letters" are questionable, the intention of the publisher who collated them together is clear in its scope: by gathering these texts, the publisher acted like a collector and the readers were his potential awed visitors. By providing witnesses, these anonymous authors insisted on the truth of their narrative; similarly, the audience of a dissection in an anatomical theater certified the truth of the knowledge gathered directly from the body. As Paula Findlen has noted, museums and collections fit into an expanded culture by emphasizing sensory experience as a means to understand and possess knowledge, "anatomical demonstrations were an important part of the experimental life of the museum," she writes, "attracting the same people who crowded into the anatomy theaters in search of a scientific spectacle."[75] The collections' visitors sought a similar first-hand experience in witnessing dissections, looking for truth by *seeing* the actual dissection. Some anatomical theaters, such as Leiden's, also housed anatomical collections during the winter months. The anatomical dissections were directly related to the collection, not only because of the physical proximity of the two during winter months, but also because the collection continued the dissection.[76] The anatomical experience, the revealing of the true knowledge of the body during dissection, was thus prolonged and refined by the collection—whereas private anatomical collections and collections of curiosities often carried the stamp of truth beyond the theater.

The visual experience of a collection was encountered both in the north and in the south for *Wunderkammern*, but the presence of anatomical collections linked to theaters of anatomy was much more prevalent in the north. Indeed, the Italian conception of the post-mortem body saw the body as an object of commemoration, as it was believed that the soul departed the body immediately after death occurred. This belief was antagonistic to the northern view of the body as a site of decay paralleled by the gradual leaving of the soul.[77] The consequent anatomical collections, or lack thereof in Italy, attested to the influence these two opposing views had on the ideas of life and death, and therefore on the presence and use of anatomical collections. Whereas the Italians emphasized the identity of the deceased person with its spirit, the northerners conflated these two identities and saw vitality in the corpse itself. As a consequence, descriptions of the anatomical theater at Bologna did not even mention anatomical collections, but rather emphasized the classical architectural structure, the busts of illustrious physicians, and the grand ceiling decorations.[78] Even though anatomical museums were founded in Italy, their numbers and ratios to museums in general were less than half the ones in Holland.[79]

The primacy of the sense of vision in the quest for truth may be seen in dissections and collections of curiosities alike. Before Vesalius, Berengario da Carpi (1460–1530) established the importance of the *anathomia sensibilis* and thus implemented an epistemological shift in the demonstration, acquisition, and transmission of knowledge—insisting that true knowledge was mostly gained by seeing rather than by reading or hearing.[80] Therefore, in Italy, public dissections became associated with a discourse related to true knowledge, as they occurred in locales meant to enhance visual access. This access was also crucial for the performative aspect of anatomical dissections occurring in theaters outfitted for the occasion, particularly during Carnival. Seeing the dissection meant participating in this visual acquisition of knowledge and the expansion of the public from medical students only to more common attendants assured this knowledge was widely spread, turning witnesses into active contributors.[81]

Just as dissections served as epistemological maquettes for the knowledge tied to a normalized body, portraits of individuals with abnormal bodies provided the best sensorial model to transmit knowledge about these anatomically anomalous bodies. Portraits of physically different humans, however, were still distinct from their engraved and printed equivalent in treatises on monsters, or single leaf *avvisi*. Whereas treatises such as Paré's or Aldrovandi's dealt with images of monsters—often anonymous ones—as additional evidence for their textual assertions, portraits stood as independent visual creations representing distinct individuals and speaking to relationships existing between patron/commissioner and subject/monster. They were neither mere traditional portraits, nor systematic scientific illustrations, nor solely *mirabilia*. For instance, the idealization—and at times allegorization—present in these portraits distinguished them from scientific records like Liceti's, which mostly if not solely focused on cataloguing physical traits. While comparable in subject matter to visual documents that highlighted the bizarre, portraits of physically irregular beings integrated an aspect absent from these visual records: namely, they highlighted the tension between idealization and likeness specific to the genre of portraiture.[82] In addition, they existed independently from textual explanations, as they inherently incorporated a visual subtext meant to serve as scientific truth. Furthermore, the intentional pictorial language employed in these portraits (compositions, references, and formal elements) was the same one used in canonical court portraiture—despite the *Wunderkammer*-quality of their subjects. They also incorporated a function typical of courtly portraits, that of commemoration since we know many patrons, in fact, felt affection toward their monstrous courtly subjects. Illustrations of collections such as Ferdinando Cospi's (1606–1685), produced eight years before his death, served as visual

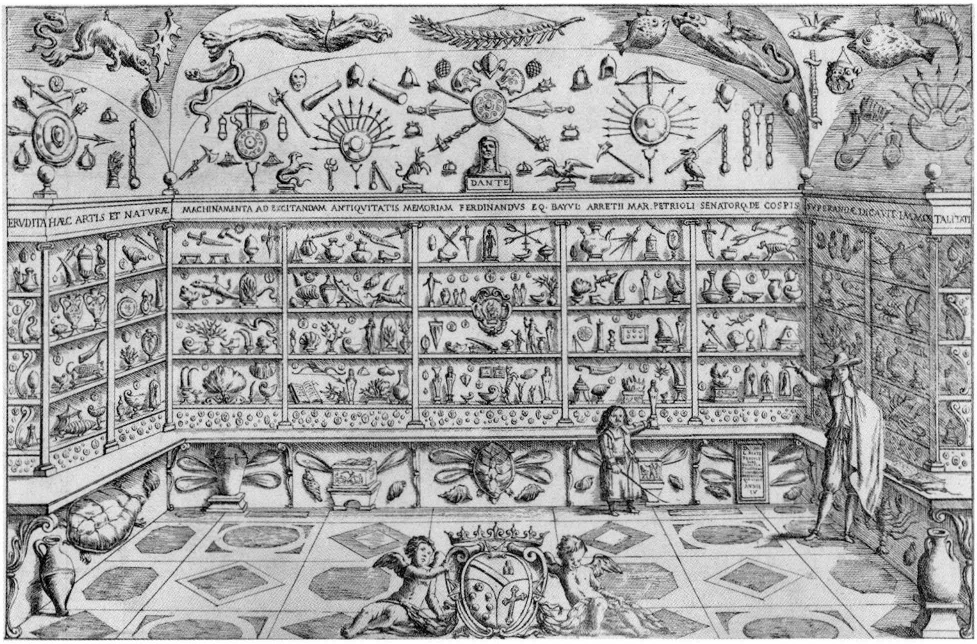
DANTE
ERVDITA HÆC ARTIS ET NATVRÆ
MACHINAMENTA AD EXCITANDAM ANTIQVITATIS MEMORIAM FERDINANDVS EQ. BAYVL ARRETII MAR. PETRIOLI SENATORQ. DE COSPIS

Figure 1.11. Lorenzo Legati, title page of the collection of *Marchese Ferdinando Cospi*, 1677, © The Trustees of The British Museum, London

testimony to the greatness of his collection; in this engraving, the parallel between the representation of the dwarf and his status as a collectible was glaringly evident (Fig. 1.11). The convergence of Sebastiano Biaviati's (Cospi's dwarf) portrait as an individual and his implied role as a guide to the collection to which he belonged—as indicated by his gesturing toward other objects and looking at the viewer—validated his dichotomous role and served as proof of his existence in both realms. Yet, portraits of monsters were not mere extensions of curiosity collections, but they existed as a combination of two worlds: they applied visual court conventions to cabinets of curiosity possessions.

Understandably, the popularity of monsters within scientific circles and court culture was the main driving force behind the production and ownership of their portraits. Since these portraits were painted to resemble the authentic sitters, the motivation behind their production could be linked to the fascination with the bodies of these specific individuals.[83] Moreover, this interest was attributed to growing attention paid to the natural sciences and to the prestige associated with such scientifically codified rarities, which ensured that collecting monsters was not debased or frivolous, but a suitable pursuit. However, portraits added another dimension to the mere wonder experienced when viewing a monstrous body or a monstrous being in a collection. They allowed the viewer to stare at length and with impunity, leisurely, and without discomfort. They also called upon the conventional senses of the viewer who recognized the setting—an official courtly portrait—but could not directly associate himself or herself with the subject, most often anyway. Akin to staring into distorted mirrors, these portraits afforded both wonder and uncertainty to the viewer, who was taught to trust his or her sight. While the exploration of the monstrous body could provide scientific knowledge, the official framing of the portrait—literally and figuratively—made this body of knowledge a vexed one. These portraits played with the anatomical *nosce te ipsum* by questioning it; they positioned the viewer in a visually doubtful scenario where inserting himself or herself inside this independent visual conversation became increasingly uncomfortable.[84] Precisely because of the abundant implications embedded in portraits of anatomically deformed individuals, it is necessary to appreciate and disentangle the complexities that live within these portraits. Monsters in visual representations have been addressed by scholars in art history, history of science, and social history; however, without fail, all the authors justify the production of these images as indices of courtly wit and humor, or as vague references to collections of curiosities only.[85] To understand the production and the impact of these portraits, it is essential to examine the nascent scientific impulses determined to categorize natural phenomena, the court culture in which monsters lived and performed, and the growing interest in the unusual. Whereas each type of physically anomalous person studied in this book gives rise to different questions regarding a specific individual's positions in a particular court, his or her status as a collectible object, and his or her participation as a subject of medical inquiry, many vectors remain common.

Italian princely courts, for instance, offer numerous unexplored avenues of inquiry for appreciating the social and intellectual position of monstrous subjects. Early modern courts were notoriously rigid and strict environments, where the slightest deviation became a matter of comment. It is precisely this rigidity that increased the courts' need for others; they provided a less defined and more open human space in the intense normative and regulated behavior imposed by courts. This conflict between normative court regulations and relief through upturned aesthetics is apparent in the portraits central to this book's examinations. The notion of Renaissance individuality has also not been adequately used to explain the role of monstrous subjects at court and their subsequent portraits. The Burckhardtian concept of the rise of the individual has usually justified the aggrandizement of personalities during the Renaissance, yet the humor associated with such a perception has been disregarded to explain these portraits, which seem to contradict such a notion. Peter Burke's view of the comic in early modern Italy offers a fruitful way to highlight the role of physically different bodies at court, within a discourse of Renaissance individuality. Indeed, among other illustrations, Burke relates the example of a joke played on a fat carpenter by the architect Filippo Brunelleschi (1377–1446). By doing so, he insists that this *beffa*—a practical joke or trick—fit perfectly with the idea of identity in an age of individualism as described by Jacob Burckhardt.[86]

People whose bodies had monstrous qualities, therefore, were full participants in the typical notion of Burckhardtian Renaissance identity; they were not mere anonymous curiosities, but rather individuals who rose within the courts that welcomed and used them. The court of Mantua stands as both a counterexample to courtly rigidity and as a perfect instance of the intersection of physical deformity and identity. It was considered bad luck to have a ruling duke who lacked a hump in his back; the court's identity was thus defined by the physical deformity of its ruler.[87] In Ferrara, some of the Este dukes legally adopted dwarves and giants, then insisted they be educated.[88] Physical deformity was thus an inherent part of most princely courts. The question is therefore not why were court portraits of monsters painted in the early modern period, but rather what would happen if we removed these monstrous subjects and their portraits from court histories. Could these portraits be omitted from the visual tradition of courtly portraiture, given said deformed sitters' strong social and intellectual presence at court? They were integral to the way elites defined themselves, and they provided the essential exceptions needed to reinforce a canon of high normalcy essential for established courts to survive.

By incorporating monstrous subjects into the controlled vocabulary of anatomical knowledge, anatomists, artists, and early modern scientists not only provided an alternate way of understanding human bodies, but they also expanded what constituted cultural conformity. Ultimately, the resulting texts and images dealing with bodies of anatomically abnormal individuals speak to the lack of linear cultural hegemony and highlight intellectual exchanges inevitable during a time of self-fashioning and scientific developments. Early modern audiences' fascination with monstrous bodies was articulated through a vocabulary of difference that allowed norms to define themselves against their own boundaries. The reciprocity between monsters and normative human beings grew in a discourse of social regulation and scientific discoveries. The treatises on monsters intervened in this discourse as active visual markers of such interactions, whereas the subjects of these works confronted the viewers with the reality of their monstrous anomalies and with the actuality of their human presence. They did so most visibly in the courts that invited, purchased, and displayed them.

Notes

[1] For the dissection of monsters I am particularly referring to Colombo's dissection of a hermaphrodite—though the other anatomically unusual bodies he dissected could fall into this same category—and to Agnolo Bronzino's participation in the dissection of conjoined twins at the Palazzo Rucellai in 1538. See Zakiya Hanafi, *The Monster in the Machine: Magic, Medicine, and the Marvelous in the Time of the Scientific Revolution* (Durham and London: Duke University Press, 2000), 18–21.

[2] While they can often overlap, I use monstrosity to denote the condition or fact of being monstrous, and monstrousness as the qualities attached to being monstrous. This differentiation is one based on the *Oxford English Dictionary* demarcation.

[3] For instance, in his encyclopedic work on animals, Conrad Gesner borrowed images from earlier German sources and from biblical texts and combined them with recently discovered animals from the new world. See Conrad Gesner, *Historiae animalium* (Frankfurt: H. Laurent, 1620) where the author describes a beast from the new world (title page of book I), a unicorn (book I, page 689), and a salamander (book II, page 80).

[4] For a detailed discussion and description of the pamphlet and its interpretation, see Jennifer Spinks, *Monstrous Births and Visual Culture in Sixteenth-century Germany* (London: Pickering & Chatto, 2009), 59–79.

[5] Andrea Carlino, "Strani corpi. Come farsi une ragione dei mostri nel XVI secolo," in *Phantastische Lebensräume, Phantome und Phantasmen* (Marburg an der Lahn: Basilisken-Press, 1997).

[6] Isidore Geoffroy Saint-Hilaire, *Histoire générale et particulière des anomalies de l'organisation chez l'homme et les animaux, ouvrage comprenant des recherches sur les caractères, la classification, l'influence physiologique et pathologique, les rapports généraux, les lois et les causes des monstruosités, des variétés de vices de conformation, ou Traité de tératologie*, 3 vols. (Paris: J.-B. Baillière, Libraire de l'Académie Royale de Médecine, 1832).

[7] Entry is found in Katharine Park and Lorraine Daston, *Wonders and the Order of Nature 1150–1750* (New York: Zone Books, 1998), 177 and is taken from Luca Landucci, *A Florentine Diary from 1450 to 1516 by Luca Landucci, Continued by an Anonymous Writer till 1542 with Notes by Iodoco Del Badia*, trans. Alice de Rosen Jervis (New York: E.P. Dutton and Co., 1927), 249–50 (translation slightly altered for accuracy); Italian text in idem, *Diario fiorentino dal 1450–1516*, ed. Iodoco Del Badia (Florence: G.C. Sansoni, 1883), 314.

[8] For more details on the monster of Ravenna, see Ottavia Niccoli, *Prophecy and People in Renaissance Italy*, trans. Lydia G. Cochrane (Chicago: University of Chicago Press, 1990), 31–51.

[9] J.B. deC. M. Saunders and Charles D. O'Malley, *The Illustrations from the Works of Andreas Vesalius of Brussels* (New York: Dover Publications, 1950), 204. For a detailed biography of Vesalius and his numerous productions and publications, 9–40.

[10] Ibid., 40–41.

[11] For centuries, the lecturer would read Galenic texts from the chair in Latin, while the pointer directed the audience's gaze to the supposed part of the body being discussed. The only person touching the corpse was the barber-surgeon whose knowledge of the actual body was considerable, but who often did not understand the Latin words being read. Consequently, discrepancies occurred between textual descriptions and the parts of the body being dissected. For a discussion of Vesalius's acquisition of actual bodies in the hope of eliminating such inconsistencies, see Jonathan Sawday, *The Body Emblazoned: Dissection and the Human Body in Early Modern Culture* (London and New York: Routledge, 1995), 195.

[12] Julie V. Hansen and Suzanne Porter, *The Physician's Art: Representations of Art and Medicine* (Durham: Duke University Medical Center Library and Duke University Museum of Art, 1999), 32.

[13] Bernard Schultz, *Art and Anatomy in Renaissance Italy* (Ann Arbor: UMI Research Press, 1985), 11.

[14] Ibid., 13 and Nancy Siraisi, *Medieval and Early Renaissance Medicine: An Introduction to Knowledge and Practice* (Chicago: University of Chicago Press, 1990).

[15] Lawrence Conrad et al. *The Western Medical Tradition 800 B.C. to A.D. 1800* (Cambridge: Cambridge University Press, 1995), 66–67.

[16] Ibid., 60.

[17] Andrea Carlino, *Books of the Body: Anatomical Ritual and Renaissance Learning* (Chicago and London: University of Chicago Press, 1999), 2.

[18] For a translation and annotation of Vesalius's *Fabrica*, see the wonderful project (in progress) undertaken by Daniel H. Garrison and Malcom Hast: http://vesalius.northwestern.edu.

[19] Conrad et al., *The Western Medical Tradition*, 278.

[20] Katharine Park, *Secrets of Women: Gender, Generation, and the Origins of Human Dissection* (New York: Zone Books, 2006), 207–59. The discussions on the *Fabrica* are numerous and it is not the goal of this chapter to address all of them. The reason Park's assessment of the *Fabrica* is noted here relates to the ways in which the viewer accessed the knowledge presented and how this method finds echoes in portraits of monsters: the balance between truth and distance, as well as the reaffirming of the viewer's superior position is a strong parallel, particularly when considering the fact that the dissected bodies were corpses of criminals facing additional punishment post mortem.

[21] Ibid.

[22] Carlino, *Books of the Body*, 43.

[23] See for instance Glenn Harcourt, "Andreas Vesalius and the Anatomy of Antique Sculpture," *Representations* 17 (Winter 1987): 28–61.

[24] While Vesalius does make some comparative anatomical and visual analyses in the *Fabrica* (in his discussion on skulls, for instance), he mostly seeks to establish an ideal anatomical norm.

[25] Andrew Cunningham, *The Anatomical Renaissance: The Resurrection of the Anatomical Projects of the Ancients* (Aldershot: Scholar Press, 1997), 88: "Vesalius represents a further stage in the revival of Galen's anatomy in that he taught the world to see a different Galenic body; and he taught anatomists, physicians and philosophers to adopt a new ambition with respect to the Ancients of anatomy."

[26] Paula Findlen, *Possessing Nature: Museums, Collecting, and Scientific Culture in Early Modern Italy* (Berkeley, Los Angeles, and London: University of California Press, 1994), 194–208 in particular.

[27] Pierre Boaistuau, *Histoires prodigieuses* (Paris: Robert le Mangnier, 1566). Some of the chapter titles are: "Nabuchodonosor," "Diables qui conçoivent," "Monstre ayant ailes & les pieds d'oyseau engendré du temps du Pape Iule second & du Roy Louys douziesme," or "Filles collées."

[28] Ibid., preface following the dedication: "Monseigneur, entre toutes les choses qui se peuvent contempler soubs la concavité des cieux, il ne se voit rien qui plus efeuille l'esprit humain, qui ravisse plus les sens, qui plus espouvente, qui engendre plus grande admiration ou terreur aux creatures, que les monstres, prodiges & abomination, sequels nous voyons les erreures de nature ou seulement preposterées, renuersées, mutilées & tronquées, mais (qui plus est) nous y decouvrons le plus souvent un secret iugement & fleau de l'ire de Dieu, par l'object des choses qui se presentent lequel nous faict sentir la violence de sa iustice si aspre, que nous sommes contrains d'entrer en nous mesmes, frapper au marteau de nostre conscience, esplucher noz vices, & avoir en horreur nos meffaicts, specialement quand nous lisons aux histories, sacrées & prophanes, que quelquefois les Elemens on esté Heraulx, Trompettes, ministres & executeurs de la iustice de Dieu."

[29] In the sixteenth century, the term "prodige" referred to a miracle, sign, or extraordinary event, of a magical or supernatural type.

[30] Additionally writing a book in the vernacular would also widen—popularize—the audience able to read Paré's work. Ambroise Paré, *Des monstres et prodiges* (Paris: G. Buon, 1585), 25e livre, préface au lecteur, eij verso: "Or disent-ils que je ne devoy escrire en François, & que par ce

moyen la Medecine en seroit tenue à mespris: ce qui me semble le contraire: car ce que j'en ay faict, est plustost pour la magnifier & honorer."

[31] Ibid., 1020: "Monstres sont des choses qui apparoissent outre le cours de Nature (&sont le plus souuent signes de quelques malheurs à advenir) comme un enfant qui naist avec un seul bras, un autre qui aura deux testes, & autres members outre l'ordinaire. Prodiges, ce sont des choses qui viennent du tout contre Nature, comme une femme qui enfentera un serpent, ou un chien, ou autre chose tout contre Nature. [...] Les mutilez, ce sont aveugles, borgnes, bossus, boiteux, ou ayant six doigts a la main ou aux pieds, ou moins de cinq ou joincts ensembles, ou les bras trop courts, ou le nez trop enfoncé comme ont les camus, ou avoir les levres grosses et renversées [...] ou toute autre chose contre Nature."

[32] Daston and Park, *Wonders*, 146.

[33] Paré, *Des monstres et prodiges*, 1027.

[34] Ibid.: "Figure de deux gemeaux n'ayans qu'une seule teste."

[35] Ibid., 1036: "Figure d'un enfant monstrueux, de defaut de la semence en deue quantité."

[36] I. Norwich, "A Consultation between Andreas Vesalius and Ambroise Paré at the Deathbed of Henri II, King of France, 15 July 1559," *SAMJ* 80, no. 5 (1991): 245–47.

[37] Daston and Park, *Wonders*, 173–214 and 175–76 in particular for the different perceptions of monsters.

[38] Paré, *Monstres et prodiges*, 1030.

[39] Norman R. Smith, "Portentous Births and the Monstrous Imagination in Renaissance Culture," in *Marvels, Monsters, and Miracles: Studies in the Medieval and Early Modern Imaginations*, ed. Timothy S. Jones and David A. Sprunger (Kalamazoo: Board of the Medieval Institute, 2002), 270.

[40] Paré, *Monstres et prodiges*, 1020: "un être que l'on monstre." The humanization used in the term "être" is notable.

[41] Ibid., 1045: "furent portées par plusieurs villes d'Italie" and "le peuple qui était fort ardent de voir ce nouveau spectacle de nature."

[42] Félix Gaffiot, *Dictionnaire Latin–Français: Le Grand Gaffiot* (Paris: Hachette, 2000) and Emile Benveniste, *Vocabulaire des institutions indo-européennes*, vols. 1 and 2 (Paris: Edition de Minuit, 1969).

[43] Fortunio Liceti, *De monstrorum natura, caussis et differentiis: Libri Duo, Aeneis iconibus ornate et aucti* (Padua: Paolo Frambotti, 1634), preface: monsters "quoque unicuique alteri monstrantur."

[44] Fortunio Liceti, in *Description anatomique des Parties de la Femme qui servent à la Generation; avec un Traité des monstres, de leur Causes, de leur Nature, & de leur differences: Et une description anatomique de la disposition surprenante de quelques Parties Externes, & Internes de Deux Enfans Nés dans la Ville de Gand Capitale des Flandres le 28 Avril 1703 &c. &c.*, par Mons.r Jean Palfyn, Anatomist & Chirurgien de la Ville de Gand, Desquels ouvrages on peut considerer comme une Suite de l'Accouchement des Femmes par Mons.r Mauriceau (Leiden: Chez la Veuve Bastiaan Schouten, 1708). Interestingly, this French version pairs the cause of monsters with a treatise on female reproductive parts, thus accentuating the generative emphasis of the book. In the preface to Liceti's translation: "Comme donc il n'y a rien de tout ce qui vit sous le Soleil, qui cause plus de surprise & d'admiration que les Monstres; Ce n'est pas sans raison que les hommes desirent si universellement de connoitre leur Essence."

[45] Michel Foucault, *The Order of Things: An Archeology of the Human Sciences* (New York: Random House, 1994), 156–57.

[46] In total, Liceti gives ten different categories of monsters and explains each one by using case studies. Furthermore, Liceti's treatise is actually written in Latin and therefore borrows from a more traditional medical textual tradition.

[47] Realdo Colombo, *De re anatomica: Libri XV* (Venice: Nicholas Bevilacqua, 1559).

[48] Robert J. Moes and C.D. O'Malley, "Realdo Colombo: 'On Those Things Rarely Found in Anatomy': An Annotated Translation from the *De Re Anatomica* (1559)," *Bulletin of the History of Medicine* 34, no. 6 (November–December 1960): 508. Colombo replaced Vesalius temporarily as the chair of surgery and anatomy on January 19, 1543 and permanently in 1544.

[49] I am grateful to Katharine Park who suggested to me that the opposition between medicine and the wonderful might be a misleading one, particularly when looking at works by physicians on medical *mirabilia*, such as Benivieni or Paré. I am also very indebted to Andrea Carlino who generously shared this article and discussed his research with me. Andrea Carlino, "Strani corpi. Come farsi une ragione dei mostri nel XVI secolo," *Phantastische Lebensräume, Phantome und Phantasmen* (Marburg an der Lahn: Basilisken-Press, 1997), 143: "during the Renaissance they were perceived and understood in many different ways: monsters were prodigies and natural wonders, monsters were signs of future catastrophes, they were used for religious and political propaganda. At the same time, they started to be conceived and studied into a medical framework. [...] My claim is that Colombo's approach to monstrous subjects through anatomical dissections induced him to conceive their morphological 'differences' as anatomical abnormalities. This approach signifies inscribing monstrosity in pathology, therefore evacuating the merely teratological and superstitious conception still operating in texts produced by other doctors and anatomists such as Ambroise Paré."

[50] Colombo, *De re anatomica*, 268.

[51] Isidore Geoffroy Saint-Hilaire, *Histoire générale et particulière des anomalies de l'organisation chez l'homme et les animaux, ouvrage comprenant des recherches sur les caractères, la classification, l'influence physiologique et pathologique, les rapports généraux, les lois et les causes des monstruosités, des variétés et vices de conformation ou traité de teratologie* (Paris: Baillière, 1832–36).

[52] Ibid., vol. 1, x in the preface: "J'ai cherché et je crois avoir réussi à démontrer que l'ensemble de nos connaissances sur les anomalies, ou pour employer dès à présent le nom que je lui donne dans cet ouvrage, la *tératologie* ne peut plus être considérée comme une section de l'anatomie pathologique; qu'on ne saurait non plus voir en elle un simple rameau, ni de la physiologie, ni de l'anatomie philosophique, ni de l'embryogénie, ni de la zoologie; qu'elle a avec toutes ces sciences des rapports presque également intimes, sans pouvoir être confondue avec aucune d'elles; qu'elle constitue par conséquent une branche particulière, un *science* distincte, dans le sens spécial qu'on a donné à ce mot."

[53] Ibid., vol. 1, 1, footnote referring to the first time the author uses the term "tératologie": "Je n'ignore pas que je m'écarte de l'opinion de tous les anatomistes, en considérant l'ensemble des nos connaissances sur les monstruosités comme une science distincte, comme un branche spéciale de la grande science de l'organisation: mais je crois pouvoir dire que cette innovation, importante pour les progrès futurs de la théorie des anomalies, et la création d'un mot nouveau, qui en est la conséquence nécessaire, seront complètement justifiées dans la suite de cet ouvrage."

[54] Ibid., vol. 1, xij: "Aussi ai-je constamment cherché à déduire des faits tératologiques, les conséquences générales et les applications qui résultent de leur étude, et n'ai-je jamais perdu de vue le but principal que je m'étais proposé en commençant cet ouvrage; celui d'arriver, par l'étude des anomalies, de leurs caractères, de leur influence sur l'organisation, de leur mode de production et de leurs

lois, à la connaissance plus exacte et plus approfondie des modifications de l'ordre normal, de leur essence, de leur raison d'existence, et des principes auxquels peut se rattacher leur infinie variété."

[55] Cesare Taruffi, *Storia della teratologia* (Bologna: Regia Tipografia, 1881–1886), vol. 1, 117 for the theological discussion and 141 for the mythological one.

[56] I am being purposefully broad by using the term "representation." Often, the inclusion of an engraving of a monster, for instance, was accompanied by a textual description of its origins and physical appearance, or a poem relating the state of this particular being. The actual representation of a monster might thus include a visual one alone, or a visual one together with a textual one.

[57] Findlen, *Possessing Nature*, 1.

[58] Adalgisa Lugli, "Inquiry as Collection: The Athanasius Kircher Museum in Rome," *RES* 12 (Autumn 1986): 109.

[59] Daston and Park, *Wonders*, 22.

[60] Martin Kemp, "'Wrought by No Artist's Hand': The Natural, the Artificial, the Exotic, and the Scientific in Some Artifacts from the Renaissance," in *Reframing the Renaissance: Visual Culture in Europe and Latin America 1450–1650*, ed. Claire Farago (New Haven and London: Yale University Press, 1995), 185.

[61] Findlen, *Possessing Nature*, 209–10, and Julie V. Hansen, "Resurrecting Death: Anatomical Art in the Cabinet of Dr. Frederick Ruysch," *Art Bulletin* 78 (December 1996): 667.

[62] For a discussion on various Italian classical collections of antiquities, their early origins, their social explication, and their purpose, see Francis Haskell and Nicholas Penny, *Taste and the Antique: The Lure of Classical Sculpture 1500–1900* (New Haven and London: Yale University Press, 1981).

[63] Philipp Blom, *To Have and to Hold: An Intimate History of Collectors and Collecting* (Woodstock and New York: The Overlook Press, 2002), 15–16.

[64] For a detailed account, various examples of such collections, and thoughts about collecting and collections in the early modern period, see Daston and Park, *Wonders*, chapters I, II, IV, and VII in particular; Findlen, *Possessing Nature*; Kemp, "'Wrought by No Artist's Hand'"; Joy Kenseth, ed., *The Age of the Marvelous* (Hanover: Hood Museum of Art, 1991); Lugli, "Inquiry as Collection," 109–124; Krzysztof Pomian, *Collectors and Curiosities: Paris and Venice 1500–1800* (Cambridge: Polity Press, 1990); Valerio Rivosecchi, *Esotismo in Roma Barocca* (Rome: Bulzoni Editore, 1982); Ingrid D. Rowland, *The Ecstatic Journey: Athanasius Kircher in Baroque Rome* (Chicago: University of Chicago Libraries, 2000); Julius von Schlosser, "Italienische Kuriositätenkammern," *Die Kunst- und Wunderkammern der Spätrenaissance* (Leipzig: Klinkhardt & Biermann, 1908); and for a comprehensive look at the history of collecting see Arthur MacGregor, *Curiosity and Enlightenment: Collectors and Collections from the Sixteenth to the Nineteenth Century* (New Haven and London: Yale University Press, 2007).

[65] Giuseppe Olmi, "Il collezionismo scientifico," in *Il teatro della natura di Ulisse Aldrovandi*, ed. Raffaella Simili (Bologna: Editrice Compositori, 2001), 20.

[66] The translation of Aldrovandi's own description is found in Daston and Park, *Wonders*, 154, note 3.

[67] Findlen, *Possessing Nature*, 60.

[68] Ibid., 199. Also see Giuseppe Olmi, *Ulisse Aldrovandi: Scienza e natura nel secondo cinquecento* (Trent: UNIcoop, 1976) and Sandra Pattaro Tugnoli, *La formazione scientifica e il "Discorso naturale" di Ulisse Aldrovandi* (Trent: UNIcoop, 1977).

[69] Jacobs, *The Living Image*, 140–41.

[70] Tobia Aldini, naturalist and prefect of the Farnese gardens, includes humans among the other marvels of the cardinal's court. Tobia Aldini, *Exactissima descriptio rariorum quarandarum plantarum quae continentur Romae in Horto Farnesiano* (Rome: Typis Iacobi Mascardi, 1625), 10, as cited in Roberto Zapperi, "Arrigo le Velu, Pietro le Fou, Amon le Nain et autres bêtes: Autour d'un tableau d'Agostino Carrache," *Annales: Économies – Sociétés – Civilisations* 40, no. 2 (March–April 1985): 310 and 324, note 11. Arrigo is referred to as a "mirabilia inte alia mirabilia."

[71] In this instance, one may think of the influence held by an image printed in a widely distributed *avviso* versus a text published in a small collection of narrational letters meant for a literate public. The gathering of these constructed letters could be akin to the propagation of urban myth types of stories.

[72] The first letter is found in *Recueil de Mélanges in quattro* (Paris: Chez la Veuve d'Anthoine Coulon, 1649), vol. 50, separation 17. It is titled "La naissance d'un monstre espouvantable, engendré d'une belle & jeune femme, native de Mark, à deux lieues de Calais, le vingt-troisième Fevrier 1649." The second letter is part of the same *Recueil de Mélanges in quattro*, and is in vol. 50, separation 20. It is titled "Memoire concernant les arts et les sciences presenté à Monseigneur le Dauphin" and is dated February 1, 1672.

[73] In the 1649 letter: "[J]e vous ferois icy la description de la naissance espouvantable d'un Monstre tres effroyable, arrivé à Mark, à deux lieues de Calais, & proche de nostre demeure. [...]. Sçachez-donc, cher Cousin, que la fille de Quelin Soufré, fut mariée apres Pasques à un jeune Lorain de nation, lequel faisoit icy l'homme prudent remply de sagesse. [...] Sa femme ainsi demeurée seule fut saisie de mal le 19 Fevrier & par des cris espouvantable, rendoit bien tesmoignage que son corps souffroit grands douleurs. Elle fut dans ce tourment jusqu'au 23. Fevrier à midy: & avec l'ayde de Servais Cardon, Chirurgien, qui luy fit incision, elle se delivra d'un enfant."

[74] The same stratagem is used in a letter dated to 1672: "Pour satisfaire la curiosité de ceux à qui vous avez parlé de cet enfant prodigieux, dont je vous ay déja écrit quelque chose, je vous en vais mander toutes les circonstances. Le 28 Septembre 1667. Nicole Vallée femme de Noël Marchand, demeurant à la Beausserie sur la Paroisse de la Chapelle Huon au Diocese du Mans, à un quart-de-lieuë de Courten-Vau, accoucha d'un garçon qui avoit en naissant une grabde chevelure blonde. [...] Sa mere le voulut nourrir elle même, & l'éleva jusqu'à trois ans & demy environ; car il mourut le 21 Avril 1671. [...] Mr. Pousset Curé de la Chapelle Huon, le pere & la mere de l'enfan, & tous les voisins sont aussi bien que moy témoins de ce prodige."

[75] Findlen, *Possessing Nature*, 194–240 and 209 in particular.

[76] Th.H. Lunsingh Scheurleer and G.H.M. Posthumus Meyjes, eds., *Leiden University in the Seventeenth Century: An Exchange of Learning* (Leiden: Universitaire pers Leiden / E.J. Brill, 1975).

[77] Katharine Park, "The Life of the Corpse: Division and Dissection in Late Medieval Europe," *Journal of the History of Medicine and Allied Sciences* 50 (1995): 119.

[78] Giovanni Martinotti, "L'Anatomia pubblica a Bologna," *L'Illustrazione medica italiana* 5 (1923): 25–29.

[79] F.J. Cole, *History of the Anatomical Museum* (Liverpool and London: The University Press and Constable & Company, 1914), 311, where we see that up to 1850 the ratio of *total number of museums founded / anatomical museums founded* is 50/14 Holland and 44/7 for Italy.

[80] Rafael Mandressi, *Textes scientifiques et savoirs sur le corps à l'époque moderne*, seminar, École des hautes études en sciences sociales, Paris, 22 November 2005. For a great discussion on the primacy of vision and Berengario da Carpi's epistemological model, see Rafael Mandressi, *Le regard de l'anatomiste: Dissection et invention du corps en Occident* (Paris: Editions du Seuil, 2003).

It is important to note that vision did not work to the exclusion of other senses in the anatomical acquisition of knowledge; in fact, partnered with the sense of touch, it became even stronger.

[81] For the discussion on Carnival, anatomy, and performance, see Giovanna Ferrari, "Public Anatomy Lessons and the Carnival: The Anatomy Theatre of Bologna," *Past and Present* 117 (1987): 50–106.

[82] Such documents were often engravings representing the actual collection. See Ferrante Imperato, *Dell'historia naturale* (1672); Benedetto Ceruti and Andrea Chiocco, *Musaeum Francisci Calceolari Iunioris Veronensis* (1662); Lorenzo Legati, *Museo Cospiano annesso a quello del famoso Ulisse Aldrovandi e donato alla sua patria dall'illustrissimo Signor Ferdinando Cospi* (1677); and Ulisse Aldrovandi's illustrations in *Monstrorum historia* (1642).

[83] Here, one can think of David Freedberg's argument about verisimilitude and how images "activate emotional engagement." See David Freedberg, *The Power of Images: Studies in the History and Theory of Response* (Chicago and London: University of Chicago Press, 1991), 200 and chapter 9 in particular.

[84] Jacobs, *The Living Image*, chapter 5, "*Nosce te ipsum*: Narcissus, Mirrors, and Monsters," particularly 134, 137, 153, 160, and 166.

[85] For instance see Paul Barolsky, *Infinite Jest: Wit and Humor in Italian Renaissance Art* (Columbia and London: University of Missouri Press, 1978); Giovanna Galli, "Strano è bello," *Stile Arte* 63 (November 2002); Christiane Hertel, "Hairy Issues: Portraits of Petrus Gonsalvus and His Family in Archduke Ferdinand II's *Kunstkammer* and Their Contexts," *Journal of the History of Collections* 13, no. 1 (2001): 1–22; James Holderbaum, "A Bronze by Giovanni Bologna and a Painting by Bronzino," *The Burlington Magazine* 98 (December 1956): 439–45; Alberto Manguel, "Lavinia Fontana: The Image as Understanding," in *Reading Pictures: A History of Love and Hate* (New York: Random House, 2000); Robin Leigh O'Bryan, *The Dwarf in Italian Renaissance Iconography*, unpublished thesis (San Diego State University, 1991); E. Tietze-Conrat, *Dwarfs and Jesters in Art* (New York: Phaidon, 1957); Barry Wind, *"A Foul and Pestilent Congregation": Images of "Freaks" in Baroque Art* (Brookfield: Ashgate, 1998); and Roberto Zapperi, "Arrigo le Velu, Pietro le Fou, Amon le Nain et autres bêtes: Autour d'un tableau d'Agostino Carrache," *Annales: Économies – Sociétés – Civilisations* 40, no. 2 (March–April 1985): 307–27.

[86] Peter Burke, *Varieties of Cultural History* (Ithaca: Cornell, 1997), 83. Burke also discusses the limits of such *beffe* and how they played into the social culture of shame and honor: "The *beffa* was often not 'pure' amusement but a means of humiliating, shaming, and indeed of socially annihilating rivals and enemies. This was a culture in which honour and shame were leading values. [...] The point to underline, at least for the period 1350–1550, is the widespread participation—both as jokers and victims—of princes and peasants, men and women, clergy and laity, young and old."

[87] I am grateful to Ed Goldberg for relating this fascinating fact to me during a conversation in the Archivio di Stato di Firenze in October 2004. I am also very indebted to Molly Bourne for sharing her immense knowledge of the Mantuan archives and referring me to sources discussing the famous Gonzaga hump. Dario Franchini et al., *La Scienza a Corte: Collezionismo Eclettico Natura e Immagine a Mantova fra Rinascimento e Manierismo* (Rome: Bulzoni Editore, 1979), 101–114 and Attilio Zanca, "Mostri nelle leggende popolare," in *I naifs e l'arte popolare* (Rome, 1975), 28–30.

[88] Guido Guerzoni graciously shared some of his research with me while he was at the Villa I Tatti and I am indebted to him for this intriguing piece of information. This conversation happened in October 2004 as well.

Chapter 2

Renaissance Portrait and Intellectual Frame

COURTS AND THEIR SOCIAL SETTINGS were the reason and the sites for the production of countless portraits of rulers. The parameters that allowed the court to function as a ruling organ also shaped its social expression, informed by the intellectual expansions patronized by influential courtiers. From scientific discoveries, to the creation of artistic institutions, the court served as a stage where such developments found visible articulations. By taking the court as its center, this chapter examines the role monsters played in such regulated social spaces. As an ambiguous presence, subjects who had visibly different bodies allowed courtiers to find relief from their strictly ruled lives through a distorted mirror that, ironically, reflected more human qualities than the personae these courtiers were meant to assume. These human qualities, sometimes exaggerated in visual portrayals or grotesquely mocked in performances, allowed courts to reinforce strict behavioral standards on their non-monstrous subjects by providing them with an escape. However, portraying dwarves or hirsutes presented a challenge to contemporary theoretical discourses that emphasized perfected aesthetic ideals over realistic demonstrations. Yet, hiding their deformities did not fit the reason for their presence at court since it was this precise physical deformity that allowed them to enter the court. Consequently, this chapter also briefly addresses the limitations of the common interpretive framework of Renaissance portraiture; the primacy of art academies in determining the visual parameters of courtly images in the sixteenth century; and how, in fact, images of monstrous beings subverted the prevalent art theoretical discourse on representation. In addition, these portraits invoke visual studies that are generally relegated to the realm of scientific illustrations, such as *imagines contrafactae*, *foglie volante*, or eclectic collections gathered in bound printed volumes.[1] However, it is by employing the particular epistemology that stems from producing and circulating such visual productions that scholarship on early modern portraiture can break the restrictive edifice that has defined it.

❧ ❧ ❧

The court, as a social center, controlled the individual freedom of courtiers; they had to adhere to written principles meant to emphasize the concept of *civiltà* and thus suppress behavioral aspects that did not fit within this normative regime.[2] Most courtiers set the stage for a created image of themselves that paralleled the ruler's image at court. The pressure of social conventions established by court etiquette incited courtiers not only to adopt rigid behavioral standards while at court, but also to emulate such dispositions in more private realms, so as to establish their congruence with the established order of rulership.[3] Whereas these written and spoken rules of performative actions were meant to assert and promote kingship through theatricality, display, and emulation, they also allowed for the subversion of authority through a similar, but inverted, vocabulary.[4] This is precisely where dwarves, hirsutes, or other particularly favored deformed individuals served as *negative* barometers, providing the visual and social contrast needed to counterpoint the self-presentation of courtiers.

Courtiers scrutinized the behavioral performance adopted by other members of the court. A prominent courtier therefore needed to study social discourses carefully and produce external affects that would not only determine his or her status at court, but allow said status to adopt an upward trajectory. These tenets dictated how portraits of courtiers were painted and, subsequently, how academies—often tied directly to courts or to prominent court members—and artists developed paradigms that justified certain aesthetic preferences. Although produced in the same locale, portraits of anatomically intriguing sitters in fact challenged intellectual rationalizations for the visualization of power and the articulation of taste in these courts. It is in the dialectical relation set by *ritrarre* and *imitare* that the subversion offered by portraits of abnormal beings finds its most striking expression.

Most discussions of Renaissance portraiture dwell on the tension between *ritrarre* and *imitare*, terms that were central to the debates surrounding the development of visual arts in the sixteenth century. At the source of most sixteenth-century art treatises and debates lay Leon Battista Alberti's (1404–1472) *Della Pittura* (1435). Considered the first modern treatise on the theory of painting, Alberti's writing and its many interpretations have shaped the discourse on Renaissance painting from the fifteenth to the twenty-first century. Though based on antique texts, *Della Pittura* also included concerns and thoughts on contemporaneous art practices. The idea of likeness and representation found its first clear articulation in the beginning of Book One. The Florentine humanist states: "No one will deny that things which are not visible do not concern the painter, for he strives to represent only the things that are seen."[5] However, in Alberti's elaboration on *istoria* in Book Two, verisimilitude is qualified as ancillary to the dignity that should be emphasized by the artist (however artificially constructed):

> The obscene parts of the body and all those that are not very pleasing to look at, should be covered with clothing or leaves or the hand. [...] Plutarch tells how the ancient painters, when painting kings who had some physical defect, did not wish this to appear to have been overlooked, but they corrected it as far as possible while still maintaining the likeness. Therefore, I would have decency and modesty observed in every 'historia', in such a way that ugly things are either omitted or emended.[6]

The appearance of the represented subject was for Alberti grounded in actual observation, and likeness an important quality for the overall effect of the painting. However, Alberti was not a pure empiricist—in fact he was one of the first Renaissance theorists to propose a balance between likeness and idealization. For him, material reality and ideal representations needed to tally with each other to visually perfect the idea of *istoria* and demonstrate the artist's *invenzione*.[7]

While basing their writings on *Della Pittura*'s main concepts, many sixteenth-century art theorists developed a distinction between *imitare* and *ritrarre*. The difference between the terms is best explained by Vincenzo Danti (1530–1576) in *Il Primo libro del trattato delle perfette proporzioni* (1567):

> By the term *ritrarre* I mean to make something exactly as another thing is seen to be; and by the term *imitare* I similarly understand that it is to make a thing not only as another has seen the thing to be [when that thing is imperfect], but to make it as it would have to be in order to be of complete perfection.[8]

But the relationship between the two terms was a source of continued dispute in the Cinquecento, particularly as artists increasingly determined their own intellectual positions. Giovan Battista Armenini (1530–1609), for instance, remained concerned with the problem posed by Alberti and his inquiries make evident not only the differences between *ritrarre* and *imitare*, but they also highlight the subsequent intellectual constructions emanating from these two theoretical concepts. Armenini started by questioning the emphasis on external visual appearances for the production of portraiture. This led him to interrogate the meanings of both *ritrarre* and *imitare*. For him, *ritrarre* only implied the record of the sitter's physical likeness through the accurate use of color, composition, and line; *imitare*, on the other hand, surpassed the mediocrity born from the mere use of *ritrarre* and allowed the artist to transcend simple documentation of the visible.[9] By *imitando* the artist applied his skills, as well as his intellect in order to capture not only the sitter's outer likeness, but also to hint at the subject's character and to do so in a perfected artistic manner. This *maniera*, according to Giorgio Vasari (1511–1574), was the combination of the artist's mastery of three sets of aesthetic skills: order, harmony, and his *invenzione*. Later, and along the same lines, Giovan Paolo Lomazzo (1538–1600) highly recommended applying the same stylistic criteria of decorum and propriety to the art of portraiture as those used in grand classical compositions. He therefore reinforced the idea of *imitare* and *bella maniera*, but still acknowledged the need for *ritrarre* as a stepping-stone for *imitare*, which in turn promoted *invenzione*.[10]

Ideally, then, the artist could start by using nature and then move beyond his sensible perception to incorporate intellectual elements that would perfect his creation. Because of the emphasis placed on enhanced artistic invention, Pliny's story of Alexander the Great and Apelles became a common point of reference in sixteenth-century art theory.[11] According to Pliny, Alexander the Great gave his mistress Campaspe to his painter after realizing that Apelles had fallen in love with her; he was assured of Apelles's fidelity to her likeness and was content to have instead the perfected portrait of his former mistress. Alexander's satisfaction with the image of his mistress, rather than with her physical presence, was seen as a confirmation of the artist's abilities to perfect nature through his creative capacity. Pliny's story conflates with its varied theoretical analyses in the sixteenth-century, which led to the tendency to equate the portrayal with the sitter.[12] Enhancing, yet not disregarding, likeness became the leading theoretical motivation for sixteenth-century portraiture.

Art theorists in the sixteenth-century did more than speculate on actual art production. Their writings also affected, and in turn were influenced by, art practice in the Cinquecento. The *paragone* debate is a particularly telling example of the mutual interaction between ideas and images and is relevant for the way in which portraits of monsters are a visible application of theoretical discourses. The most famous, and first, example of *paragone* was found in Leonardo da Vinci's (1452–1519) *Treatise on Painting* (1480–1516), in which Leonardo argued for the superiority of painting over sculpture, poetry, and music.[13] A surprising choice for his time, Leonardo's decision to defend painting seems to have stemmed from the artist's struggle to demonstrate his respectable social status.[14] His main argument for the superiority of painting was its scientific aspect and its affiliation with the field of optics.[15] Part of Leonardo's argument rested upon the fact that the painter could imitate works of nature directly without mediation, as opposed to the other arts such as poetry or ekphrasis.[16] For him, painting represented a direct connection to nature, whereas poetry entailed a once-removed description of nature.[17] The idea of imitation lay at the core of the *paragone* debate, and here we see an inchoate dialogue between *ritrarre* and *imitare*. But in addition to setting intellectual parameters for this debate, Leonardo also expanded it and argued for a more wide-ranging view on the arts in general—an idea later developed by Cinquecento theorists.[18]

Almost half a century after Leonardo, Benedetto Varchi (1503–1565) became one of the most eminent theorists on the *paragone*, restarting the debate years after it had been abandoned and adding new philosophical elements to it.[19] In 1550, he delivered and published his *Due Lezzioni* and provided the foundation for many of Vasari's theoretical statements.[20] The repeated comparison between the different art forms allowed artists and theorists alike to converse about notions such as *disegno*, *imitazione*, or *invenzione*. The *paragone* debate had come to define the tension between *ritrarre* and *imitare*.

It is crucial to note that the rhetorical articulations of the *paragone* debate construct a problematic relation between likeness and idealization. In some cases these terms are opposed, and in others they are similar. This unresolved tension finds echoes in twentieth-century scholarship on Renaissance painting and portraiture in particular. Indeed, the balance between likeness and idealization mirrors the balance between *ritrarre* and *imitare*, mostly in terms of the analogous contrast between outer appearance and inner character. Whereas likeness seems to emphasize outer appearance, idealization tends to reveal the inner character of the sitter. Modern scholarship has interpreted Renaissance portraiture as the pursuit of inner character as revealed by the outer appearance of the sitter. Thus, physical likeness has been considered a necessary, but secondary element to the ultimate goal of the portrait: the presentation of inner character. In common court portraits, then, the physical integrity of the subjects proclaimed their inner wholeness. In 1860, Jacob Burckhardt (1818–1897) established in his *Civilisation of the Renaissance in Italy* a line of thought that has framed most scholarship on Renaissance culture and portraiture to date. Burckhardt's insistence on the rise of the individual, and on unique personalities in the Italian Renaissance is essential to the study of Renaissance portraiture, and thus for the examination of portraits of monsters produced in the early modern period.[21] The implications of Burckhardt's argument were manifold: he positioned the individual, not the community, as the central axis around which Renaissance thought and culture pivoted—thus implicitly positioning art production around the same axis. Consequently, scholars of Renaissance portraiture have often read it as a visualization of this central Burckhardtian idea: the rise of the individual and the "awakening of personality."[22] Burckhardt wrote the first modern, coherent synthesis of Italian Renaissance culture—one that divided the era into a variety of themes such as the state, the revival of antiquity, festivals, and religion. Throughout his work, Burckhardt dealt with the Renaissance as a distinct chronological, social, political, and cultural break. This emphasis underlined most of his discussions, including that of Renaissance individuality. Indeed, Burckhardt presented the Renaissance individual as a decidedly new and separate—though linked—entity from the community, religion, or race to which he might have belonged; he also defined the Renaissance individual as clearly distinct from the medieval man, therefore disregarding notions of historical and social continuity. He described the Renaissance as the era of the self-made and self-taught man—and hence, as the most propitious period for the dawning of self-consciousness. Starting with the Italian states, and the ways in which they allowed for the rise of the individual by lifting a "veil," Burckhardt then addressed issues relevant for smaller early modern communities, and eventually focused on the individual per se. The combination of his ideas gave rise to the ubiquitous early modern concept of self-fashioning.[23] In terms of portraiture, Burckhardt believed—in line with the importance of avowed individuality for the early modern person—the prominence of the individual depended on whether the uniqueness of the sitter was conveyed successfully to the viewer. The sitter's distinctiveness could be emphasized through the portrait's physical resemblance to the sitter, particularly since physical likeness was believed to reveal the character of the subject. The sitter could be, and *should* be according to Burckhardt, unique in his or her character. The idea of uniqueness, however, seems to have been co-opted by many scholars to omit the ways in which portraits of monsters could, in fact, serve to represent a take—and an expansion—on Burckhardtian ideas.

Art historians have deployed Burckhardt's argument about the rise of individuality to explain the reemergence and re-definition of portraiture as a genre in the Renaissance.[24]

Modern scholarship on Renaissance portraiture is thus not fully or adequately equipped to deal with portraits of monstrous individuals, simply because studies that address portraiture rarely question the canonical tradition that positions Renaissance portraits as explicit statements on the sitter's personality. This approach tends to suggest that outward likeness serves a precise and unique function: the revelation of the sitter's persona and the emphasis on the sitter's social qualities. Portraits of physically abnormal sitters, however, present the viewer with a series of complications that require a larger investigative framework. They break the linear connection between external appearance and internal character, since the physical traits of a monstrous individual do not necessarily speak to his or her inner character. By focusing on the physical anomaly of the sitter, the artist suppressed the distinction between inner and outer states, or at least questioned it. These portraits existed because of, and were composed around, the sitters' unusual bodies; the character of the monstrous subject was addressed subsequently to the overt visual interest held by his or her body. The persona of the monstrous sitter was not the principal goal of his or her portrait, as stated by both early modern art theorists and modern scholars. The mere existence of these portraits, therefore, underlines the shortcomings of a homogeneous approach to early modern portraiture.

While inherently emphasizing external features, court portraits of anatomically abnormal individuals were not devoid of idealization. Motivated by their own sense of aesthetics, academic training, cultural history, or the stipulations of a patron, artists might, and often did, manipulate their supposedly faithful observations. Indeed, empirical and objective portraits were not appropriate for a courtly setting, as the viewing audience expected a certain degree of aesthetic covering, regardless of the true features of the painted subject. This complex layering of interactions made for an even more complex process of production and viewership. Commemoration or authoritative presentation, though not absent, were not the primary goals of most of the portraits discussed in this book; yet, human sentiments were more relevant to portraits of dwarves, hirsutes, and various other human monsters than has been previously assumed.

Idealization in portraits of anatomically curious subjects is as significant an element as it is in mainstream Renaissance court portraiture, though its objectives may be more varied than the simple acceptance of courtly aesthetics and character enhancement. Idealization in these portrayals could be interpreted as a shield against the visual violation of the audience, rather than as a complete negation of the human qualities of the portrait.[25] In this sense, the idealization prevented the viewers from associating their own selves *directly* with the abnormal bodies they were seeing or to possess the marvelous subject as their own object. Viewers were invited to look, to feel wonder, and to *question* their own selves, much like the experience they would assume during an anatomical dissection or a visit into a collection of curiosities.

The Renaissance portrait recorded an encounter between the sitter and the artist. The agencies of the artist, the sitter, and the patron therefore are elements that constitute the critical formative parts of a portrait. Agency and the qualities of interaction can be gauged through an analysis of levels of idealization, the wishes of the patron, and the purpose and function of the portrait. But portraits of physically anomalous people are more difficult to frame in a similar fashion, because of the uncertain status of the sitters themselves and of the display mechanisms activated post-production. In rare cases the topic of agency applies to the sitter, but in most cases, the sitter had no voice in his or her representation.[26] Whereas the usual patron-as-sitter/artist gave the sitter some say in the creative process, in these portraits the process was driven primarily by the artist and patron. Active constructions of the self are thus less apparent in portraits of sitters who were anatomically abnormal. Portraits of physically different court subjects stand in direct contrast to typical court portraits, then, because the sitter's agency is often elided. These portraits also make strong statements regarding the sitters' social status. The scholarship on individual works depicting monstrous individuals sporadically addresses the ways in which each portrait might hint toward the position of the specific subject at court. But no consistent interpretative framework has been devised for the study of social statements made by portraits of monsters, nor does the literature on court artists and their productions provide a structure for analyzing the reason for producing such portraits.[27] This stems from the fact that court portraits have been studied as statements of the individuality and social status of the artist, as well as the sitter. But the social status of the sitter is, at best, ambiguous in portraits of individuals with extraordinary bodies. And the status of the artist is of no great concern in these works because, in general, the artist is not tying his or her social standing to that of the sitter, for obvious reasons, but rather to that of the patron who is very rarely the subject of such portraits.[28]

The main questions regarding portraits of physically different individuals are thus: What role do these portraits play in capturing the social status of the sitter and of the patron? How was the relationship between mimesis and idealization implemented? Did it allow the character of the "collectible" subject/object to come through? The social status at issue was usually that of the patron of the portrait or "owner" of the physically deformed individual being portrayed. By commissioning a portrait, the patron would assert his or her social standing twice: first, by visualizing his or her possession; and second, by collecting, owning, and displaying a symbol of his or her high social status.[29] Portraits of monsters particularly emphasized this ambiguous status of the sitter. Portraits such as that of Cosimo I de'Medici's (1519–1574) dwarf Morgante by Bronzino (1503–1572) painted around 1547 (Plate 1) speak to his station in life as a court jester, but it also reveals the tension between his identity as a generic figure of jest (by virtue of his physical qualities) and his identity as a unique and recognizable dwarf in the court of Cosimo I and as the Medici patriarch's faithful companion. In the case of *Morgante*, the painting reflected the social status of the patron who owned and commissioned the portrait, since

> [t]he adoption of the dwarf as a visible symbol of princely magnificence by [Renaissance] courts has far reaching implications for the social and artistic development of Renaissance Italy. The dwarf's conspicuous appearance in court festivities and imagery transmitted ideas of status and nobility, thereby influencing public perceptions that equated the dwarf with courtly prestige.[30]

It also added to Morgante's status as well, albeit on a secondary level. Indeed, the fact that Bronzino represented the dwarf in this manner elevated his subject's status from a mere joke to that of a unique individual.

Similarly, Andrea Sacchi's (1599–1661) 1641 portrait of the castrato Marc'Antonio Pasqualini (Plate 3) deals with the issue of status. In Marc'Antonio Pasqualini's portrait, the strongest statement relating to social status seems to be the one made about the castrato's—the actual sitter and the patron of this painting—social prominence. Whereas Pasqualini's portrait implicitly points to the castrato's ties to his courtly patron, it explicitly highlights the social status of the singer; the patron's social eminence is only an ancillary part of the painting. However, one could argue that a castrato was also a courtly "possession." Among the rare castrati that succeeded in becoming famous singers, there were those who had to sacrifice their freedom to live under the oppressive auspices of their patrons. Choirs did offer a less restrained personal environment for castrati, yet they did not have the same appeal as courtly settings, which could give castrati greater fame and fortune.[31] Thus the portrait, commissioned as a gift to Cardinal Barberini, was as much a statement about the patron's status as it was about the castrato's own social standing.

Falling between a *Morgante*-type of painting and a portrait akin to that of Pasqualini, Lavinia Fontana's (1552–1614) portrait of Antoinette Gonsalvus (1595) (Plate 2) places the social status of the subject in a dialogue with that of the patron who commissioned the portrait. A young girl with congenital hypertrichosis—the excessive growth of hair all over her body—Antoinette Gonsalvus became a monster worthy of attention and thus of portrayal. As a hirsute girl, she was associated with supernatural and mythical beasts like wild men and satyrs. The portrait of Antoinette Gonsalvus, along with other portraits of her family members, follows a visual tradition reserved for members of the highest social spheres.[32] The composition of the painting, particularly the typical courtly three-quarter length, as well as the details of the dress, strongly indicate the social status of Antoinette, a social position also substantiated by biographical information. An interesting and complex work, this painting is a rare portrait that balances the sitter's status against the patron's, while still touching upon the feral qualities of the little girl. But, on its surface, Fontana's painting humanizes Antoinette and associates her with other young noble women of Bologna.

A systematic study of Renaissance portraits of others and otherness opens a dialogue between the genre of portraiture, Cinquecento and Seicento art theory, the history of collecting, anatomical inquiries, and the study of social codes. By addressing the social, historical, scientific, and visual vectors that drive such a study, some of the rigid art theoretical devices that have served to frame early modern portraiture and therefore portraits of unusual sitters produced in the sixteenth and seventeenth centuries may be expanded. Ultimately, the factors that led to the commission, painting, and viewership of portraits of anatomically deformed individuals reveal and parallel the intricate intellectual settings in which they were produced.

Notes

[1] Andrea Carlino makes a fascinating point about artists as visual witnesses and the function of such visual scientific collections in "Fatti contraffatti tra curiosità e scienza: Note su Konrad Gesner e la collezione di fogli volanti di Johann Jacob Wick," *Arte + Architettura in Svizzera* 57, no. 1 (2006): 37–44.

[2] Norbert Elias, *The Civilizing Process*, trans. Edmund Jephcott (New York: Urizen Books, 1978), 53.

[3] Norbert Elias, *The Court Society* (New York: Pantheon Books, 1983), 88.

[4] Thomas da Costa Kauffmann, "Images of Rule: Issues of Interpretation," *Art Journal* 48, no. 2 (1989): 119.

[5] Leon Battista Alberti, *On Painting and Sculpture: The Latin Texts of De Pictura and De Statua*, ed. and trans. Cecil Grayson (London: Phaidon, 1972), 36.

[6] Ibid., 79 and 81.

[7] As "the artful presentation of narrative and the control of the number and appropriate actions of depicted figures." Fredrika H. Jacobs, *Defining the Renaissance Virtuosa: Women Artists and the Language of Art History and Criticism* (Cambridge: Cambridge University Press, 1997), 55.

[8] Vincenzo Danti, *Il primo libro del trattato delle perfette proporzioni*, ed. Paola Barocchi, in *Scritti d'arte del Cinquecento*, vol. 1 (Milan and Naples: Riccardo Ricciardi Editore, 1960), 241; as translated in Jacobs, *Defining the Renaissance Virtuosa*, 45.

[9] For the explanation on the opposition and hierarchical disposition of *ritrarre* and *imitare* for portraiture, see Jacobs, *Defining the Renaissance Virtuosa*, 44–45.

[10] Giovan Paolo Lomazzo, in *Scritti d'arte del Cinquecento*, vol. 3, ed. Paola Barocchi (Milan and Naples: Riccardo Ricciardi Editore, 1977), 2737.

[11] Pliny the Elder, *Natural History*, trans. H. Rackham (Cambridge, MA: Harvard University Press, 1956–66), sections 35.95 and 35.86.

[12] Mary Rogers, ed., *Fashioning Identities in Renaissance Art* (Aldershot and Brookfield: Ashgate, 2000), xiii: "[Rupert Shepherd] discusses the conflation of the image with its prototype, that, predicated upon an aesthetic of naturalism, was in part grounded in Pliny's anecdotes of the dogs, and birds, and even other artists, who were deceived by the realism of a painting into confusing it with life. Contemporary ekphrasis also played a role in 'shaping the perceptions of those who produced (the works of art) and consumed them.' In portraiture there was certainly a tendency to equate the portrayal with the sitter."

[13] Leatrice Mendelsohn, *Paragoni: Benedetto Varchi's "Due Lezzioni" and Cinquecento Art Theory* (Ann Arbor: UMI Press, 1982), xx. I here use the phrase *Treatise on Painting* loosely since there was no *actual* treatise written by Leonardo himself. His notes where posthumously arranged by Francesco Melzi. For different arguments, analyses, and hypotheses about the organization and production of Leonardo's writings on art, see Claire Farago, ed., *Leonardo's Writings and Theory of Art* (New York and London: Garland Publishing, 1999).

[14] Mendelsohn, *Paragoni*, 38.

[15] Farago, *Leonardo da Vinci's Paragone: A Critical Interpretation with a New Edition of the Text in the Codex Urbinas* (Leiden and New York: E.J. Brill, 1992), 92: Leonardo's "defense of painting [was] that it [was] a science, based on perspective and defined as the branch of optics that represents things on a flat surface."

[16] Michael, W. Kwakkelstein, *Leonardo da Vinci as a Physiognomist: Theory and Drawing Practice* (Leiden: Primavera Pers, 1994), 80–81: "Leonardo praises the painter above the poet for his ability to imitate the works of nature directly, without having to resort to disciplines that are not really his."

[17] Farago, *Leonardo da Vinci's Paragone*, 92.

[18] Mendelsohn, *Paragoni*, 38: "Leonardo's *paragone* marked a turning point away from Medieval scholasticism towards a more expansive view of the arts. His definitions were both progressive and retrospective, combining aspects of Medieval and Antique theories with the Quattrocento search for objective data. He injected new life into old formulas. Leonardo's most important contribution was to set up a series of proofs to justify his contention that art was a form of cognition."

[19] David Summers, *Michelangelo and the Language of Art* (Princeton: Princeton University Press, 1981), 269: "After the High Renaissance, interest in the issue subsided, and little is heard of it again until 1548 when Benedetto Varchi, always drawn to airy disputes and ignited by the general interest in art theory that began to stir around the middle of the century, took up the old arguments, greatly amplified them, and pursued them to heights of philosophical elaboration unknown before."

[20] Mendelsohn, *Paragoni*, xx.

[21] In her study of portraiture for instance, Mary Rogers points to Burckhardt's precedent, *Fashioning Identities*, xiii: "According to the classic argument of Jacob Burckhardt, the development of the individual was the defining characteristic of the man of the Italian Renaissance, who, schooled by the culture of classical antiquity, became newly conscious of his personal as distinct from his various group identities."

[22] Jacob Burckhardt, *The Civilisation of Renaissance Italy*, trans. S.G.C. Middlemore (London: George Allen & Unwin, 1921), 129. The author uses the phrase "awakening of personality" to describe the ways "man became a spiritual individual and recognized himself as such" thanks to the political circumstances of Italy.

[23] Ibid., 129–68. It is, however, essential to note that these individuals were given expression within a group. So, whereas Burckhardt highlights the self-awareness of the individual, such consciousness could only exist inside the parameters set by an early modern community.

[24] Most scholars have emphasized the importance of idealization and commemoration, albeit with distinctive nuances such as the viewer's participation in the activation of a portrait of the dialectical tension between appearance and representation, for instance. For a small sampling of canonical studies related to these thoughts, please see John Pope-Hennessy, *The Portrait of the Renaissance* (New York: Bollingen Foundation, 1966); Robert W. Hanning and David Rosand,

Castiglione: The Ideal and the Real in Renaissance Culture (New Haven and London: Yale University Press, 1983); Jodi Cranston, *The Poetics of Portraiture in Italian Renaissance* (Cambridge: Cambridge University Press, 2000); Harry Berger, Jr., *Fictions of the Pose: Rembrandt against the Italian Renaissance* (Stanford: Stanford University Press, 2000).

[25] Berger, *Fictions of the Pose*, 112, in relation to some portraits by Bronzino: "also, idealization is a way to protect the portrait from violation. The more mimetic the portrait is, the more human, and thus the more violable."

[26] This assumption is based on the lack of evidence found in contracts. Indeed, it seems that patrons who commissioned the portraits made decisions on behalf of the physically different sitters whose voice is not present in these contracts.

[27] See, for example, Michael Warnke, *L'Artiste et la cour: Aux origines de l'artiste moderne* (Paris: Éditions de la Maison des Sciences de l'Homme, 1989).

[28] The last chapter of this book addresses what happens when, in fact, the patron and the sitter *are* the same person.

[29] Nicholas Mann and Luke Syson, *The Image of the Individual: Portrait in the Renaissance* (London: British Museum Press, 1998), 67: "Renaissance portrait collections are susceptible to a mode of analysis which construes them as vehicles for individual *fama*, the means of self-aggrandisment and, when they appear outside aristocratic circles, a 'bourgeois' appropriation of princely habit."

[30] Robin Leigh O'Bryan has clearly demonstrated what was associated with the possession and the display—representational or physical—of a dwarf in a princely or regal court. See Robin Leigh O'Bryan, *The Dwarf in Italian Renaissance Iconography*, unpublished thesis (San Diego State University, 1991), 65.

[31] John Rosselli, "From Princely Service to the Open Market: Singers on Italian Opera and Their Patrons, 1600–1850," *Cambridge Opera Journal* 1, no. 1 (1989): 113–37.

[32] Christiane Hertel, "Hairy Issues: Portraits of Petrus Gonsalvus and His Family in Archduke Ferdinand II's *Kunstkammer* and Their Contexts," *Journal of the History of Collections* 13, no. 1 (2001): 4–5.

Chapter 3

Perfected Miniatures: Dwarves at Court

DWARVES HELD COMPLEX POSITIONS IN courts. Whereas they served as cultural markers of the eminent social spheres in which they lived, their physical deformities often prohibited them from being treated as full members of the court. Despite these restrictions, they occupied an odd position of privilege. Their presence reinforced the controlled standards and rules of the environments in which they lived, precisely because it remained on the margins. To depict dwarves, whose presence at court was central to its complete identity, was to visually affirm their existence and role there. Their portraits established a discourse between physical difference and the ideals of early modern court life. In addition, the portraits confirm the growing popularity of dwarves living in many European courts. Their bodies possessed physical qualities that dictated their actual presence at court and ultimately their portraits served a similar function. The Florentine court surrounding the Medici family provides a fertile ground for the investigation of the parallels between the lives of dwarves as favored court monsters and their subsequent visual presence in officially sanctioned portraits.

The Medici established themselves as the ruling family of Florence and, as such, adopted many regal indices, including the possession and employment of dwarves. Furthermore, ducal secretaries documented every activity related to the ducal court and recorded all correspondence dealing with the Medici with utmost attention. Therefore, the abundance of period documents allow for a thorough examination of court life and its subsequent visual production during Medici rule. These documents—both visual and textual—allow for one particular dwarf to rise to the surface with more attention: Morgante, Cosimo I de'Medici's (1519–1574) favored dwarf. Bronzino's *Morgante* is therefore used here to decipher the dichotomous position of dwarves at the Florentine ducal court and in satellite or separate courts in northern Italy and parts of France. These individuals benefited from the court's educational, intellectual, and social advantages, but they were required to retain their marginal and wondrous qualities by participating in grotesque entertainments. Dwarves introduced the notion of difference into courtly vocabulary and daily life, yet the flawed human space they embodied also allowed courts to reassert their rigid standards of normality. Taken as a paradigm, Bronzino's *Morgante* demonstrates how physical difference was categorized and interpreted through the presence of dwarves at court.

In 1893, the historian Cosimo Conti first made the connection between an entry in a 1553 Medici inventory and a double-sided portrait of a dwarf in the Uffizi.[1] This painting was Agnolo Bronzino's (1503–1572) portrayal of Morgante (Plate 1). Bronzino's choice of subject was not exceptional for his time since dwarves were a common feature of sixteenth-century court life. However, his depiction of Morgante is unusual because it refers simultaneously to scientific discourses, art theoretical debates, ducal self-fashioning, and social activities at the Medici court. A double-sided canvas, Bronzino's portrait shows Morgante in the nude on both sides. In the front, the dwarf is facing the viewer and gazing toward the owl he holds on his right hand. The owl, identified as a combination of a little owl and a long eared owl is tied to a cord Morgante grasps in his left hand.[2] Another bird—a Eurasian jay—flies on the upper right side of the canvas, while two butterflies fly at the level of his knees. Noticeably, one of the butterflies is covering Morgante's genitals. The plain, but recognizable background is barely changed—with the addition of a tree instead of a stump and the visible rock formation framing the entire scene—in the back of this canvas, where we see Morgante's rear side, his head turned toward the viewer. In his right hand, the dwarf holds several dead birds tied together and in his left hand, the spears that allowed him to kill those birds and a string attached to an owl. The birds range from a house sparrow to a European robin.[3] The owl, different from the one represented on the front side of the canvas, is perched on Morgante's left shoulder and throws a piercing gaze at the viewer.

In the seventeenth century, the front of this double-sided canvas was heavily painted over, so as to turn the inexplicable unclad body of the dwarf into the more acceptable mythological figure of Bacchus (Fig. 3.1). Until its restoration completed in 2010, the front of the canvas depicted a dwarf, Morgante's head and genitals were covered with grapes and grape-leaves, and he was shown holding a glass in his right hand and a pitcher in his left. Following the ruling of Cosimo I, Morgante's popularity might well have faded and he may have lost his monopoly as a favored court dwarf. It would thus have been awkward for the subsequent households to keep a double-sided, lifesize representation of a naked deformed being whose fame had waned and thus whose emblematic authority had shifted. It was easy to hide the back of the canvas by framing it, but the front needed to be visually rearranged so as to fit the sensibilities of the family, as well as that of their visitors—especially since Morgante was no longer a daily presence in Florence. Painting over the front of the canvas provided an easy solution, as it would allow the family to keep and exhibit a work painted by the renowned court artist Bronzino. Most catalogues thus refer to the scene in the front as a Bacchanal scene, and mention no allegorical references for the rear view portrait using instead a descriptive series of nouns, such as "Morgante with an owl on his shoulder."[4]

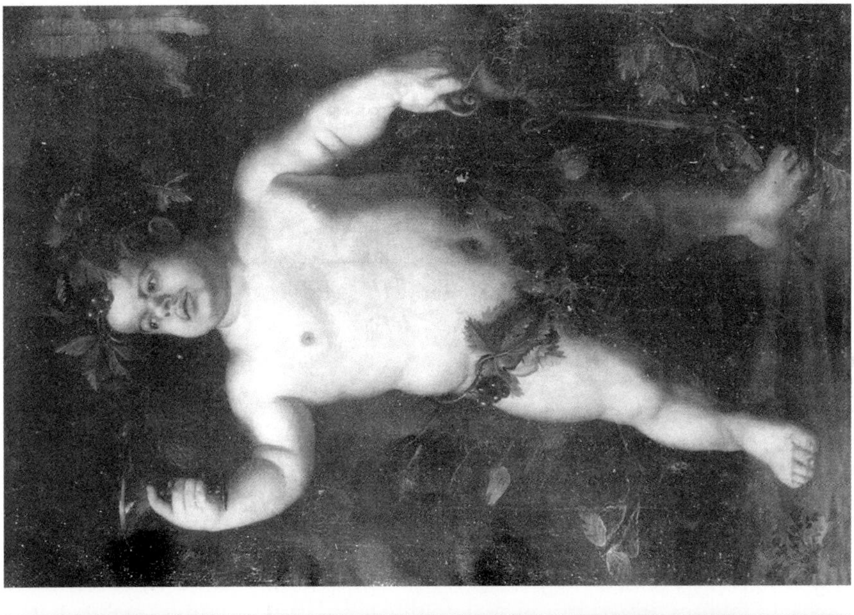

Figure 3.1 (*verso and recto*). Agnolo Bronzino, *Portrait of Morgante*, pre-restoration, ca. 1547, Galleria degli Uffizi, Florence

It is important to add a parenthetical note here regarding the geographical life of the *Morgante*. The Medici made the Palazzo Pitti one of their main residences shortly after Eleonora di Toledo (1522–1562) bought it from Luca Pitti in 1549. The moving of the *Morgante* was thus certainly made from the Palazzo Vecchio to the Palazzo Pitti first, while Eleonora was still alongside her husband. The portrait may have then moved to Poggio Imperiale shortly after Maria-Maddalena bought it in 1617. She was known for using many *guardarobe* items to furnish and decorate her new palazzo and, incidentally, 1617 is approximately the date when the front of the canvas was turned into a more acceptable and generic, if still odd, Bacchus.[5]

In addition to letters, references in records of the *guardarobe* of princely establishments, and entries in records of payment, many visual works attest the popularity of dwarves in Renaissance courts.[6] From Andrea Mantegna's (1431–1506) fresco in the *camera degli sposi* in Mantua (1474), to Giovanni Stradano's (1523–1605) tapestry of the *Boar Hunt* (ca. 1574), or to Lavinia Fontana's (1552–1614) *Visit of the Queen of Sheba*, dwarves were included in countless works as conventional symbols of the courtly milieus. Bronzino's work is, however, more unusual than most of these representations because it treats the subject of the dwarf independently. Executed sometime before 1553 and toward the end of Bronzino's most productive years at the court of Cosimo I, this portrait was part of the Duke's program to restore and redecorate his many residences.[7] Most catalogue entries made before the modern restoration of *Morgante* focus on its relation to Cosimo I's famous dwarf; its unusual double-sided canvas; and its mention in the 1553 and (more extensive) 1587 Medici inventories.[8] Bronzino scholarship has amply discussed the ways in which this portrait demonstrates the artist's attempt to establish the superiority of painting over sculpture as a response to Benedetto Varchi's *inchiesta* and the *paragone* discourse.[9] In these terms, Morgante's double-sided portrait has been analyzed as a rhetorical exercise. Indeed, by showing a male figure in the round, and through different views, Bronzino allegedly succeeded in proving that painting was not only equal to, but greater than sculpture.[10] Morgante's portrait has also been considered a burlesque *clin d'oeil* to Bronzino's allegorical portrait of Cosimo I in the nude as Orpheus (Plate 4).[11] The dwarf's portrait has been linked to the idea that crude humor and jest were in fact practiced and appreciated in most Renaissance European courts.[12] By mocking the ideal body of Cosimo I, Morgante's defective body in the nude highlighted a type of raw irony based on vulgarizing Cosimo's aesthetic ideals. Bronzino's *Morgante* has, overall, been positioned by most scholars as a typical depiction of a dwarf as court possession, as curiosity, and as part of courtly banter.[13]

What has generally been overlooked, however, is that this portrait also and primarily speaks to the dialectical position of individuals like Morgante in Italian courts. Featuring both explicit and ambiguous references to monsters at court, Morgante himself, the Medici family, anatomical inquiries, and collecting practices, this Bronzino painting opens new paths for exploring the intellectual and social boundaries of the court milieu by way of this marginal signpost.

Morgante's own persona is undeniably central to the construction and understanding of Bronzino's portrait. Furthermore, his biography is essential to defining the status of dwarves at court in a more general sense, even if the particulars of his life remain specific to Morgante alone. His name was based on the name of the giant in Luigi Pulci's 1478 *Morgante Maggiore*, published under the auspices of Lucrezia Tornabuoni. The irony in naming a dwarf after a giant turned the name Morgante into a rather popular moniker and several other Medici dwarves carried that same name, one that highlighted the comical aspect lying in such a pun. The precise dates of Morgante's life are debatable, as are the precise dates during which he was in the service of Cosimo I de'Medici. Even the first possible acknowledgment of Morgante is dubious. Although the Medici Archives Project assumes that a 1544 document concerning a bird hunt refers to the famous dwarf, Detlef Heikamp posits that the first true assertion of Morgante's presence at court dates to 1548.[14] Heikamp uses a visual account to justify this date. During his work on the Palazzo Vecchio between 1555 and 1565, Giorgio Vasari (1511–1574) designed and oversaw many of the decorations and the paintings that today stand as the palazzo's final and cohesive visual product. On the first floor, in the quarters of Leo X is the *Sala di Cosimo*. One of the roundels, positioned in the center of the right wall as one enters the room, shows Cosimo as a superintendent overseeing the construction of Elba's fortification projects (Fig. 3.2).[15] From the bottom left part of this roundel, the head of Morgante emerges. No more than his right shoulder and a right profile of his head are visible, yet we may recognize the dwarf because the image is almost a copy—with an added piece of clothing—of Bronzino's portrait, which certainly served as a model.

We know that Cosimo went to Elba in 1548, and the *tondo* itself bears the inscription "ANNO MDXXXXVIII" on its side, confirming the date. Considering the age at which a jester or a dwarf could be officially listed in *giornale di entrata e uscita* or in *guardarobe* as part of the court, we may infer that Morgante was beyond puberty when he became Cosimo's favored companion. The steady presence of a dwarf with his *signore* might not have been unusual at court, but Morgante would have held a place at court for a few years before Cosimo may have wished for his presence to be recorded by his side on official functions such as the visit to Elba.[16] Since there is a *terminus post quem* date of 1548 for Morgante's presence at court, it may be assumed that Morgante was probably born around 1530.

As for Morgante's death, Antonfrancesco Grazzini ("il Lasca," 1503–1584) gives a chronological clue, since he wrote an ode to commemorate it.[17] We know that Grazzini died on February 18, 1584; this date may thus stand as a tentative *terminus ante quem* for Morgante's death. A lifespan of fifty to sixty years is feasible for an achondroplastic dwarf in the sixteenth century considering the medical conditions that would have been

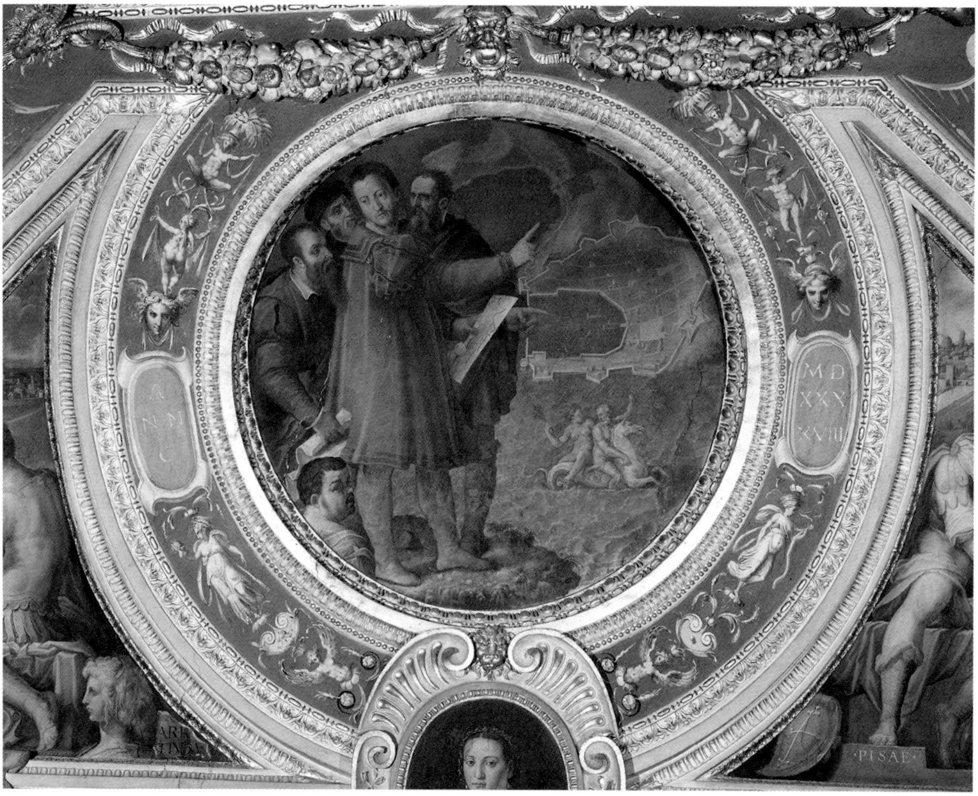

Figure 3.2. Giorgio Vasari, *Cosimo I de'Medici as a Superintendent in Elba*, 1555–65, Palazzo Vecchio, Florence. Scala/Art Resource, New York

a part of Morgante's life as an achondroplastic dwarf.[18] In addition, these dates correspond loosely to the reign of Cosimo I de'Medici, which lasted from 1537 until 1574.

It is important to note the conflation that has often been made between Morgante and another court dwarf, Pietro Barbino. Giorgio Vasari clearly differentiates the two. First, he mentions Bronzino's depiction of Morgante:

> Bronzino then made for Duke Cosimo a full-length portrait of the dwarf Morgante, nude, and in two ways—namely, on one side of the picture the front, and on the other the back, with the bizarre and monstrous members which that dwarf has; which picture, of its kind, is beautiful and marvelous.[19]

Then, later in his biographies, Vasari briefly discusses Valerio Cioli's (1529–1599) sculptures of both Morgante and Pietro Barbino, hence clearly presenting the two dwarves as separate entities:

> The Duke has also caused the same Valerio to make a nude statue of the dwarf Morgante in marble, which has proved so beautiful and so like the reality, that probably there has never been seen another monster so well wrought, nor one executed with such diligence, lifelike and faithful to nature. In like manner, he has caused him to execute the statue of Pietro, called Barbino, a gifted dwarf, well-lettered and a very gentle spirit, and a favourite of our Duke.[20]

Vasari's writings are not the only evidence supporting the dissociation of Morgante from Barbino. The reliability of Vasari is confirmed by visual observations. Cioli's statues of *Morgante as Silenus* (Fig. 3.3) and *Pietro Barbino* (Fig. 3.4) as part of a fountain in the Boboli gardens evidently depict two different individuals who bear no resemblance to one another, aside from their short stature; indeed, Morgante's torso was particularly distinctive. Though both dwarves lived in and served at Cosimo's court during roughly the same years, they were separate and distinct members of the court. Because more information is available on Morgante and because his life sparked the interest of writers, painters, sculptors, and courtiers alike, this chapter concerns itself mainly with Morgante as a paradigmatic late-Renaissance court dwarf.

Morgante's true name is somewhat clearer than his life dates. Detlef Heikamp has unearthed a document that not only gives Morgante's real name, but also his geographical origin; furthermore, it establishes a precedent for the juridical personhood for dwarves, as discussed later in this chapter. In 1555, Cosimo gave his dwarf a ducal privilege by bequeathing him a farm in the province of Arezzo. In the document that seals the legacy Morgante is to receive from the Grand Duke, Cosimo refers to Morgante as: "Braccio *(a)* nuncupato Morgante Bartholi de Podio Fornionis et de Statu illustrissimi domini Cesaris Alydosii domini Castri nuncupati del Rio, nano ducalis palatii nostri ac servitori nostro nobis dilectissimo salutem et omne bonum."[21] From this document it can be determined that Morgante's proper name was in fact Braccio di Bartolo, and that he came from Poggio Fornione in the province of Bologna.

Not all anatomical anomalies were seen as equally fascinating to the various courts of Europe; at nearly every court, however, the most prized deformed individuals were, like Morgante, dwarves.[22] Bronzino inserted a telling element that refers to Morgante's currency as an object: southern swallowtail butterflies.[23] The butterflies are original to the painting and identifiable as insects common in the summer months of June and July in the southern Tuscan region of Italy. By juxtaposing the dwarf next to a recognizable regional insect found in many cabinets of curiosities, Bronzino's commentary was twofold. First, he identified the geographical region in which Morgante lived; many viewers might have encountered such a butterfly during a visit to Florence and Tuscany. Second, Bronzino equated the collectible status of Morgante with that of a popular, collectible insect—leaving no doubt to the desirability of owning a dwarf like Morgante. The association of dwarves with collectible objects was a common occurrence. Furthermore, period sources also described dwarves as being akin to animals, because it was believed that their

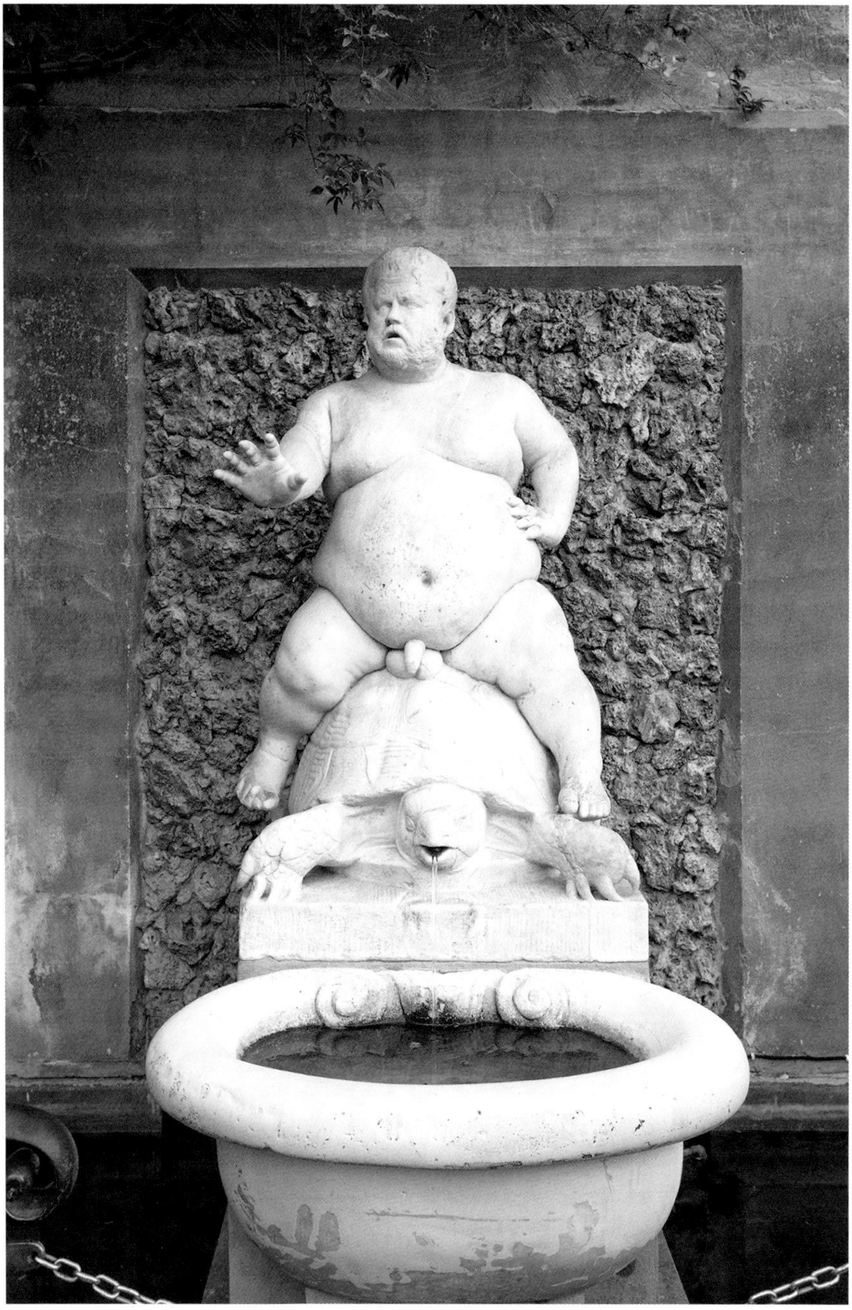

Figure 3.3. Valerio Cioli, *Morgante as Silenus*, ca. 1560, Boboli Gardens, Florence. Vanni Archive/Art Resource, NY

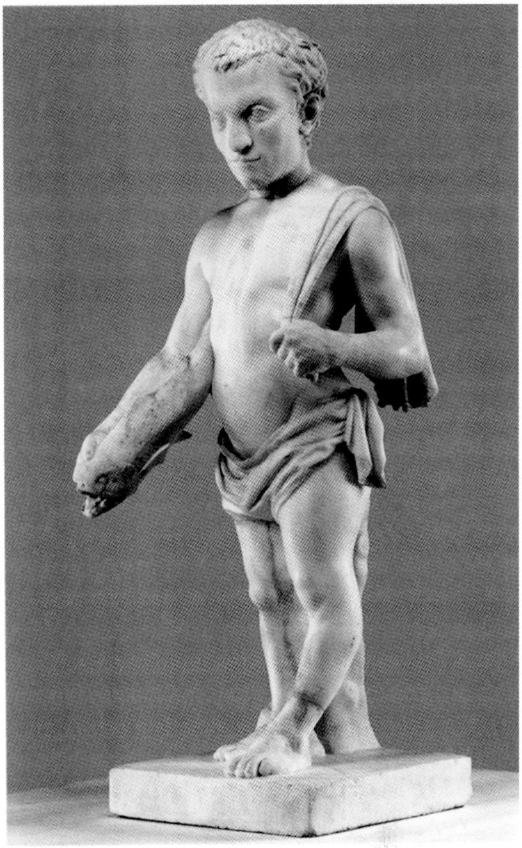

Figure 3.4. Valerio Cioli, *Pietro Barbino*, ca. 1560, Museo Giardino di Boboli, Florence, after Touba Ghadessi, *Il* Nano Morgante *di Agnolo Bronzino – Un dipinto "a due dritti" restaurato*, 2012

parents failed to pass on to them a fully developed human soul. Paracelsus conjectured that even though dwarves were born from humans, they did not inherit the souls of their parents; dwarves were partly equated to animals, and like exotic or rare ones, were prized collectible items.[24]

This bestial connection was visually asserted and repeated in various representations associating dwarves and dogs. For instance, from Antonis Mor's 1549–1553 *Cardinal Granvella's Dwarf and a Dog*, to Girolamo Macchietti's *Dwarf with a Dog and Boy*, from a preliminary drawing for the *Martyrdom of Saint Lawrence* done in 1572 (Fig. 3.5), to Agostino Carracci's 1598 *Composition with Figures and Animals*: *Hairy Harry, Mad Peter and Tiny Amon* (Plate 5), to Karel van Mander's 1650 *Court Dwarf Giacomo Favorchi*, and to Francesco Trevisani's 1705 *Banquet of Anthony and Cleopatra*, dwarves were almost invariably shown accompanied by dogs. In addition to the association of dogs with licentiousness and the fact that the juxtaposition of a dog to a dwarf would visually demonstrate the smaller size of the latter, it is their connection to faithfulness that seems also *à propos* in these representations. Indeed, as topoi of loyalty, they spoke to the close nature of the relationship between the miniature humans and their patrons. Just like dogs, dwarves would stay faithful to the courtiers who owned them. The visual and symbolic association between dwarves and dogs finds its roots in Egyptian early dynastic courts (2920–2770 BCE), where stelae of dwarves and dogs were not only similar in appearance, but also carved with great attention. This, according to Véronique Dasen, "confirms that the short men had a special place in the household, and, as markers of prestige, may have had a similar position to that of favourite dogs."[25] It is as collectible marvels that dwarves found their ways into courts, even if eventually they served other capacities thanks to the loyalty they showed to their patrons.

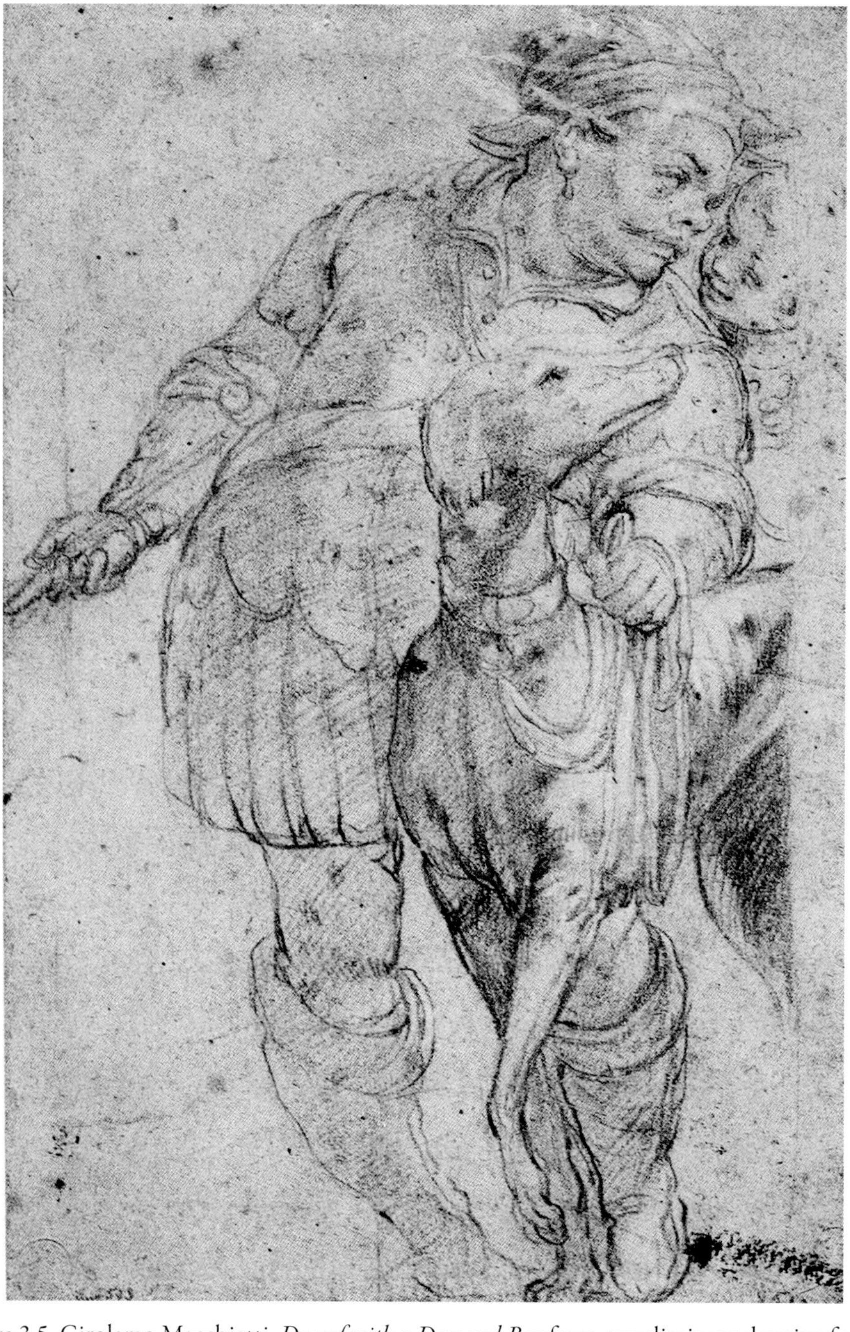

Figure 3.5. Girolamo Macchietti, *Dwarf with a Dog and Boy* from a preliminary drawing for the *Martyrdom of Saint Lawrence*, ca. 1572–73, Palais des Beaux-Arts, Lille, after Touba Ghadessi, *The Medici, Michelangelo, and the Art of Late Renaissance Florence*, 2003

Dwarves were also offered as presents from one court to the other, a practice that made them valuable diplomatic assets.[26] This is particularly apparent in the Medici court. From February of 1581 to December of that year, several letters from the agent of Bianca Cappello (1548–1587, Grand Duchess of Tuscany 1579–1587), Alberto Bolognetti, described the perfect female dwarf he found for Cappello in Warsaw; the *nana* is described as having great "proportions" and being "very beautiful."[27] The *nana*'s travels through Cracow and Vienna were fully documented and she provided a concrete, material link between Anna Jagiellon, Queen of Poland (1523–1596), and the Grand Duchess of Florence. Though not a central participant in the diplomatic relations between Tuscany and the Polish-Lithuanian Commonwealth, this marginal individual, as well as the other accompanying dwarves that followed her on the way to Florence, acquired much greater dimensions due to the importance of the tie she established between the two courts during a time of war.[28]

On a less political note, dwarves also carried gifts and messages from courts to their satellites or to other independent courts. This tradition persisted and there are accounts of dwarves bearing presents or correspondence throughout the seventeenth century. For instance a letter from the Duchess of Mantua Caterina de Medici-Gonzaga (1593–1627) to her brother Cosimo II de'Medici (1590–1621), dated to 1618, mentions Morgante—a different one from Bronzino's painted subject.[29] Also, on September 8, 1621, Caterina wrote to announce that she sent her dwarf, also named Morgante, back to Grand Duchess Maria Magdalena von Habsburg-de'Medici (1589–1631) and apologized that he returned late.[30] Caterina had retained Morgante in Mantua, planning to send unspecified gifts with him to the Medici court, but ultimately decided to wait for a safer way to deliver the presents and sent Morgante empty-handed.[31] Interestingly, the whole letter pertains to the dwarf's situation. The mention of Morgante is neither an afterthought nor a last-minute added paragraph. The centrality of this marginal individual in the correspondence of two prominent women attests to the increased presence and participation of dwarves in courtly matters.

Letters revolving entirely around the subject of dwarves are no exceptions in various courts and at various times, as the presence and exchange of these courtly marvels was a pivotal element of discussion in many of these settings. Chancellor Gabriele Calzoni, a Gonzaga resident in Venice, wrote a long letter to Duke Guglielmo Gonzaga (1538–1587) on September 28, 1583, discussing the many qualities of a dwarf the Duke might enjoy and the reasons this dwarf should be brought to Mantua—for instance, the *nano*'s good proportions, his ability to speak Italian and to read French and Spanish.[32] Interestingly, Calzoni refers to the dwarf as another "Morgantino," reiterating not only the popularity of our Morgante, but also the weight of implication this his name bore in various courts. In a fascinating epistolary exchange, we see Isabella d'Este (1474–1539) mentioning her wish to send a dwarf to Renée de France (daughter of Louis XII, married to Isabella's nephew Ercole II d'Este), and more intriguingly we read of Isabella's attempts at breeding dwarves. Indeed, Isabella opens her letter to Renée by stating that

> four years ago I promised the most illustrious Madama Renata that I would give her Excellency the first fruit to issue from my race of little dwarves, by which I meant a female. As your Ladyship knows, two years ago a little girl was born. Though we cannot hope she will stay so small as my Delia, she will nonetheless no doubt remain a dwarf, and given her beauty, she deserves to be treasured.[33]

Isabella not only owned dwarves, but she attempted to reproduce them, thus adding a personal stamp to a valuable commodity meant to function as a self-fashioning element that allowed her to demonstrate courtly grace and play with popular fascinations.

As court dwellers, dwarves dressed in regal costumes and participated in elaborate ceremonies. Several entries in records of the *guardaroba* and letters to secretaries verify the sartorial importance given to the appearance of dwarves in the Medici court. Eleonora di Toledo ordered various garments for court dwarves Lodovico, Filippino, and Gianmaria, including luxurious silk garments.[34] A letter from 1543 to the ducal major-domo Pierfrancesco Riccio mentions, less typically, leather garments for one of the dwarves.[35] Around the same time, the major-domo received a letter from Vincenzo Ferrini also mentioning the need for black silk clothes and accessories meant for the dwarf Filippino.[36] Though most of the correspondence regarding dwarves' clothing was written to and from secretaries or, more prestigiously, Medici women, there is evidence of Medici patriarchs' knowledge of such garment matters. In 1565, Cosimo I wrote to authorize diverse payments, including expenditure related to clothing for the dwarf Gradasso.[37] The sartorial importance given to court dwarves undoubtedly related to the original reason behind their presence at court: they were court dwellers *because* of their physical appearance. Emphasizing the features (through dress) that allowed them to exist within the confines of a palazzo therefore only seemed logical.[38] Also, the normalizing function of clothing cast their abnormalities in relief; indeed, clothed, a dwarf resembled any courtier, but for his or her abnormally short body that subsequently held accrued significance.

Aside from their visible presence at courts during festivities, dwarves could also serve an understated role as part of the court's retinue through less celebratory tasks. Just like pages, they had access to intimate spheres of the courtier's lives; however, unlike pages who entered the court in their early teens, dwarves could defend themselves like adults.[39] In addition, dwarves were allowed to be more irreverent toward the courtier they served and had more intimate access to the courtier's personal affairs.[40]

As described by Tommaso Garzoni, the close interaction of the dwarves with his or her *signore* or *signora* was a highly visible and celebrated one. The dwarf was present for most of the courtier's activities and thus garnered knowledge regarding the courtier's likes and dislikes, thoughts, and external relationships.[41] The physical proximity of the dwarves to the family they served was confirmed not only by many documents stating their actual closeness, but also through juxtapositions found in records of *guardarobe*. One telling example is seen in an inventory dating from 1587. Within a category entitled "Quadri di pittura," not surprisingly, a list of paintings owned by the Medici family is noted. In this list, a portrait of a dwarf is recorded on the same page and in the same terms as portraits of Medici family members such as Cosimo Il Vecchio or the Prince of Savoy. In fact, this portrait, catalogued simply as "un Ritratto in tela d'un nano senza ornam.," stood between an entry recording the portrait of the Queen of France and the portrait of an anonymous man.[42]

This Queen of France may have been Catherine de'Medici Valois. She, in fact, provides a great example of how central dwarves were in a sovereign's life. After François I (1494–1547) and Pope Clement VII (1475–1534) decided that Catherine de'Medici (1519–1589) was to be wedded to Henri d'Orléans (1519–1559), future Henri II of France, the French court administration recorded all her possessions. Among these, a dwarf, Jehan de Nano, was listed as a "vallet de chambre."[43] This inventory of goods was continually updated through the years, and inevitably, Jehan de Nano appeared repeatedly as Catherine de'Medici's "vallet de chambre."[44] Interestingly, Jehan's records were not separated from those of his vallet counterparts in the *garde robe* documents. The only reference made to Jehan's physical deformity, and thus to his particular position at court, was through his suffix. Furthermore, the date when this *garde robe* started preceded the arrival of the future Catherine de'Medici to France; it is therefore likely that Jehan was in Rome with the bride-to-be and followed her to French soil after she married Henri d'Orléans in 1533. Not only did Jehan follow Catherine to France, but there is also evidence that he was well cared for. The same aforementioned inventory lists specific coat garments made for children, yet this list is dated from 1532 before Catherine and Henri were even married.[45] The child-size clothing may easily have been prepared for a dwarf, since no children would have been in the immediate care of Catherine and there would have been no need for her to register them as part of her own *garde robe*.[46] And, again, no distinction is made between the dwarf's clothing and Catherine's various linens and dresses. This lack of separation and emphasis is notable since it stands in opposition to the belief that dwarves were a representation of the world turned upside down and were thus treated in a special manner. These records silently indicate that they were, in fact, a necessary and normal part of courtly spheres and, like other members of the court retinue, had their needs accommodated. Further documents point to a strong connection between the Queen of France and her dwarves. Dated to 1602, a record of succession based on her previous inventories establishes the bequests that Catherine de'Medici Valois left to various members of her family, her retinue, and court workers.[47] Again, without differentiation, the beneficiaries of her possessions—including her dwarves—are listed next to the amount of money or belongings they are to receive. From the noblewoman Gabrielle de Rochechouart to Noel Rousseau, *ecuyer de cuisine* (kitchen attendant), the list of beneficiaries is surprisingly homogenous in its written presentation. It is therefore not unexpected that a René Rondeau, *tailleur des nains* (tailor for her dwarves) is found between Suzanne Carron, *veuve de defunct* Pierre Godet, *luy vivant Paintre & Vallet de Chambre* (the widow of a painter and court attendant), and Mathurin Brossier, *Sommier du garde-manger* (a clerk who dealt with household food).[48] Undifferentiated from that of his court counterparts, René Rondeau's trade is notable for its inventoried normality. In the same vein, and in this same record of succession, a Damoiselle Jeanne Petit is listed as one of Catherine's direct attendants—once again, not separated from her counterparts at court, and her miniature stature only indicated by the 'petit' following her name.[49] The unique reaction that the dwarf's presence might have provoked at court is erased in the mundane reality of inventoried goods linked to people. Indeed, the absence of emotional wonder we encounter in records such as these might be closer to the quotidian interactions that existed between the dwarves and their masters.

Dwarves were thus prized—and extremely visible—members of powerful courts. They were undoubtedly appreciated by their wealthy patrons and they existed mostly to satisfy the needs and pleasures of these patrons for whom they were among many types of objects that demonstrated princely wealth or knowledge.[50] The dwarves and their portraits were therefore part of collections that enhanced the status of the self and the family, and acted as figurative manifestations of the ideology of rule.[51] The appearance assumed by a familial authority was codified and formed a specific rhetoric of power, if this family was indeed at the head of the constructed system of rule. In order to control the highest positions in this arbitrary—yet highly rigid—structure, the Medici family devised a formation of authority based on their own standards. They also employed recognizable marks of ruling nobility legible to both the families they hoped to emulate and the ones they wished to subvert. It is as part of this self-fashioning process that dwarves became an essential instrument of the Medici's ruling ambitions. Indeed, they adopted visible signs of sovereignty that echoed the practices of established noble circles in early modern European courts; one such pursuit was the collecting and displaying of dwarves like Morgante. Morgante—as a recognizable dwarf—embodied a microcosmic ideal of a ruling topos the Medici wanted to locate and promote, which they did very actively through visual representations such as Bronzino's portrait. Thus Morgante's representation on a double-sided canvas stands not only as a visual testament to this famed *nano*, but also as a mirror to Cosimo's noble aspirations. His princely image became linked to that of a deformed individual, and indeed it was perhaps in this type of juxtaposition that his lordship became most visible.

Most portraits of dwarves pointed to unknown individuals and to their role as entertaining, and often anonymous, companions to the ducal retinue and courtiers. However, before discussing how this portrait was a strong indication of the importance of a specific dwarf at the court of Cosimo I de'Medici, let us turn to the ways in which Bronzino's portrayal of the dwarf Morgante occupied a significant position in the articulation of a central axis in Cinquecento art theory. The *paragone* debate, sparked by Leonardo da Vinci's writings, remained part of the contemporary cultural discussion during the time Bronzino produced most of his works under the auspices of Cosimo I.[52] The *paragone* of the Italian Renaissance stressed the differences between arts, setting painting and sculpture against one another. This debate still had currency in the mid-sixteenth century, especially in a setting such as a court, where physical differences were emphasized rather than downplayed.[53] Though Bronzino was part of the Compagnia di San Luca by 1538, the Accademia del Disegno (founded in 1563) would gather all the arts under the umbrella of *disegno* and therefore make debates such as the *paragone* obsolete.[54] Indeed, by promoting methods and practice based on several artistic forums, the Accademia del Disegno centralized and unified varied artistic discourses.[55] Bronzino was active, along with other art theorists, in the formation of cultural and intellectual debates regarding the arts in general throughout the 1530s.[56] In fact, Bronzino participated in discussions dealing with the primacy of the arts quite directly—for in the 1540s he wrote letters to Benedetto Varchi (1503–1565), Cosimo's court historian and art critic, pertaining to the primacy of the arts.[57] In an *inchiesta* made in 1546, Benedetto Varchi, complimented Bronzino's poetic and artistic talents, but in his *Lezzioni*, lectures meant to define the arts, he also questioned the relative merits of painting and sculpture.[58] Bronzino replied to Varchi's *inchiesta* in an unfinished letter in which he surprisingly offered seven arguments in favor of sculpture over painting.[59] Because this letter was never completed, there are no writings from Bronzino that elaborate on his opinion regarding the superiority of painting over sculpture. However, Bronzino's *Morgante* may be read as the conclusion of his letter to Varchi, a coda to his defense of sculpture. In this painting, indeed, we see a direct, if delayed, response to Varchi: rather than write a counter-argument for the supremacy of painting over sculpture, he visually articulated it through this portrait.[60] According to Deborah Parker, "in depicting the dwarf's front and back, Bronzino archly displays painting's ability to show, as does sculpture, more than one perspective of the human body."[61] In addition to the ability to show more than one perspective on the human body, *Morgante* also demonstrates painting's ability to avoid one of sculpture's defects, namely the impossibility of simultaneously showing both a rear and a front view with a face.[62] By slightly varying the angles and multiple views of his portrait, Bronzino succeeded in overcoming this flaw and thus proved painting superior to sculpture. Sefy Hendler, interestingly, stretches this idea further by noting that Bronzino not only proves painting's supremacy to sculpture, but also added a fourth dimension to his work, that of time. Indeed, the flying butterflies on the front of the canvas and their absence in the back, as well as Morgante's varying facial hair in the front and in the back reveal the existence of time as an inherent component of this double-sided portrait.[63]

Due to the central place Bronzino's *Morgante* holds in the application of the *paragone* theory to the practice of painting, we may arrive at a more precise dating of this portrait. *Morgante* has a *terminus ante quem* of 1553, since it is specifically mentioned in a *Guardaroba Medicea* document dating from 1553.[64] However, because of the 1546 date of Varchi's *inchiesta*, it is probable that Bronzino painted the work sooner than 1553. In fact, a date of 1546 to 1548 would also correlate with two other chronological indications. The first lies in the action represented in Bronzino's portrait. Most of the bird-hunting activities in Cosimo's court are recorded in the 1540s, and notably around 1544. The fact that Bronzino would choose to represent the famed dwarf by associating him with a bird hunt may in fact point to a popular activity performed by Morgante around 1545, rather than many years later. The second chronological indication is based on the underdrawing of the *Morgante*. Bronzino drew a *quadrattura* on both sides of the canvas, so as to accurately depict the proportions of the dwarf's body. Once he completed the torso, he drew the rest of the body free hand, with no *pentimenti* or re-positionings; it was a sure hand. Similarly, the painting itself does not show many corrections—nor could it have supported them. Because *Morgante* is painted on a single canvas, one which is overly worked on both sides, numerous additions and corrections might have ruined the fragile ground.[65] It is therefore possible to assume that the making of *Morgante* was not a lengthy process—and, indeed, if done as a visual response to Varchi's 1546 *inchiesta*, it was probably produced shortly thereafter. Additionally, we know that Morgante was a ubiquitous figure around Cosimo by 1548. As mentioned previously, Vasari painted the dwarf at the side of the Medici ruler during his visit to Elba—dated 1548—in a roundel decorating the quarters of Leo X in the Sala di Cosimo (Fig. 3.2).[66] The production of Vasari's painting dates to around 1556, yet this roundel demonstrates that Morgante was a famous and recognizable individual by 1548; since Vasari copied Bronzino's painting of Morgante for his roundel, it is feasible to assume an approximate date of 1547–1548 for Bronzino's double-sided canvas.[67] It is worth noting that Morgante's established appearance in this court tableau, set in 1548, is as his own portrait. Finally, Bronzino painted the portrait of Morgante following Cosimo's request—one that would have required some exchange of money to seal the commission.[68] However, in a *giornale di entrata e di uscita* recording expenses and contracts between 1549 and 1553, no mention is made of such a contract.[69] Bronzino only started to receive an annual stipend from Cosimo de'Medici in the 1550s, which means that individual contracts and details of commissions would have been recorded at least until then.[70] We can thus assume that the request made to the court artist occurred and was settled before 1549.

Having determined a chronology both for Morgante and for his portrait by Bronzino, it is interesting to see it in a dialogue with earlier produced portraits such as that of Cosimo de'Medici's 1539 portrait as Orpheus (Plate 4). In addition to discussing how portraits of dwarves adopt and burlesque the poses of princely and regal compositions, Campbell also describes the particulars that applied to Bronzino's commission to paint the court dwarf.[71] The dialogue between *Cosimo I as Orpheus* and *Morgante* is one that is more complex than a mere reference and occurs on several levels. Painted between 1537 and 1539, this nude portrait of Cosimo I highlights the head of the Medici family's qualities as a faithful husband, strong lover, successful politician, and head of a future strong dynasty. Bronzino chose the myth of Orpheus and Eurydice to illustrate the love between Cosimo I and Eleonora di Toledo (who was either betrothed or recently-wed to Cosimo at the time of production). In most versions of the myth, Orpheus loses Eurydice forever because his fervent ardor for her forces him to look at his lover while she leaves Hades, thus breaking the deal Orpheus made with Pluto and Proserpina for the return of Eurydice. However, medieval versions of the myth gave the lovers a happy ending, making Bronzino's choice a logical one.[72] As Orpheus, Cosimo is represented holding a contemporaneous *lira da braccio* in his left hand and a bow in his right one; in the immediate background, Cerberus appears tamed and we assume it is because Cosimo/Orpheus has already played music to appease him.[73] Bronzino highlights the sexual nature of his portrayal in several ways: the *lira*'s yonic attributes are accentuated by the juxtaposition of the erect phallic bow emerging from between Cosimo's legs; the reddened cheeks and lips of Cosimo/Orpheus point to a coital visualization; and his direct, erotic gaze at the viewer turn us into Eleonora/Eurydice, invited to join her lover Cosimo/Orpheus. But Bronzino also inserted political commentaries in this painting. The nudity of Cosimo/Orpheus is not meant to be merely supplementary to the passionate mythological narrative of lovers lost and found, but it overtly refers to another mythological figure, that of Hercules. In fact, the bust Bronzino painted is modeled after the famed *Belvedere Torso*, thus making Cosimo into a hybrid figure combining the loving body of a faithful husband—Orpheus—to the strong political body of a civic leader—Hercules.[74] This strong, heroic body is one that can reproduce and produce strong heirs, thus establishing a dynastic claim to power and avoiding extinction. This hyper-idealization of the male body is one that finds immediate—but opposite—equivalencies in Bronzino's portrayal of Morgante. Indeed, Morgante's body is decisively not ideal: the curvature of his shortened limbs, every unseemly skin fold, and his enlarged abdomen are all carefully depicted as being far from a perfected Renaissance body. The reason for his nudity is far from allegorical—it is meant to allow the viewer impunity in staring at a deformed wondrous body. The back of the canvas is perhaps closest in tone to Cosimo's portrait. Indeed, Bronzino shows the dwarf turning his head toward the viewer and in a sense mimicking Cosimo's pose as Orpheus, gazing back at Eurydice. However, Morgante's pose and facial expression are neither erotic nor inviting. If we are Eleonora/Eurydice in Cosimo's portrait, then, given the activity performed by the dwarf and the owl staring at us, we are the hunted game in Morgante's portrait. Cosimo's bow also finds resonance in the rods held by Morgante.[75] Whereas Cosimo's bow speaks to his strong virility, Morgante's rods are visually separated from his body and are used as accessories to kill, rather than as a tool used to tame an enemy diplomatically through soothing music. Morgante's crudeness is here placed in contrast to the refinement of Cosimo's method of subdual. The pairing of these two paintings speaks loudly to the necessity of dwarves at court. Indeed, Morgante serves as a foil to the perfect courtly body of Cosimo, metaphorically and literally; in a sense, Bronzino's portrait confirms the qualities of an ideal courtier by demonstrating its opposite—but related—mirror image. Through the imperfections of Morgante, we see the greatness of Cosimo. *Morgante* has thus been seen as a satirical visual pun on Cosimo's allegorical portrait, and previous scholarship has agreed that the details of this ironic and humorous work were commissioned and specified by Cosimo himself.[76] According to Campbell, this portrait corroborates Paul Barolsky's claim regarding the appreciation of humor and jest at the court of Cosimo.[77] It is also interesting to note that earlier scholarship on Bronzino's *Morgante* has seen this representation of Morgante as an excuse for the artist's life-studies of freaks, which is in opposition to what has been said in more recent studies on the matter.[78]

The entertaining elements essential to the livelihood of a dwarf often found their way into visual representations. Whether entertaining, dancing, hunting, or acting in staged fights, dwarves performed many activities for the pleasure of their patrons. One of the many qualities Alberto Bolognetti describes to Bianca Cappello, regarding the traveling *nana* and her sister, has to do with their ability to "be witty, sing, and do thousands of [other] things."[79] A typically entertaining spectacle took place in Cosimo's presence in 1544, a dwarf—most likely Morgante—fought naked with a monkey and was declared victorious after the Duke stopped the dwarf from killing the monkey.[80] The ubiquitous nudity of Morgante is significant. Just like his double-sided portrait serves as a foil to the perfected body of Cosimo I, his generic nudity allowed Morgante to be immediately perceived as an "other." Visually, he embodied the crudeness of *ritrarre* and allowed courtiers to surpass it and to be idealized via *imitare*. It is the flaws of Morgante's body—most visible in his bare state—that activated a reverse discourse of rigid perfection so prevalent at court. Such demonstrations were not uncommon. For instance, at the court of Philip the Good, during a feast celebrating the duke's marriage to Isabella, daughter of King John I of Portugal in 1430, the Burgundian court giant Hans engaged in a mock battle with Isabella's dwarf, Madame d'Or.[81] The grotesque aspects of court dwarves themselves were highlighted to comic effect by many artists who, instead of recording their exact characteristics, emphasized their comical features to remind viewers of the place dwarves held at court as jesters and entertainers, first and foremost.[82] Still at the court of Philip the Good, the tradition of inserting live beings in pies became common practice; this custom was carried out for two centuries and, in the eighteenth century, a pie concealed a dwarf during a banquet given in honor of Charles I and Queen Henrietta by the Duke of Buckingham.[83] The amusing entertainment inherent in watching a miniature human being—Jeffrey Hudson—emerge from an edible pastry was an essential quality for the livelihood of dwarves at court. Any visual narrative that emphasized it was a welcome nod to their positions as court entertainers. What artists visually added to the appearances of dwarves was often akin to satirical commentaries using known facts and/or legends. In fact, even the name chosen for dwarves and the ironic connotations attached to them reflected a common practice. Odoardo Farnese's (1573–1626) and Catherine de'Medici Valois's court dwarves, for example, were both named Rodomonte—a joking reference to the epic, brave, and chivalrous heroes of Boiardo and Ariosto.[84] The name Rodomonte was appropriately shortened to Amon, a verbal parallel to the size of the dwarf. Farnese's Amon actually appears in a portrait done by Agostino Carracci in 1598 and titled *Composition with Figures and Animals: Hairy Harry, Mad Peter and Tiny Amon* (Plate 5). This portrait groups together a dwarf, a buffoon, and a hirsute man, along with dogs, monkeys, and a parrot. The documents left about the dwarf Amon tell us that he was part of Cardinal Farnese's retinue and assigned caring for the dogs used for court hunting.[85] His close visual connection with one of the dogs calls upon both his life occupation and the common trope of faithfulness carried by dwarves and dogs alike. Not unlike Bronzino's portrait of Morgante, this painting combines social commentaries with popular beliefs and actual realities. Centered around the hirsute, the portrait shows the buffoon to his left and the dwarf to his right, a monkey on his left shoulder, a dog on his lap, his paw held by the second monkey seated on the ground. Only the buffoon's head and collar are visible, evidently because his normal body presented no interest to the painter or the viewer. On the other hand, both the bodies of the hirsute and of the dwarf are fully depicted, with careful attention paid to the unusual size of the dwarf and the hair on the body of the hirsute. Amon leans on his large dog, while a parrot on his left hand eats fruit offered by the hirsute. Roberto Zapperi has convincingly argued that this painting not only speaks to the interest held by various courts in possessing and displaying wonders such as dwarves and hirsutes, but he also states that this composition presents an ideal view of the world, achieved mostly by animals, where feuds are absent. In this ideal world, physically abnormal individuals such as dwarves and hirsutes are superior to normative human beings since they do not care about difference in appearances and origins and they participate in upholding social peace.[86] Most notably, Zapperi points to the fact that this painting was probably not commissioned by Cardinal Farnese, but was rather a self-initiated work by Agostino Carracci or a painting suggested by one of the sitters. This would imply an incredible amount of agency on the part of subjects who were often listed as objects belonging to courtiers; it also problematizes the complex iconography employed by Carracci, one that is based on Democritus's ideals regarding the superiority of beasts over humans. Would dwarves or hirsutes associate themselves so openly with the animal kingdom as to shadow their full human aspects and present themselves as liminal creatures? Regardless, few comical factors find their way in this representation.[87] In this sense, it follows the tone set by Bronzino is his painting of Morgante.

The back view of *Morgante* depicts the dwarf, an owl on his shoulder, rods on his left side, and dead birds on his right hand. The iconography of the owl on Morgante's shoulder is not clear. Cesare Ripa's *Iconologia* does not elucidate this mystery, as an owl perched on a shoulder referred most likely to superstition, which does not seem to be relevant here.[88] Literary romances often associated magical powers with dwarves and the association of the owl with a dwarf may indeed refer to the supernatural power he possessed. However, it is not the case here, precisely because of the narrative attached to the totality of the attributes surrounding and held by Morgante. Catalogues do not clarify the significance of the owl to a great extent, either. Most likely, this image referred to the activity of hunting, which seems to have been a popular activity for dwarves to perform, including Morgante. A document from Lorenzo Pagni, dated 1544, relates the story of a dwarf catching birds at the Medici court.[89] His mention of an owl is informative, as the document presents a telling instance of a Medici court practice: bird hunting performed by dwarves. The presence of the owl on Morgante's shoulder may thus refer to one of these bird hunts, whereas the type of game he is holding in his right hand could help identify the specific hunt Bronzino's work is intended to reference. In addition, the three spears Morgante is holding are spears used for bird hunting; the spears were presumably used to stab and recover the smaller fowl, caught because of the owl who served as bait and who is tied by a string to Morgante's hand.[90] Through these realistic details, Morgante is identifiable and is situated within a narrative of actual court activity rather than an imaginary grotesque world.

Deborah Parker has made a persuasive and thorough interpretation of Bronzino's *capitoli* in relation to his visual productions. She argues that the birds in Morgante's hand and the owl on his shoulder point to the phallic attributes of the dwarf, since the owl was a common euphemism for the phallus of a sodomite and was used by Bronzino in his poetry.[91] The birds may, in fact, also refer to a common hunt scene. Bronzino painted the hunting spears with extreme precision; in addition, owls were used to attract birds, such as the one depicted in Morgante's hands. The effort to represent details identifiable with bird hunts described in ducal correspondence makes a strong case for Bronzino's intention to record an actual event that took place in the Medici gardens. Whereas it was often the case that dwarves' sexual organs were atrophied as well, the various representations of Morgante in the nude—and the Boboli garden sculpture in particular—suggest that Morgante was actually not suffering from this atrophy.[92] If indeed, as Parker suggests, this owl refers to the generous dimensions of Morgante's "appendages," then Bronzino might have been playing on a sexual pun regarding dwarves as lecherous persons. This double-sided canvas is essentially a before- and after-the bird hunt scene, but one that may hold a sexual dimension as well.

The sexual subtext of this double-sided painting also finds articulation in the narrative unfolded by the sequence of the portrait. The front side of the painting shows an active owl, a bird in flight, and southern swallowtail butterflies in motion. Most conspicuously, one of the butterflies serves as a "fig leaf" for Morgante, yet it highlights, rather than covers, his genitals. On the back of the canvas, the motion has stopped, the owl is rested, and the birds are dead, flaccid. In lieu of Morgante's covered genitals, we see the spears—paralleling *Cosimo I as Orpheus*'s phallic bow—held by the dwarf. As Sefy Hendler has suggested, the presence of the monarch butterflies in the front of the canvas, and their absence in the back, suggest two distinct moments in the narrative of this double-sided canvas; so does the fact that Morgante is beardless in the front but not in the back of the canvas.[93] Time, framed by the elements mentioned above, occupies a crucial role in Bronzino's composition as it not only identifies the narrative of the hunt, but it also points to the pre- and post-coital implication of this portrait. The hunt is an actual one, as well as metaphorical one thanks to the wide understanding of Bronzino's puns about birds and the centrality of the genital-covering butterfly. Indeed, the term *parpaglione* in old Tuscan referred to a butterfly, but it also finds resonance in the verb *sparpagliare*.[94] Morgante's ability to "scatter" and "disseminate" is one that alluded to the dwarf's propensity to successfully finish a sexual act.[95] The rhetorical convention used for decorum is in fact subverted by signaling to the viewer what needs to be revealed: Morgante's genitals and capacity to function as a sexual being is central to his identity.

The placement of the painting in the Palazzo Vecchio supports the idea that *Morgante* was not just a random burlesque portrait, or merely the visual manifestation of a collectible curiosity. The portrait was placed in the Palazzo della Signoria in a vestibule set above newly built rooms.[96] This room was intended for guests and foreigners visiting Cosimo I. Consequently the works placed in this room were meant to speak to and about Cosimo I and the Medici family. The other works in the room were maps, a globe, paintings of the Madonna and Child, and diverse official portraits. Why then would Morgante's portrait be included in this room? Cosimo I may have wanted to place a portrait of his dwarf in this context simply to demonstrate his possessions or to display a complex visual retort, but the painting also stood in for the court's particular practices. In this room, Morgante was given a legible identity that linked him to the court and the court to him. There is little doubt that if Morgante had not been recognizable as an individual belonging to, and partly defining, the Medici court, Cosimo I would have hesitated to place him in a room where his own identity was at stake.[97] The visual association of Morgante and Cosimo I in the decoration of the Palazzo Vecchio was a strong and repeated one. Even outside of the Palazzo Vecchio and of Florence, Morgante's tie to Cosimo was strong: we know that, in addition to Elba, Morgante was known in—and probably accompanied Cosimo to—Siena, Rome, Bologna, Ferrara, and Venice.[98] Indeed, in the absence of Cosimo I, a representation of Morgante alone might have stood as a type of *impresa* for the Medici patriarch. Furthermore, the original frame of the *Morgante* was hinged, which encouraged the viewer to activate the painting in order to look at both of its sides.[99] Such a close relationship with the companion of Cosimo I suggests the viewer's active engagement with the Medici court *via* this painting. Because of the temporal dimension Bronzino painted in this portrait, the viewer's engagement with the painting, and consequently with Cosimo I's court, was temporal as well as visual; the viewer would therefore be aware of his/her own temporal part in the narrative of the Medici court signified by the *Morgante*.

Interestingly, comical subtexts are also absent from other visual representations of dwarves in the Palazzo Vecchio. In the *Sala dei Cinquecento*, for example, on the wall facing the main access to the room, one sees a mural representing the war between Florence and Siena. The first episode, on the left of this wall, is the *Presa del Forte presso la Porta Camollia di Siena* (Fig. 3.6). Painted by Vasari, Naldini, and Stradano, this grand-scale composition shows the action that occurred during the night of January 26 and January 27, 1553, when the Marchese di Marignano brought down the fortifications of Siena and penetrated the city.[100]

Notably, to the right of the Marchese, a dwarf in full military garb holds a lantern.[101] Vasari chose to depict him in the forefront of the action, almost to the middle of the frame, as one of the most visible characters of the entire composition. Far from embodying any type of comic relief or playing with a possibly humorous aspect of this belligerent situation, the Marchese's dwarf is present during a serious situation, and depicted in a serious manner. Here again, the dwarf is certainly not depicted as a comical element, but as a loyal companion who based his actions on that of his *signore*.

In addition to his possible reference to an event happening in real time—the hunt—Bronzino also focused on the real anatomical details specific to an achondroplastic dwarf. Bronzino's interest in anatomy was well known to his peers. This assumption is substantiated by a 1565 document written by Alessandro Allori, one of his students, that describes in detail the specifics of Bronzino's interest in the body.[102] In a dialogue on *disegno*, Allori mentions not only Bronzino's interest in human anatomy, but also his significant knowledge in the practice of dissection.[103] Bronzino's knowledge of dissection may not have stemmed from direct experience, but rather from reading Vesalius and Valverde, and perhaps from attending semi-public dissections. In fact, it is very likely that Bronzino did indeed attend a dissection performed in Pisa by Vesalius in 1544, since Cosimo himself was present during at least one of them.[104] This interest in anatomy apparently stayed with Bronzino, for although the dissections occurred in 1544, his interest in anatomy and Vesalius was still noted in 1565. It may well have been Vesalius's influence that led Bronzino to observe this dwarf so directly. Vesalius published his *De humani corporis fabrica* in 1543; Bronzino, certainly aware of the Vesalian emphasis on physical observation, seems to have translated this into an ethos of direct observation turned on the body of Morgante. He treated Morgante's physical aspects as one might treat any anatomical object of inquiry, therefore recording the individual and the non-ideal physical features of the dwarf as naturalistically as possible. Far from a generic or anonymous body, Morgante's physique became under Bronzino's hand a unique site of inquiry. In this visual "dissection" of Morgante's body, the artist invested an abstract idea of anatomical knowledge with the material reality of Morgante's body—even turning this body over for the viewer.[105]

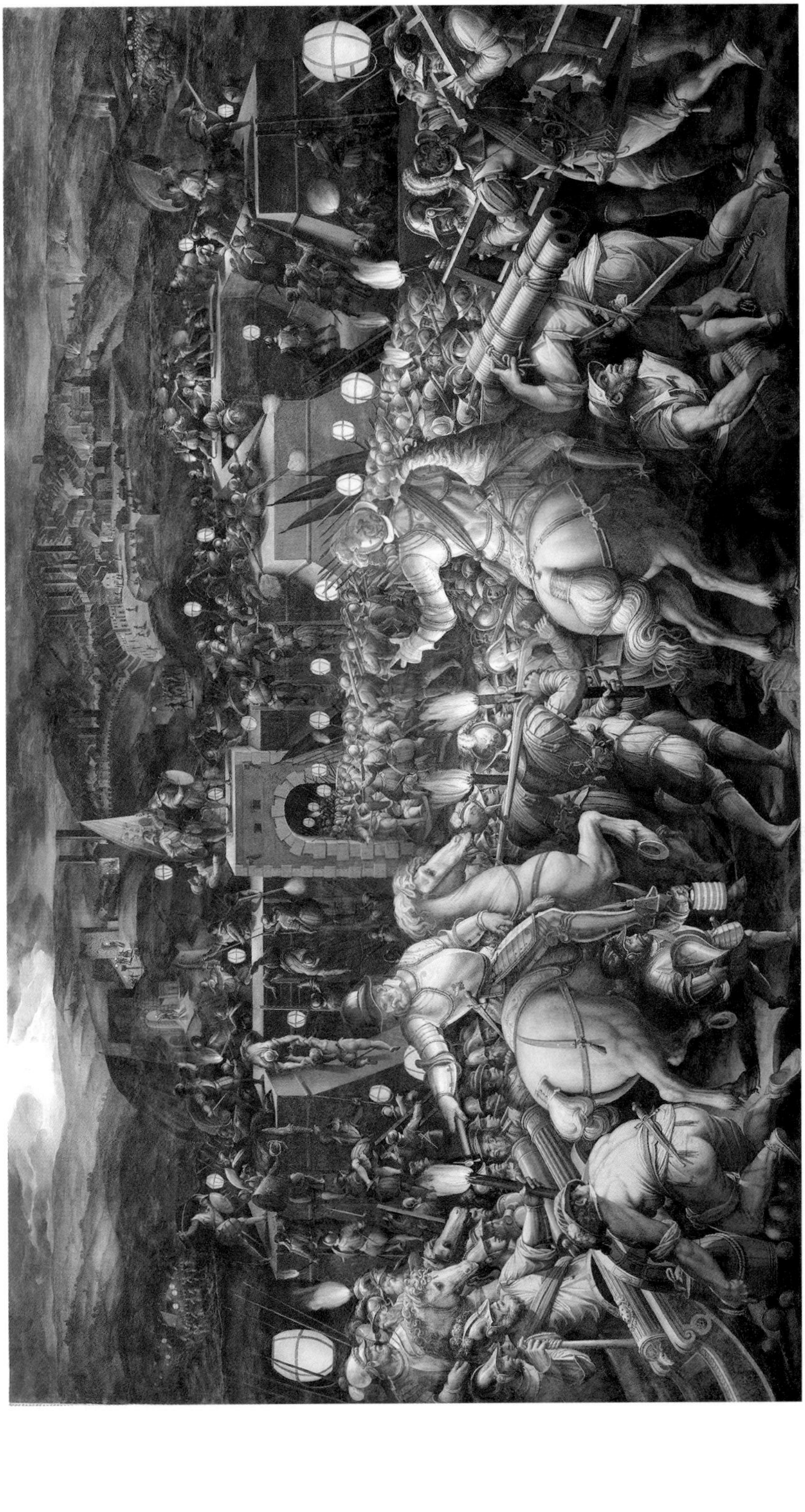

Figure 3.6. Giorgio Vasari, Giovan Battista Naldini, and Giovanni Stradano, *Presa del Forte presso la Porta Camollia di Siena*, ca. 1556, Palazzo Vecchio, Florence

Bronzino's effort to depict Morgante realistically is visually supported by his accurate curvatures and shapes of the limbs and his visual features—different in the front and in the back, since Morgante has a beard and fine moustache in the rear view. This realism is further underscored by the size of the painting: 150 cm by 100 cm, a height and width that roughly corresponds to that of a dwarf with achondroplasia.[106] If Morgante were indeed an achondroplastic dwarf, his height would be around 131 ± 5.6 cm.[107] This height suggests that Bronzino's portrait is in fact life-size, particularly since it corresponds to the dimensions of Cioli's statue in the Boboli garden that is also reputed to be life-size.[108] The precision of these measurements serves as a second confirmation that the artist wished to pursue anatomical accuracy over and above grotesque exaggeration.

The proportions of dwarves were inherently related to their success as collectible items and, consequently, as court dwellers. In an era that discussed aesthetics and manner as actual currency, visual proportions for dwarves were real commodities. Preference was given to dwarves who did not have large discrepancies between limbs, head, and torso, even though most achondroplastic dwarves did have a prominent chest. Emphasizing Morgante's anatomical features was a visual way to assert the reasons for his arrival to the Medici court in the first place: his miniature body heralded proportions that fit the aesthetic preferences of the courtiers who wanted him there.[109] Interestingly, the proportions and aesthetics of dwarves functioned on a reverse level and, the more emphasized their short stature was, the more unattractive they seemed, the more valuable they became. What was unsightly for a regular-sized courtier became beautiful for a dwarf.[110] The example of Bianca Capello's female dwarf is also very telling in this regard. In his letter to the Granduchessa, Bolognetti emphasized the beautiful proportions of the *nana* and the fact that finding such proportions in a dwarf took a long time and kept him from sending her a dwarf sooner.[111] Another revealing example is found in the writings of Pietro Francesco Scarabelli, author of the catalogue of Settala's museum. Scarabelli referred to Marchese Ferdinando Cospi's (1606–1686) collection, particularly to a *nana* who worked for him. The dwarf, Angelica Biaviati, was the sister of Sebastiano Biaviati; both were in the service of the Marchese, but only Angelica was described as being very well proportioned and having perfect symmetry.[112]

Naturalistic renderings of dwarves based on direct observations translated to visualizations that highlighted their humanity; indeed, these were tied to the ways in which the humanity of dwarves—or lack thereof—became legible through the documents establishing their unresolved juridical personhood. One of the few courtly documents speaking directly to dwarves' juridical personhood relates the tale of an adulterous dwarf who underwent a trial and was ridiculed publicly.[113] After discussing Cosimo I's health, Bartolomeo Concini, writing to Piero di Francesco Usimbardi, describes an event that gave great pleasure to the Grand Duke. The episode concerned a dwarf who was sent to prison and tried for adultery; the dwarf was condemned and had to ride a donkey, seated backwards, and holding a placard declaring his disloyal offense. The presence of another dwarf, Magnifichino, is also mentioned, alongside that of ministers of justice.[114] Not only is the mention of the trial and cause for condemnation important, but the reference to the presence of ministers of justice also implies inclusive trial proceedings. This indicates that, at least in some instances, dwarves appear to have enjoyed the same legal rights and obligations as any Florentine citizen. They could be prosecuted, and were granted the right to present their defense.[115] Another noteworthy event involved the incarceration of a dwarf. On July 10, 1535, Alessandro de'Medici asked for clemency for his imprisoned dwarf, Francesco, from the Duke of Mantua.[116] The fact that the dwarf was imprisoned speaks to his legal responsibility—and thus to the possibility of his juridical personhood—whereas Alessandro's request confirms the status of the dwarf as a member of his entourage, deserving of the same rights and graces. Similarly, Lorenzo Pagni wrote to Agnolo di Matteo Niccolini to complain about the brutal manners of Pirro Colonna toward a member of the ducal retinue, a dwarf, presumably Morgante.[117] It is fascinating to note, here, that Colonna reacted so violently because he believed the dwarf brought him poor luck. An even greater indicator of juridical personhood was the legal ability to possess land. In 1555, Cosimo wrote a legal document giving Morgante a farm in the province of Arezzo; not only did Cosimo's bequest grant Morgante full legal status, but the mention of Morgante's wife and legitimate sons as heirs of his property also confirmed the legal rights of dwarves to marry and bear legally recognized children on whom they could confer property.[118] Though Morgante might not have had the right to access and sit in a politically official position, his status was similar to that of a fully recognized citizen—which meant he had the right to appear before a tribunal to defend his rights, the right to ownership of private property, and he retained basic civil rights.[119]

Morgante not only received property, clothes, and gifts, but he was also paid a retainer. An order of payment sent by Cosimo in 1573 requested that the administrators of the Florentine Monte di Pietà pay Morgante ten scudi, probably every year or twice a year.[120] The recognition of Morgante's ability to handle a sum of money, and indeed to be paid at all, was another way to grant him legal personhood. Nor was Morgante an exception. Sebastiano Biaviati and his sister Angelica Biaviati, the two dwarves who belonged to the Marchese Ferdinando Cospi, were, according to Lorenzo Legati, both on salary.[121] These individual cases are more telling than what we learn from Paolo Zacchia's (1584–1659) treatise on medico-legal questions. Paolo Zacchia, physician to the popes, devoted a great part of his life to exploring the relation between medical questions and their medical and legal applications. The result was a large compendium organized by themes and dealing with specific cases. Even though Zacchia did devote a *liber* to the question of monsters' legal rights, the terms were often too general to apply to dwarves.[122] The questions presented, as well as the cases introduced, were more functional for other types of monsters, such as hirsutes or hermaphrodites.

Morgante's position is one that highlighted the parallels between his status as a curiosity at court with his status as a human being with particularly interesting anatomical features. The interest in Morgante's person and in Morgante as an oddity is confirmed because of the numerous depictions of Morgante that followed Bronzino's portrait. From Valerio Cioli's ca. 1565 *Morgante as Silenus* to Giovanni Stradano's series on the coronation of Cosimo from the 1540s (Fig. 3.7), and from Jean Boulogne's (1529–1608)—known as Giambologna—numerous bronze statuettes of Morgante blowing a cornetto (1570) (Fig. 3.8), or riding a barrel (before 1582) (Fig. 3.9), one can get a sense of Morgante's continued importance at the Medici court. Repeatedly, artists found the dwarf to be an inspiring sitter, one who allowed them to use *invenzione* and demonstrate their mastery of *imitare* via close *ritrarre*. For the production of *Morgante on a Dragon* (1582) (Fig. 3.10), Giambologna worked with the Granducal goldsmith Lorenzo della Nera to produce a model to be placed on a fountain.[123] *Morgante on a Barrel* is based on the model with a dragon, but *Morgante Blowing a Cornetto* is another original composition that has several variants. One of these shows Morgante standing up, his left hand resting on a cane-like rod and his right hand holding the cornetto to his mouth. The stance of the dwarf reminds the viewer of the front side of Bronzino's portrait, with similar body curvatures and overall shape.[124] This similarity underlines two significant

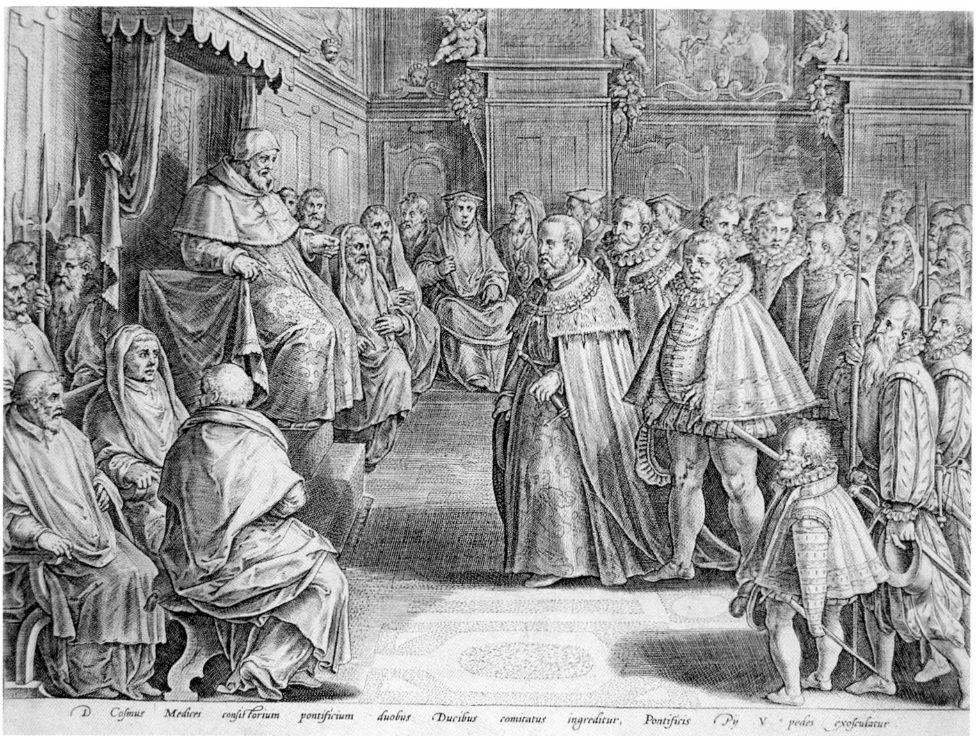

Figure 3.7. Giovanni Stradano, *The Papal Meeting of Cosimo I de'Medici* from the *Procession* series, 1540s, © The Trustees of The British Museum, London

points: first, Morgante's body remained a site of visual investigation for many years; second Bronzino's painting continued to generate subsequent artistic productions for a long time. Interestingly, James Holderbaum sees other similarities between Giambologna's statuette of Morgante on a dragon and Bronzino's painting. For Holderbaum, Giambologna also strove to depict accurate features, rejecting the slightly caricatural shape of the dwarf in Cioli's marble statue. Additionally, the twisted position of Morgante's body allows the observer many viewing angles that unfold as the gaze turns around the work, thus demonstrating the true ascendency of sculpture. In doing so, he imbued his statuette with aesthetics that combined natural reality with *disegno*.[125] For both Giambologna and Bronzino, Morgante became a distinctive locus for the exploration of truth in representation and for the articulation of a visual argument emanating from art theoretical discourse. Stradano also included Morgante as a prominent part of Cosimo's retinue, depicting him in the foreground of the composition in every panel. The dwarf is not an afterthought; he is an essential part of the regal procession and celebration of Cosimo's ruling glory. If Giambologna's statuettes, by virtue of their size and themes, did not directly point to the social and political importance of the dwarf, then there is at least no comical exaggeration in these three-dimensional representations. By investing an anatomically deformed individual with a narrative—the celebration accompanying Morgante's blowing a cornetto or his participation in a festive pouring of wine when he rides a barrel—the artists and patrons visually acknowledged that a dwarf might be more than a mere comical spectacle at court.

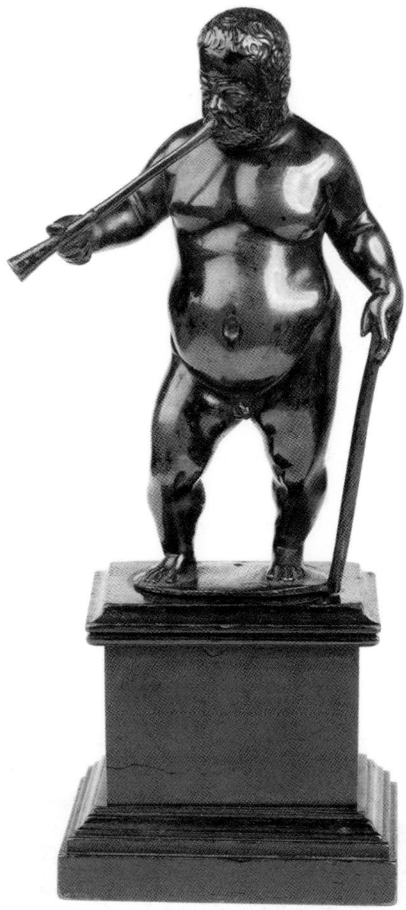

Figure 3.8. Giambologna, *Morgante Blowing a Cornetto*, ca. 1570, The Victoria and Albert Museum, London

An account published in 1762 gives a sense of how court rules operated in the sixteenth-century Medici court, which in turn allows for a better understanding of the social space that surrounded Morgante and determined the ways in which his portrayal

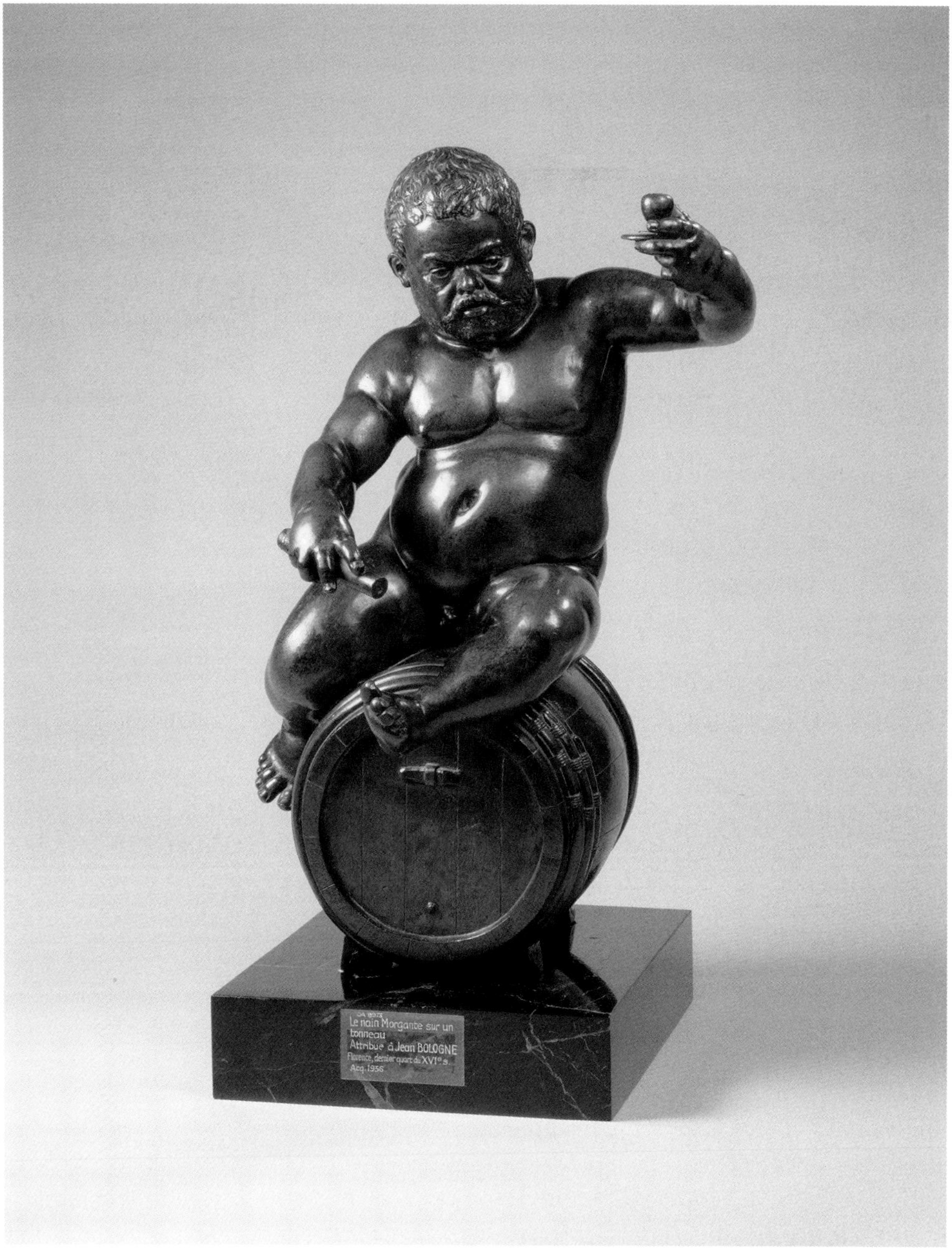

Figure 3.9. Giambologna, *Morgante on a Barrel*, ca. 1580, Musée du Louvre, Paris. RMN-Grand Palais/Art Resource, New York

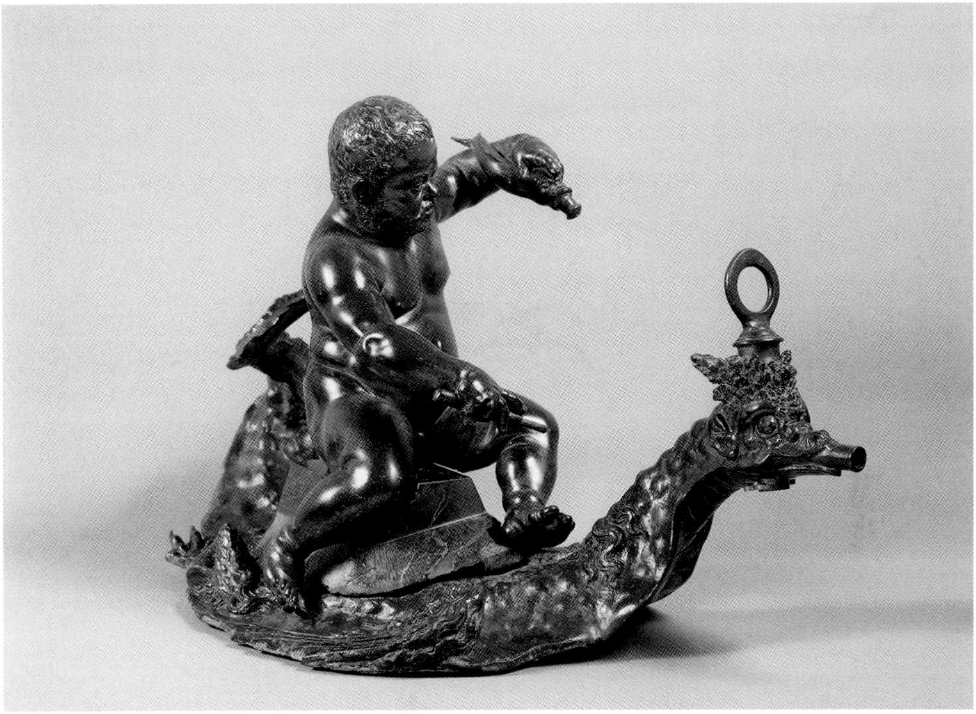

Figure 3.10. Giambologna, *Morgante on a Dragon*, 1582, Museo del Bargello, Florence. Scala/Art Resource, New York

could be deciphered. This account relates discussions that occurred between Giorgio Vasari and Francesco de'Medici (1541–1587) regarding the decorations of the Palazzo Vecchio and the image of the *Principe* that was intended to be communicated through these visual productions. Throughout the discussion, the two paid great attention to the visual details that would express the grandeur of the Medici duke within the confines of his public palazzo. In addition, the language used between Vasari and Francesco is colored with linguistic affects speaking to *civiltà*.[126] The self-constraint used by Vasari in rendering this dialogue echoes the distinctive pattern of highly controlled behavior inherent in the process of civilizing present at the Medici court.[127] Surpassing his status as an artist and becoming an intellectual *literato* at the court of Cosimo, Vasari's writings testify to the meticulous qualities necessary for a courtier's survival and success in sixteenth-century Florence.[128] His mastery of courtly behavior is exemplified by his choice of words and verbal description of the respect due to Francesco de'Medici. For instance, in Vasari's transcription of his discussion with Francesco de'Medici, most of his responses to the duke start with the acknowledgment of his title and with a sentence acknowledging the good judgment of Francesco.[129] Vasari used his skills as a courtier to promote his skills as an artist, just as, in a sense, he adapted his artistic prowess to fit the language of the Medici court.[130] It is these parameters that Bronzino as an artist and Morgante as a dwarf had to navigate in order to survive, socially and in actuality. Bronzino's portrait of the dwarf addressed not only the social position of the dwarf, but also the artist's fluency in the court's expectation and in current theoretical debates.

Finally, this fluency, and the place of *Morgante* in it, is best understood by seeing how Bronzino masterfully played with portraiture at the Medici court and how he created a successful representational vocabulary in Florence and beyond. The idealization of power represented within portraits of Medici rulers and their courtiers emphasized *ritrarre*, and used *imitare* just enough to make the ruler recognizable. Cosimo I, for instance, favored portraiture because he believed it helped him promote the Medici dynasty's superiority and establish a visual documentation of his rule.[131] As a commander in arms, he asked Bronzino to emphasize his consolidation of power over the Florentine territories and represent him in his armor in a painted portrait dated 1545 (Fig. 3.11). The visual connection made between the recognizable likeness of Cosimo I and his military costume legitimized the power of the Medici house. Similarly, Bronzino depicted Cosimo I's wife Eleonora di Toledo and their son Giovanni in his famed portrait of 1545 (Fig. 3.12).[132] As an official state portrait, this work stood as an exemplary image of Medici self-fashioning. Bronzino included numerous iconographical elements pointing to the regal position of Eleonora as the bearer of Medici sons. The elaborate details of her dress almost overshadow the likeness of her face, which is in fact overwhelmed by the overall emphasis on wealth and power—but her recognizability still remains necessary as a key element of her identity and statement of power.[133] In the same way, the courtier Luca Martini stands with a drawing of his engineering plan to drain malarial swamps on Cosimo I's territories, in a portrait Bronzino executed between 1551 and 1555 (Fig. 3.13). While an active patron of the arts and a highly visible courtier at the Medici court, Martini's identification occurs through his courtly pose and indication of expertise, as much as it does through the recognizability of his face.[134] Again, his character is conveyed through the idealization of his stance, accompanied by the mimetic emphasis on his features, which allowed viewers to identify the sitter. Even portraits of children fell within this discourse. Parental goals were to produce a good Christian and a good citizen out of a child; therefore, demonstrating the potential of the portrayed child to acquire language, reason, civility, and decorum was essential.[135] This project is visually achieved in portraits such as that of Don Garzia de'Medici, painted by Bronzino in 1550 (Fig. 3.14). Even though his facial features are similar to a later documented portrait, his identity is largely conveyed through the qualities possessed by a future responsible and civilized ruler. The elaborate red silk garment, the courtly pose, and the bare background project the image of a child infused with *gravitas* and a mirrored model of his courtier parents.[136] The qualities a future Medici courtier should possess are central to Bronzino's portrait; the actuality of the child's features come second to the construction of a visual vocabulary

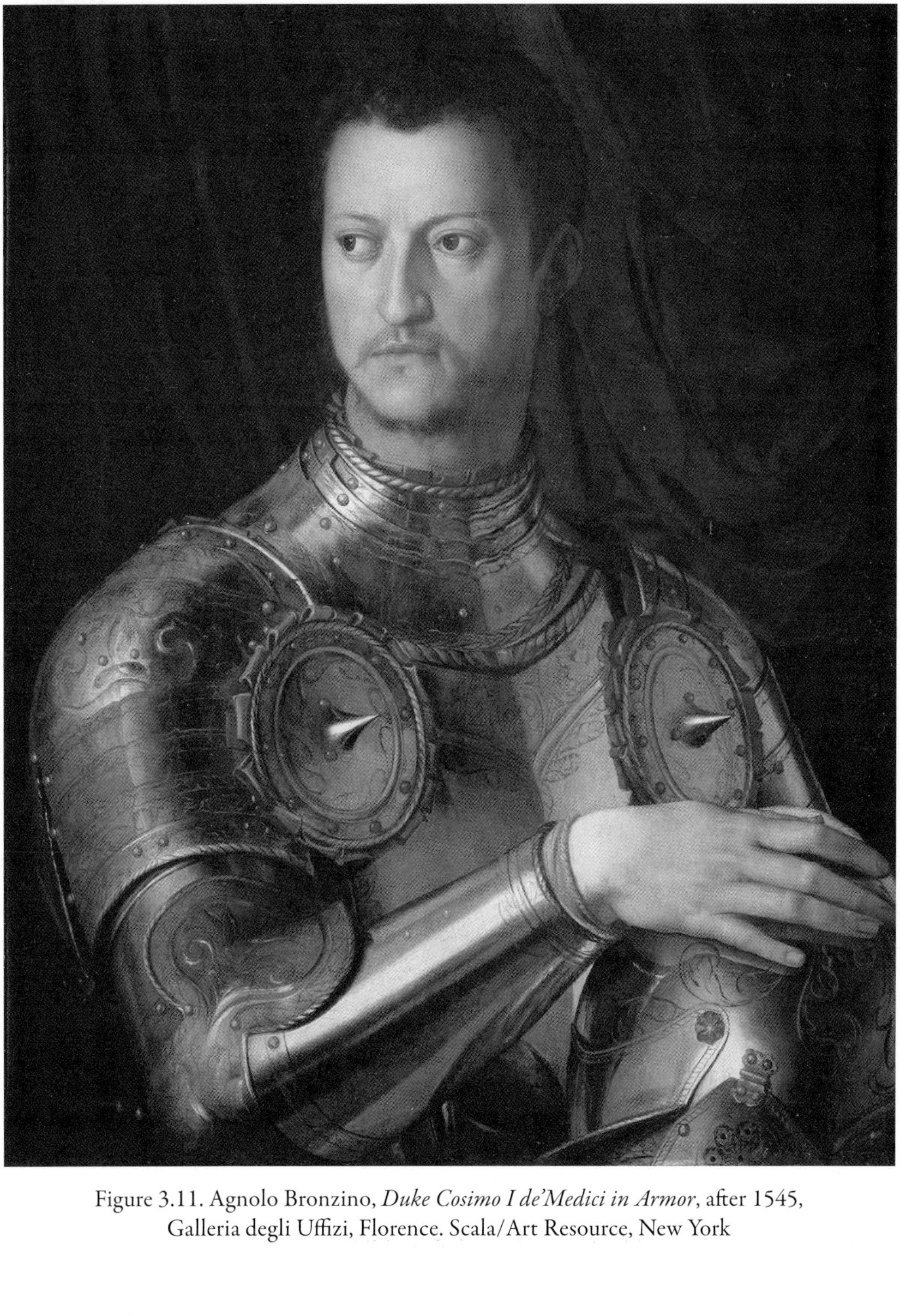

Figure 3.11. Agnolo Bronzino, *Duke Cosimo I de'Medici in Armor*, after 1545, Galleria degli Uffizi, Florence. Scala/Art Resource, New York

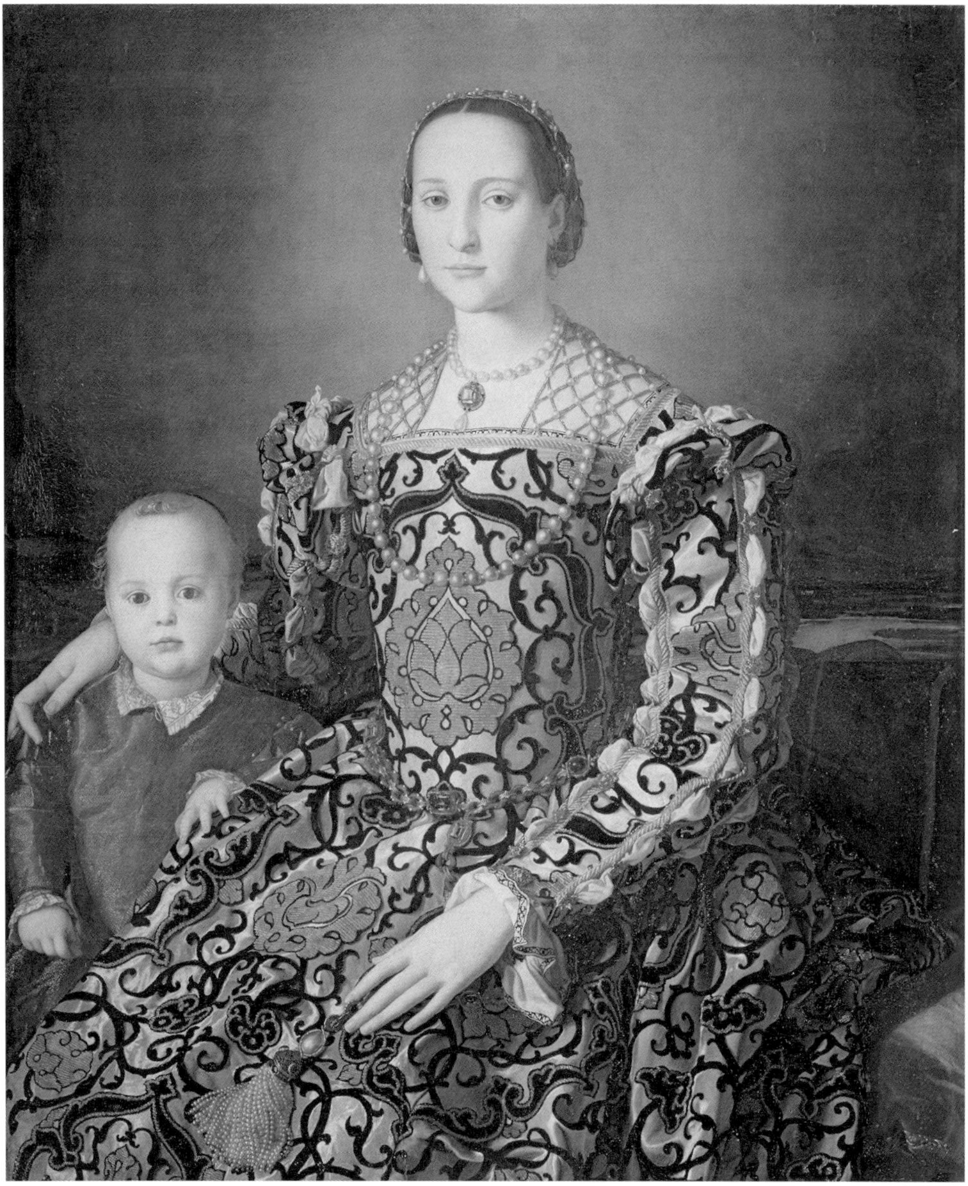

Figure 3.12. Agnolo Bronzino, *Eleonora di Toledo and Her Son Giovanni*, 1545, Galleria degli Uffizi, Florence. Scala/Art Resource, New York

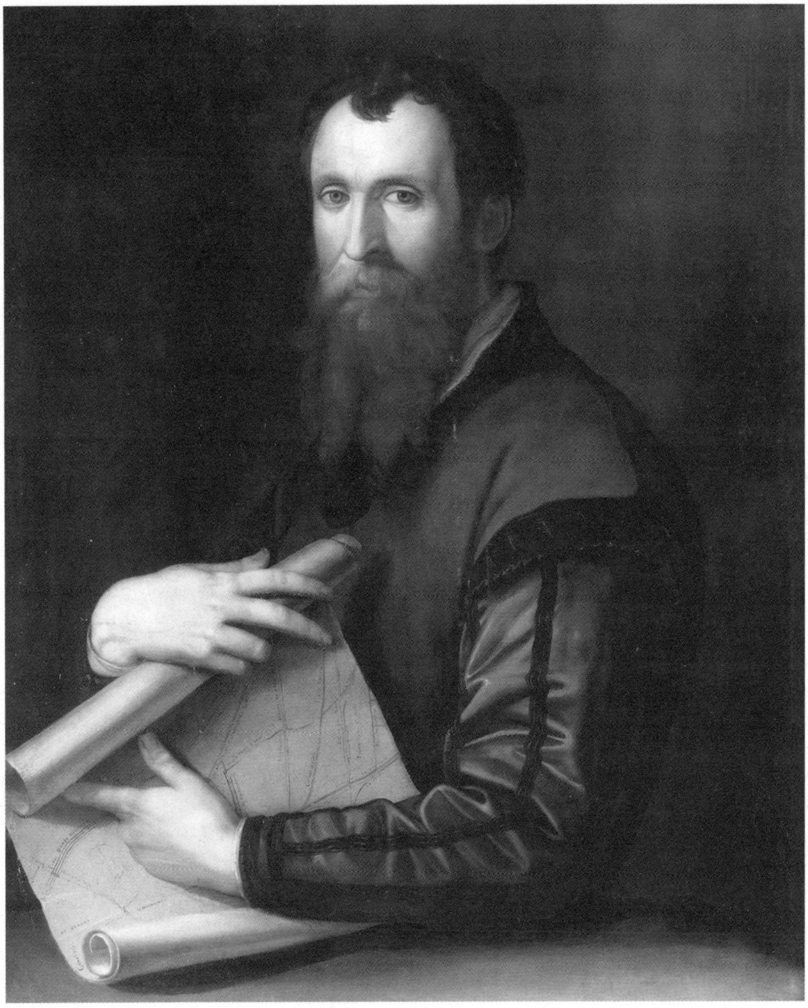

Figure 3.13. Agnolo Bronzino, *Luca Martini*, ca. 1551–55, Palazzo Pitti, Galleria Palatina, Florence

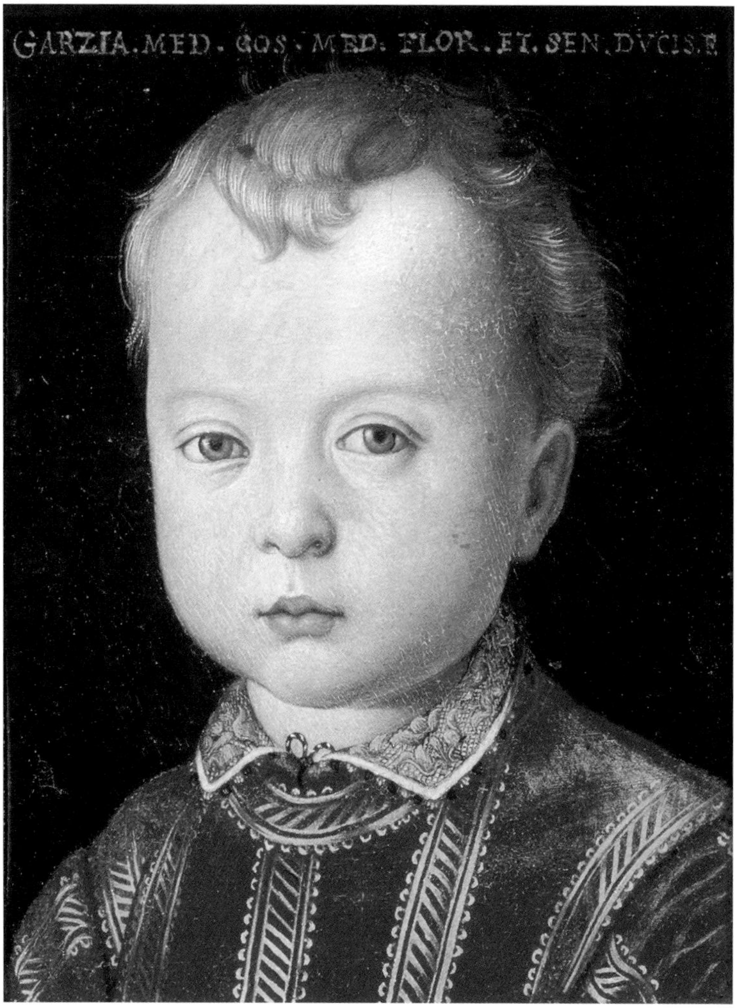

Figure 3.14. Agnolo Bronzino, *Don Garzia de'Medici*, 1550, Museo del Prado, Madrid

of Medici power. Bronzino's portrait of Morgante reversed the standard vocabulary of power and self-presentation by highlighting the dichotomy between mimesis and character. Dwarves enhanced the courtly masquerade by grotesquing it; yet, for their wit and jest to have legible currency, this mockery had to use common visual vocabulary. This vocabulary was—primarily—visible through their bodies, which their portraits emphasized. *Imitare* regained currency—in portraits similar to that of Morgante—as it was essential in making the portraits participate in an idealized court setting where visual compositions emphasized *ritrarre*.

As an ambiguous presence, dwarves allowed courtiers to find relief from their strictly ruled lives through a distorted mirror. The human qualities present in these deformed bodies, sometimes exaggerated in visual portrayals or grotesquely mocked in performances, allowed courts to reinforce strict behavioral standards on their normative subjects by providing them with an escape and a foil. Because dwarves like Morgante were an inherent part of Renaissance courts, one might therefore ask whether their presence at court was not, in fact, necessary because they helped define the very standards that they also lampooned. The presence of dwarves provided relief from strict court settings, because they were alter egos to courtiers. In some instances, however, dwarves achieved a surprisingly high degree of status. Morgante's portraits speak loudly to the position he occupied at court, but demonstrate even more obviously the human status he acquired during his stay with the Medici family. The role played by dwarves at court was particularly delicate, since their presence was not only due to their wondrous qualities as miniature versions of tall adults, but it was also dependent upon their roles as jesters of the court. This balance between the wondrous, comical, and human was a fragile one. This precarious social and legal equilibrium found resonance in their portraits, where comical components sometimes yielded to references to social prominence and legal independence. Bronzino's depiction of Morgante epitomizes the complex situation of successful dwarves at the Medici court. Initially Morgante was celebrated because of his comical deformities, yet like many other dwarves, he also transcended his droll attributes and actively engaged in quotidian court life. Bronzino made this dichotomy visually legible. The artist established his depiction on the reality of Morgante's body, but emphasized the actuality of the dwarf's life by pointing to a real event. The subsequent display of this double-sided canvas reinforced the importance of Morgante's presence at court. The written accounts, and economic and diplomatic details attached to Morgante and other dwarves at the Medicean court uphold this painting as a complex articulation of the position of dwarves at court. As an animate sign of difference, Morgante allowed for the rigid norms of courts to exist.

Notes

[1] Cosimo Conti, *La prima reggia di Cosimo I de'Medici nel Palazzo già della Signoria di Firenze* (Florence: Giuseppe Pellas, Editore, 1893), 96.

[2] Sefy Hendler, entry for Bronzino's *Morgante* in *Bronzino: Artist and Poet at the Court of the Medici*, ed. Cristina Acidini, Carlo Falciani, and Antonio Natali (Florence: Mandragora, 2010), 217. Hendler states that the owl "resembles a little owl (*Athene noctua*), but in terms of size it is reminiscent of a long-eared owl (*Asio otus*)."

[3] Sefy Hendler, among other wonderful statements about this painting, has identified the birds. They are: common chaffinch (*Fringilla coelebs*), European robin (*Erithacus rubecula*), house

sparrow (*Passer domesticus*), and maybe a Cretzschmar's bunting (*Emberiza caesia*) or an Ortolan bunting (*Emberiza hortulana*). Sefy Hendler, *Gracious and Beautiful Monster: The Literary Universe of Bronzino's Nano Morgante* (Florence: Maschietto Editore, 2016), 55.

[4] See for example Edi Baccheschi, *L'opera completa del Bronzino* (Milan: Rizzoli Editore, 1973), 109: "La tela è dipinta sui due lati; sul recto, il *Nano Morgante come Bacco*; sul verso, il *Nano Morgante con gufo su una spalla*."

[5] Lisa Goldenberg was generous with her time and with her knowledge. She discussed many inventories and administration details with me. The idea that the *Morgante* may have been moved to Poggio Imperiale and the minutiae about Maria-Maddalena were inferred thanks to her help.

[6] Beyond visual representations, epistolary correspondence in particular attests to the desire that many courtiers had in possessing dwarves as objects generating wonder. One early example is found in the writing of the English chronicler Matthew Paris who writes about a man of very short stature he found in the Isle of Wight in 1249: "he was hardly three feet tall but had ceased to grow. The queen ordered him to be taken around with her as a freak of nature to arouse astonishment of onlookers. The length of his tiny body is sixteen times that of this line." Reference taken from Lorraine Daston and Katharine Park, *Wonders and the Order of Nature 1150–1750* (New York: Zone Books, 1998), 190 citing Matthew Paris, *The Illustrated Chronicles of Matthew Paris: Observations of Thirteenth-century Life*, trans. Richard Vaughan (Cambridge: Corpus Christi College/Alan Sutton, 1993), 113.

[7] Deborah Parker, *Bronzino: Renaissance Painter as Poet* (Cambridge: Cambridge University Press, 2000), 9.

[8] See for instance Baccheschi, *L'opera completa del Bronzino*, entry 163; Andrea Emiliani, *Il Bronzino* (Busto Arsizio: Bramante Editrice, 1960), 83; and Marco Collaretta in *Palazzo Vecchio: Committenza e collezionismo medicei 1537–1610* (Florence: Electa Editrice, 1980), entry 517. For the 1587 inventory, Archivio di Stato di Firenze (ASF), Guardaroba 126, 38r: "Un quadro in tela con ornamento di noce ritrattovi Morgantaccio nudo con gufo in mano Doppio detto quadro che di dietro mostra la schiena."

[9] Parker, *Bronzino*, 15; James Holderbaum, "A Bronze by Giovanni Bologna and a Painting by Bronzino," *The Burlington Magazine* 98 (December 1956): 442; and Leatrice Mendelsohn, *Paragoni: Benedetto Varchi's "Due Lezzioni" and Cinquecento Art Theory* (Ann Arbor: UMI Press, 1982), 150.

[10] Parker, *Bronzino*, 155 and Holderbaum, "A Bronze," 442. Also, see the detailed discussion on Bronzino's academic dialogue and its significance for the *Morgante* portrait elaborated further in this chapter.

[11] Lorne Campbell, *Renaissance Portraits: European Portrait-Painting in the 14th, 15th, and 16th Centuries* (New Haven and London: Yale University Press, 1990), 145.

[12] Paul Barolsky, *Infinite Jest: Wit and Humor in Italian Renaissance Art* (Columbia and London: University of Missouri Press, 1978) and for Morgante 145 in particular: "Bronzino's work [*Morgante*] demonstrates again how the highly mannered society of the court appreciated this kind of vulgar comedy."

[13] E. Tietze-Conrat, *Dwarfs and Jesters in Art* (New York: Garden City Books, 1957); Giuseppe Bertini, "Johann Gersmueter's Portrait of a Dwarf of the Farnese Court," *Burlington Magazine* 134, no. 1068 (1992): 179; Robin Leigh O'Bryan, *The Dwarf in Italian Renaissance Iconography*, unpublished thesis (San Diego State University, 1991); Robin Leigh O'Bryan, *The Grotesque in Medici Taste and Patronage*, unpublished dissertation (University of Virginia, 2000).

[14] Detlef Heikamp. "Il Nano Morgante: Tentativo di un ritratto," in *Giambologna: Gli dei, gli eroi*, ed. Beatrice Paolozzi Strozzi and Dimitrios Zikos (Florence and Milan: Giunti, 2006), 290, footnote 14.

The 1544 reference is written by Lorenzo Pagni, a ubiquitous Medici secretary during the ducal reign of Cosimo, and is found in ASF, Mediceo del Principato (MP) 1171, 3, 147: "Il Duca [...] questa sera è stato nel giardino più d'un'hora, dove il Nano, avendo teso i panionj a quelli bossi del laberinto [labirinto] di fuora, et havendo messoli appresso la sua civetta ha preso sei o otto uccellinj con gran piacere di [...]."

[15] Ettore Allegri and Alessandro Cecchi, *Palazzo Vecchio e i Medici: Guida storica* (Florence: Studio per edizioni scelte, 1980), 146, note 4.

[16] Indeed, it was a recognized and accepted fact that the *signore* of the house would be accompanied by his dwarf almost incessantly. See Tommaso Garzoni, *La piazza universale de tutte le professioni del mondo*, ed. Paolo Cherchi and Beatrice Collina (Torino: Einaudi, 1996), 2:1306: "A questi [buffoni] oggidí si porta ogni rispetto, perché stanno all'orecchia de'signori, scalzano Sua Eccellenza caminan seco in carrozza, gli vanno dietro in compagnia, sempre gli sono alla coda, mai si parton da suo conspetto, e fanno insieme con esso una compita relatione, perché non si trova il signor senza buffone, né il buffon senza il signore."

[17] Antonfrancesco Grazzini, *Le rime burlesche, edite e inedite, di Antonfrancesco Grazzini, dette Il Lasca*, ed. Carlo Verzone (Florence: Sansoni, 1882), 317–19. The poem is titled *In morte di Morgante nano*. For a detailed annotation, please see Giuseppe Crimi and Cristiano Spila, eds., *Nanerie del Rinascimento: "La Nanea" di Michelangelo Serafini e altri versi di corte e d'accademia* (Rome: Vecchiarelli Editore, 2006), 60–66.

[18] Achondroplasia and its medical attributes are developed later in this chapter.

[19] Giorgio Vasari, *Lives of the Painters, Sculptors, and Architects*, trans. Gaston du C. de Vere (New York and Toronto: Alfred A. Knopf, 1996), 2:873.

[20] Ibid., 2:895.

[21] ASF, Pratica Segreta 186, ca. 126v, *Cosmus Medicus Dei gratia Florentie dux*. Translated: "To Morgante, the dwarf of our ducal palace and our most beloved servitor, known as Braccio di Bartolo, from Poggio Fornione and from the state of the most noble lore Cesare Alidosi, the lord of the castle known as the Castel del Rio, I wish good health and every good thing." I am grateful to Joel Relihan for his translation.

[22] This classification of dwarves is taken from Joy Kenseth, *The Age of the Marvelous* (Hanover: Hood Museum of Art, Dartmouth, 1991), 33: "Europeans most often considered natural wonders as examples of God's ingenuity; less frequently they described them as cases of 'nature errings.' A great many animal, botanical, and geological specimens were regarded as marvels, but normally the term was applied when the object was unusually large or small, extremely rare, exotic, abnormally or grotesquely shaped, or spectacularly beautiful. [...] No less fascinating to the European mind were the human prodigies: dwarves, freaks, and other human anomalies often became the subject of art and poetry and were discussed at length in natural histories. Although sometimes viewed as nature's 'mistakes,' they were most often regarded, like geniuses, as God's marvelous work and the products of his divine wisdom."

[23] I am grateful to Robert G. La France for identifying the butterfly as a southern swallowtail (*Papilio Alexanor*) and to Areli Marina for relating his expertise to me.

[24] Theophrasti Bombast ab Honenheim dicti Paracelsus, "Liber de nymphis, sylphis, pygameis et salamandris et de ceteris spiritibus," in *Operum medico-chimicorum*, 9 (Frankfurt, 1605), 54–55,

cited in Roberto Zapperi, "Arrigo le Velu, Pietro le Fou, Amon le Nain et autres bêtes: Autour d'un tableau d'Agostino Carrache," *Annales: Économies – Sociétés – Civilisations* 40, no. 2 (March–April 1985): 314 and 325, footnote 26.

25 Véronique Dasen, *Dwarfs in Ancient Egypt and Greece* (Oxford: Clarendon Press, 1993), 107.

26 Norbert Schneider, *L'art du portrait: Les plus grandes oeuvres européennes 1420–1670* (Cologne: Benedikt Taschen, 1994), 167: "Les nains étaient recherchés par les cours royales et princières comme raretés et curiosités dans toute l'Europe; ils étaient achetés, vêtus de tissues précieux, parés d'or et de bijoux et exhibés à l'occasion de représentations ou de fêtes. Ils étaient souvent offerts comme surprise ou cadeaux. Même les dignitaires de l'Eglise se conformaient à cette mode."

27 ASF, MP 5928, 106, February 2, 1581: "Finalmente hò trovato una nana, la qual di già hò qui in Varsovia, et è cosi ben proportionate che ui veramente levata questa della Regina, no hò mai veduta la più bella; ma perché i freddi sono grandi in queste parti, et non piccioli ancora per tutta la Germania, sono consigliato à non metterla al pericolo del viaggio per hora, ma aspettare à prima neva. Frà tanto la Ser.ma Regina mi fa gratia di tenersela in Corte perche impari creanze et le ho data per maestre qull'altra sua Nanina tanto gratiosa come scrissi et della quale sperano haver la sorella, ma detta sua sorella no è riuscita come si pensava [...]"; folio 187, February 15, 1581: "Per occasione che mi si porse ditrovarmi a giorni passati in corte delle Ser.ma Regina mia, Mons. Bolognetti Vescovo di Massa Nontio di S. S.t: che quivi hora si trova, mi diede a cura di condurre meco una Nana per servitio della H.V. Ser.ma er mandarla a Vienna al M.re Ambasciatore del Ser.mo Gran Duca Consorte di vra Ser.ta: Il che havendo messo mi opera hoggi che e il terzo giorno del mio arrivo a corte, la mando al s. Amb.re per on Gentilhuomo Polaco nomato S.re Giovanni Kobilmiczhi, et mi [...] lingua Cobilnisczi, Il quale mettendo a viaggio in carozza, mi credo che la fancuilla si condurra comodamente, havendola lo massime al gentilhuomo molto raccomandata, et provisi di qual cre suo bisogno per difenderla dal freddo, la puttina si domanda soffia, la quale se bene di et tenera, no dimeno, nel aspetto et ne gesti, e, assai ben grave et per 9 giorni che stata tra mi viaggio e mi casa meco mi pare che sia timorosa, obbediente, et assai ragionevol gra onde piaccia a Dio di condurla a salvamento credo fede che con il tempo la Al.za Ser.ma: ne cavera servition e trastullo, io ho reputato aspetti di mia grandissima fortuna quelta piccola occasione di potermi gratificare l'Altezza vra Ser.ma: Tuttavia se mi negotio di maggiore importanza per servitio di Vra. A. Ser.ma Io p [...]"; MP 5929, 179, August 6, 1581: "Per l'Antico mio desiderio et per l'obligo particularissimo, c'ho di servire a V.A. Ser.ma, non mancai sub. ch'io giunti in Cracovia di mettermi in prattica per trovar qualche nana degna di comparire [...] a lei. Ma'in effetto da tutti quei ss. Canonici et varÿ altri gentilhuomini et mercanti mi fù detto risolutamente ch'io non ne troverei se non in Lituania. Di più anco [...] ch'io havevo in questo negotio di gran concorrenti, cioè i ss. Principi [...] i quali per quanto mi fù referto ne facevano cercare con molta diligenza in tutte quelle parti, dove sono potentissimi. Da Cracovia poi io sono venuto quà in Varsovia dove da trè Nane in poi, che ha La ser.ma Regina, due sgarbatissime et una veramenti bel [hole in letter for word following "bel"] non se ne trova alcun altra affatto"; folio 553, December 15, 1581: "Con tutto che poi non m'occorresse andar in Lithuania, ne sia forse per occorrermi cosi presto aspettandosi qua il Re fra pochi giorni non ho pero mancato ne manco di procurer la Nana con ogni diligenza anzi n'hebbi ai giorni passati quasi firma promesse da una di questi Matroni della Ser.ma Regina la quale mi dava anco intentione che mi sarebbe condotta molto presto. Onde scrissi

al S.ore Giovanni Alberti conforme all'ordine di V.A. Ser.ma chi mi avisasse a chi potruo farla consignare in Vienna sperand'io trovar commodita di mandarla sin là dove sarà à mezza strada. Tuttavia non mi è stata mandata ancora et questa Sig.ra si scusa con la difficultà dicendo che si bene in questa parti nascono alle volti simili animali, si dura però fatica a trovarre [...] et di comparir inanzi à Prencipi grandi. Et dire, che stà in prattica d'havere una sorella d'una Nanina che hà qui la Ser.ma Regina la più bella cosuccia, la più savia, la più gratiosa, la più discreta, che si possa imaginare. Chi la guarda senza saper altro, la repute une puttina di cinqu'anni onde in vederla poi caminare, parlare, et leggere, et stare in Chiesa, come stà con tanta devotione resta stupido. Questo hò voluto dire per la speranza ch'io ho della buona riuscita di questa sua sorella Nana ancor essa et molto picciola (come mi vien detto) per la felicità di quella madre. Ondi non manco di sollecitar per havenda in tutti modi. Conchi fo fine inchinandomi humilissimamenti a V.A. Ser.ma [...]."

28 Russia entered Moscovy in 1581.

29 ASF, MP 2955, May 31, 1618, at the bottom of the letter: "Alla quale do nuova che hier sera harivorno li nani, et io lo chiari Morgante, et di nuovo fo humilissima reverenza a V.A.S [...]."

30 Because this letter dates from 1621, it is evident that the Morgante mentioned here is different from the subject painted by Bronzino.

31 ASF, MP 2952, Carteggio. Letteri della Duchessa di Mantova, September 8, 1621: "Ritorna Morgante a servir V.A. Io l'ho trattenuto qui alcuni giorni pensando di valermene oer inviarle alcune cose, ma perchè non mi sono assicurata che fossero ben condotte me le sono ritenute per miglior occasione, et intanto ho voluto far fede a V.A. [...] affunchè presso di lei resti scusato [...]."

32 Archivio di Stato di Mantova (ASMn), Archivio Gonzaga (AG) 1513, 380–81v. I am greatly indebted to Molly Bourne for these documents. Part of the letter reads: "è un altro Morgantino [...] ben proportionato, legge libri francesi e spagnuoli [...]."

33 The original Italian letter, as well as its translation, were generously given to me by Deanna Shemek. The letter, dated September 11, 1532 is written by Isabella d'Este to Diana d'Este. The original Italian reads: "Io primisi gia quatro anni sono a madama illustrissima Renata di voler dar a sua excellentia el primo fruto che usise della raza delli mei nanini, dico de femina. Et come vostra Signoria sa hormaii sono dui ani che naque una putina. La qualle anchora non dia speranza di dover restare in tutto cossi piccola come è la mia Dellia, non dimeno senza alcun dubbio rimanerà nana. Et per la belleza sua meritarà di esser tenuta cara."

34 ASF, MP 1171, 338, April 18, 1545: "Anchora le calze, giubone, saione e stringhi si detono al nano, el quale ne molto alegrò [...] La S.ra duc.a mia S.ra [Eleonora di Toledo] m'à comandato che io hordinj in Pisa [...]"; MP 1170, 262, June 10, 1543, Lorenzo Pagni to Pier Francesco Riccio: "Dice la S.ra mia Duchessa che la S.V. facci fare dua giubbonj di seta Bianca et dua para di calze bianche per Lodovico et Filippino nanj et che le mandi quanto prima può [...]"; MP 1173, 204, June 6, 1547: "nostra Signora Duchessa m'ha comandato che io scriva a V.S. che quella facci rivestire Gianmaria nano et che vengha le forme che sono in chamera del'Anna [...]."

35 ASF, MP 1, insert within folio 4, no dates, though the Medici Archives Project dates it around March 9, 1543, not signed: "Al nano se tagliato i vestimenti di cuoio [...]."

36 ASF, MP 1170a, 68, August 16, 154: "E' bisognia che la S.V. ci facci mandare 8 braccia di nastro di seta nera per la choda della S.ra Giulia e che ci sia domanj così da fare dua o 3 chamicie per Filippino [...]."

37 ASF, MP 225, 24, December 14, 1565: "et a pagare a più monasteri et ricamatori per I racmi della livrea del vestire et per il vestire di Gradasso et oro di canutiglio et parte di fattura di sue sarti [...]."

[38] Hence the inclusion of court dwarves in lists that request clothing for court personnel such as court pages, footmen, coach-drivers, and courtiers. See ASF, MP 1175, 44, December 4, 1549: "Nani: Gradasso, Morgante, Filippino, Fattapio, Atalante, Don Grillino, Gianmaria, Fiorentino della lettigha, Santone della lettigha [...]."

[39] This information was relayed in a personal conversation with Guido Guerzoni who kindly discussed his unpublished research on the differences between pages and court dwarves, October 2004.

[40] Ed Goldberg relayed these thoughts in a personal conversation in May 2006, as we were conversing about the diverse positions held by dwarves in the Medici environment.

[41] Garzoni, *La piazza universale*, 2:1306.

[42] Guardaroba Medicea, Inventari generale, 132, dated 1587–91, 124.

[43] Bibliothèque nationale de France (BNF), Garde Robe (GR), Manuscrit français (MF) 2952 (215), n.a. 9189, dated 1530, 15v.

[44] BNF, GR, MF 2952 (215), n.a. 9189 continues with dates every year, and Jehan de Nano is found on pages 25v, 51r, 65r ....

[45] BNF, GR, MF 2952 (215), n.a. 9189, 221r.

[46] While the child-size garments may have been part of a dowry inciting the future queen of France to produce heirs, the above-stated "inventaires" do not mention anything related to a dowry and the rest of the possessions listed do not relate to properties commonly given as a dowry. I am very grateful to Jacqueline Musacchio for discussing this note with me. Additionally, I am indebted to Sheila ffolliott who mentioned the possibility that these garments may in fact be for dolls, which served as models meant to allow courtiers to familiarize themselves with foreign dress. This idea would indeed make sense for the impending move of this Italian Medici woman to France. See Yassana C. Croizat, "'Living Dolls': François Ier Dresses His Women," *Renaissance Quarterly* 60, no.1 (Spring 2007): 94–130.

[47] BNF, Nouvelles Acquisitions (NA), MF 1049.

[48] BNF, NA, MF 1049, 30r.

[49] BNF, NA, MF 1049, 29v.

[50] For a full discussion on the relationships between possessing, knowing, and socially defining oneself, see Paula Findlen, *Possessing Nature: Museums, Collecting, and Scientific Culture in Early Modern Italy* (Berkeley, Los Angeles and London: University of California Press, 1994), 17–36, in particular. The possession of knowledge in the particular case of a court dwarf leads to an interesting idea regarding the statement latently made by a patron being surrounded by dwarves; indeed, dwarves' most visible power was their appearance. While the Spanish court did attribute specific supernatural powers to dwarves, this chapter intentionally chooses to omit a courtly setting that was completely different in its practice than the ones discussed here.

[51] Nicholas Mann and Luke Syson, *The Image of the Individual: Portrait in the Renaissance* (London: British Museum Press, 1998), 67.

[52] Though we should note that the reasons for Leonardo's version of the *paragone* were different than the ones debated during Bronzino's time. Indeed, "the *paragone* in Leonardo's time served a legitimate function as a vehicle for expressing the artist's struggle for higher status. In the 1540s, however, the period of the debate's greatest popularity, the artist's desire for recognition as more than a mere craftsman, while still an issue was no longer the only issue." Mendelsohn, *Paragoni*, 38.

[53] Carl Goldstein, *Teaching Art: Academies and Schools from Vasari to Albers* (Cambridge: Cambridge University Press, 1996), 225.

[54] Karen-edis Barzman, *The Florentine Academy and the Early Modern State: The Discipline of Disegno* (Cambridge: Cambridge University Press, 2000), 30.

[55] Ibid.: "Vasari's invocation of the *Accademia Fiorentina* suggests that *disegno* was to serve as an artistic analogue to the Tuscan vernacular in Medici cultural politics. An important difference was that the *Accademia del Disegno* would not promote a vernacular style or a particular artistic dialect so much as a local form of practice—that is a theoretical discourse, a method of learning, and procedures of production associated with the local schools of art, in particular, with Michelangelo."

[56] For the formation of Bronzino in the literary and visual arts and the development of Florentine academies, please see Maurice Brock, *Bronzino* (Paris: Flammarion, 2002), 7–17 in particular and Mendelsohn, *Paragoni*, 17–27.

[57] Mendelsohn, *Paragoni*, 30.

[58] Parker, *Bronzino*, 15, and Holderbaum, "A Bronze," 442.

[59] Mendelsohn, *Paragoni*, 150: "[Bronzino] begins by listing the arguments (seven in all) in favor of sculpture, but he never finishes the letter, leaving the painter's, and presumably his own point of view incomplete. Our understanding of his theoretical attitude must rest entirely on the grounds of his discussion of sculpture. After assessing the sculptor's claim to presenting an infinite number of views, Bronzino presents the painter from the *sculptor's* point of view, stressing the advantage of sculpture: 'the painter ... in each figure never offers more than one view, which he selects according to his style, Since it is sufficient if the side he exhibits has grace [abbia grazia], he does not care what it would look like from the sides which are not visible. For this reason as well, sculpture would be more difficult ... And continuing this line of reasoning, they [sculptors] say that it is far more beautiful and pleasing to find in one particular figure all the physical attributes of a man, a woman or an animal, such as the face, the chest, and the other parts, and, turning around, to discover the side and the arm and what joins them, and then from the back [to see] the spine and how the front parts correspond to those of the side and the rear and to appreciate the many beautiful relationships. Finally, moving around a statue, to be totally satisfied with seeing it as a whole.'"

[60] Ibid., 151: "Front and rear views of the figure of the dwarf Morgante, similar to one executed in bronze by Valerio Cioli, were painted on reverse side of a canvas. The object was to prove that in two painted views the beholder could see all those aspects visible to him when viewing the bronze in-the-round. Rather than simple frontal or rear views, the two poses represented are angled slightly so that aspects of the sides as well as the front and back of the figures are actually visible in both painted 'halves.'"

[61] Parker, *Bronzino*, 155.

[62] Holderbaum, "A Bronze," 442.

[63] Hendler, *Bronzino*, 217. He states that Bronzino moves "beyond the third dimension, the exclusive domain of sculpture, to place his Morgante in the fourth one: time."

[64] Conti, *La prima reggia*, 96.

[65] I am greatly indebted to Diane Kunzelman who was at the head of the restoration project of Bronzino's *Morgante*, held in the Fortezza da Basso between 1987 and 2010. Dr. Kunzelman took the time to explain to me the numerous non-invasive (IR, UV, X-ray) studies that had been done on the *Morgante* over the years, and what these studies revealed about the portrait, including the under-drawing, the fragility of the single canvas, and Bronzino's compositional process.

[66] Allegri, *Palazzo Vecchio e i Medici*, 146, note 4.

[67] The painting of this episode was suggested to Vasari by Bartoli in a letter written to him in 1556. See Karl Frey, *Der literarische Nachglass Giorgio Vasaris* (Munich: Müller, 1923–30), 1:CCXXXIV, 439.

[68] Vasari, *Lives*, 2:873.

[69] Guardaroba Medicea 18, Giornale di entrata e uscita, dates: 10 April 1549 until 18 February 1553. Throughout the *giornale* mentions are made of payments made from Cosimo to Bronzino, but not one of these records indicate that these payments were made for the *Morgante*.

[70] Barzman, *The Florentine Academy*, 30. Bronzino's annual stipend was of 150 scudi, which allowed the duke to "call upon him freely for his services."

[71] Campbell, *Renaissance Portraits*, 145: "Cosimo I, Grand Duke of Tuscany, commissioned Bronzino to paint two nude, full-length portraits of his dwarf Morgante, who presumably had to sit for them. Bronzino's canvases, framed back to back, remained in the Medici collection."

[72] Robert B. Simon, "Bronzino's 'Cosimo I de'Medici as Orpheus,'" *Philadelphia Museum of Art Bulletin* 81, no. 348 (Autumn 1985): 20.

[73] Maurice Brock notes that, while only one canine head is painted, Cerberus is identifiable as the three-headed guardian of Hades because of the initial three heads visible in Bronzino's original painting thanks to laboratory analyses. See M. Tucker, "Discoveries Made during the Treatment of Bronzino's *Cosimo I de'Medici as Orpheus*," *Philadelphia Museum of Art Bulletin* 81, no. 348 (Autumn 1985): 28–32, as cited in Brock, *Bronzino*, 171.

[74] Brock, *Bronzino*, 172–74.

[75] For a fascinating reading of Morgante's *panione*, sexual connotations, and literary ties, please see Hendler, *Gracious*, 53.

[76] Campbell looks at Vasari's description of Bronzino's work to deduce that Cosimo did indeed commission his court painter for the portrait. See Vasari, *Lives*, 2:873: "Bronzino then made for Duke Cosimo a full-length portrait of the dwarf Morgante, nude, and in two ways—namely, on one side of the picture the front, and on the other the back, with the bizarre and monstrous members which that dwarf has; which picture, of its kind, is beautiful and marvelous."

[77] Deborah Parker also supports this claim, but she does so verbally through Bronzino's own poems, rather than through his visual productions alone. See Barolsky, *Infinite Jest*,145: "Bronzino's work [*Morgante*] demonstrates again how the highly mannered society of the court appreciated this kind of vulgar comedy."

[78] Tietze-Conrat, *Dwarfs and Jesters*, 90. Tietze-Conrat clearly states that Bronzino had a particular anatomical interest for these *mostri* and that he used an allegory as a pretext to cover his life-study. Unfortunately, she presents no evidence for this assertion.

[79] ASF, MP 5928, 106, February 2, 1581: "le fare ragionare, cantare et far de loro mille prove."

[80] ASF, MP 1171, 2, 62, June 29, 1544: "[...] Hebbe un poco d'intertenimento d'una battaglia che fu fatta tre [tra] il Nano et una scimia che ha il Proveditore di qui molto brava, nella quale detto Nano rimase con due ferite, una nella spalla et l'altra nel braccio, et la scimia stroppiata nelle gambe, la quale s'arrese, domandando al Nano la vita per merzede, benchè lui non intendendo il linguaggio suo, havendola presa per le gambe di dietro, attendeva abbacchiarla del capo in terra. E se non che 'l duca mio s.re vi s'interpose, el Nano la finiva d'ammazzare. Detto Nano combattè ignudo, et non haveva altr'arme che un paro di brache che gli coprivano le vergogne. Basta che lui è restato vincitore, et ha guadagnato [scudi] X d'oro, per i quali ha impegno l'anello del Vescovo di Furlì [...]."

[81] Daston and Park, *Wonders*, 105. A discussion of gender and its impact on the lives and perception of dwarves is an important project, but one beyond the scope of the present chapter.

[82] I am referring particularly to the series of engravings done by Jacques Callot in 1616 of the Gobbi dwarves. See Daniel Ternois, *Jacques Callot: Catalogue complet de son oeuvre dessinée* (Paris: F. de Nobele, 1962); Olaf Schmidt, *"Callots fantastisch karikierte Blätter": Intermediale Inszenierungen und romantische Kunsttheorie im Werk E.T.A. Hoffmanns* (Berlin: Erich Schmidt, 2003); and Sarah B. Kirke and Britt Salvesen, *The Incisive Imagination: Jacques Callot and His Contemporaries* (Milwaukee: Milwaukee Art Museum, 2004).

[83] I am indebted to Tripp Evans for this reference. Jessica Kerwin Jenkins, *Encyclopedia of the Exquisite: An Anecdotal History of Elegant Delights* (New York: Doubleday, 2010), 201.

[84] Zapperi, "Arrigo le Velu," 309.

[85] Stato della casa dell'ill. mo sig. cardinale Farnese di felice memoria per tutto il 10 d'aprile 1589, in Archivio di Stato di Napoli, Archivio Farnesiano, 1849, as cited in Zapperi, "Arrigo le Velu," 308.

[86] Zapperi, "Arrigo le Velu," 320–21 in particular.

[87] For a further discussion of this painting and its relevance for the central character—the hirsute man Enrico, son of Petrus Gonsalvus—of the composition, please see chapter 4.

[88] Cesare Ripa, *Baroque and Rococo Pictorial Imagery: The 1758–60 Hertel Edition*, ed. Edward A. Maser (New York: Dover Publications, 1971).

[89] ASF, MP 1171, 3, 147: "Il Duca [...] questa sera è stato nel giardino più d'un'hora, dove il Nano, avendo teso i panionj a quelli bossi del laberinto [labirinto] di fuora, et havendo messoli appresso la sua civetta ha preso sei o otto uccellinj con gran piacere di [...]."

[90] Again, I am grateful to Diane Kunzelman for explaining the shape and the function of these specific rods to me.

[91] Parker, *Bronzino*, 155: "The owl is among the most common euphemisms in burlesque poetry for the phallus of a sodomite—and a term that appears frequently in Bronzino's *capitoli*. The owl in the painting may therefore express one of the painter's most outlandish puns—suggesting either that not all Morgante's appendages are small or that the dwarf is a sodomite." Though a very interesting reading of this painting could be done through Renaissance queer theories, it is beyond the scope of this chapter. For more details, see James M. Saslow, *Ganymede in the Renaissance: Homosexuality in Art and Society* (New Haven and London: Yale University Press, 1986) and Michael Rocke, *Forbidden Friendships: Homosexuality and Male Culture in Renaissance Florence* (New York: Oxford University Press, 1996).

[92] Pierre Launois, "Esquisse iconographique sur quelques nains," *Nouvelle iconographie de la Salpêtrière* 24, no. 1 (1911): 117.

[93] Hendler, *Bronzino*, 217.

[94] I am again indebted to Robert G. La France for noting the etymology and the highly meaningful connections between the visual butterflies and their sexual connotations.

[95] Jean Toscan examines various verbs that denote "throwing" as signifiers of ejaculatory acts. See Jean Toscan, *Le carnaval du langage: Le lexique érotique des poètes de l'équivoque du Burchiello à Marino (Xve–XVIIe siècles)* (Lille: Presses universitaires de Lille, 1981), 1061–64.

[96] Conti, *La prima reggia*, 96: "terrazzino sopra il ricetto delle stanze nuove della Guardaroba."

[97] I am still to find accounts of travelers who came and saw this portrait. These accounts would be precious documents and would help me understand how exactly indeed this portrait was viewed, displayed, and perceived, and to what extent the viewer's gaze activated the portrait's puns and identity.

[98] Grazzini, once again, provides valuable information in his ode to Morgante when he cites the places where the dwarf was seen: "E Siena e Roma e Bologna e Ferrara / alla sua vista rimaser stupite, / attonite e smarrite. / Ma s'ei poteva condursi a Vinegia, / quella città che pregia / virtù, valore ed ardir

più che umano, / o qualche nuovo e strano / animaletto leggiadro e ridicolo, / portava gran pericolo / di diventar gentiluomo Viniziano." Verses 57–66, in Crimi and Spila, *Nanerie del Rinascimento*, 66.

[99] Diane Kunzelmann is to be thanked for the information related to the original frame of Bronzino's painting. Furthermore, Sefy Hendler proposes to look at Bronzino's *Morgante* as an inter-active painting, precisely because of this display mechanism. Hendler, *Gracious*, 65.

[100] Allegri, *Palazzo Vecchio e i Medici*, 258, note 1.

[101] Maurizio Arfaiolio pointed this dwarf to me. I am grateful for his help.

[102] Barzman, *The Florentine Academy*, 30.

[103] Vesalius and Valverde are repeatedly mentioned, which presupposes that both artists knew the works of the two anatomists and certainly knew of them. Paola Barocchi, ed., *Scritti d'arte del Cinquecento*, vol. 2 (Milan and Naples: Riccardo Ricciardi Editore, 1971), 1950.

[104] ASF, MP 1171, 6, 286, January 22, 1544.

[105] Jonathan Sawday, *The Body Emblazoned: Dissection and the Human Body in Renaissance Culture* (London and New York: Routledge, 1995), 3, where the confrontation of the abstract idea of the body to the reality of a corpse is theorized.

[106] It is known that most court dwarves were achondroplastic dwarves, and the physical details given by Bronzino help confirm that most likely, Morgante was indeed plagued by achondroplasia. For instance, see Launois, "Esquisse iconographique sur quelques nains," 118: "Aux *nains achondroplasiques* appartient la superiorité numérique et souvent aussi celle de la laideur. On les trouve représentés dans un nombre d'objets d'art, en particulier dans les tableaux que nous ont laissés les maîtres de la Renaissance, l'Arétin, Mantegna, Veronèse, Velasquez. Ils ont été pendant longtemps les favoris des princes et des rois." It also makes sense that court dwarves would be achondroplastic since achondrolasia is the most frequent type of genetic bone growth disorder and occurs in one in every fifteen thousand to one in forty thousand live births. See Sandra J. Judd, ed., *Genetic Disorders Sourcebook* (Detroit: Omnigraphics, 2010), 158.

[107] D.W. Smith, *Recognizable Patterns of Human Malformations* (Philadelphia: W.B. Saunders, 1976), 188, and R. Wynne-Davies et al., *Atlas of Skeletal Dysplasias* (Edinburgh: Churchill Livingstone, 1985), 184, as cited in Dasen, *Dwarfs*, 10, footnote 10.

[108] Valerio Cioli da Settignano's *Morgante on a Turtoise* (commissioned in 1564 and finished before 1567) is 116 cm high, but he is seated, which means that standing up he could very well be close to the 150 cm of Bronzino's painting.

[109] It is essential to note that, in fact, achondroplastic dwarves did not have perfect proportions in a mathematical sense. Indeed, the prominent abdomen and head stood in contrast to their shortened limbs.

[110] For instance, in his ode to Morgante, Grazzini writes that the dwarf was "so unattrative that he seemed beautiful" ("e tanto brutto che pareva bello"), verse 6. Please see Crimi and Spila, *Nanerie del Rinascimento*, 61.

[111] ASF, MP 5928, 106, February 2, 1581: "Finalmente hò trovato una nana, la qual di già hò qui in Varsovia, et è cosi ben proportionate che ui veramente levata questa della Regina, no hò mai veduta la più bella."

[112] Pietro Francesco Scarabelli and Paolo Maria Terzago. *Museo, ò Galleria: Adunata del sapere, e dallo studio del Sig. Canonico Manfredo Settala nobile Milanese decritta in Latin deal Sig. Dott. Fis. Colleg. Paolo Maria Terzago. Et poi in italiano dal Sig. Pietro Francesco Scarabelli Dottor Fisico di Voghera, & dal medemo accresciuta. Et hora ristampata con l'Aggiunta di diverse cose poste*

nel fine de medemi Capi dell'Opra ed (Tortona, 1677), 6: "parimente Nana, d'egual simmetria delle membra benissimo proporzionate alla de lei satura, che non giunge a trenta oncie Romane, con tutto ch'elle sia d'età d'anni LV, vivendo col fratello al servigio del Sig. Marchese."

[113] ASF, MP 1212, 1, 114, February 22, 1573.

[114] Ibid., text: "Il Gran Duca [Cosimo I] va continuando nella buona salute, tanto che ha reso lo spirito alli medici et a tutti li altri servitori, et pur hieri stette a vedere lo spettacolo del Nano, il quale fu mandato prigione et firmatogli un processo d'adulterio, dipoi mandato sul asino a faccia a dietro con una poliza a lettere visibili che diceva per adulterio, et il Magnifichino sur un'altro asino preconizzava tutta la vita et ribalderia del Nano, al quale precedeva la tromba della iustitia che haveva tirato dietro tutto il populo. Et S. A. ne pigliava un gusto meraviglioso."

[115] This trial may have been an elaborate burlesque farce, but the satirical note points to the fact that such occurrences could in fact happen and at least problematized the possibility of juridical personhood for dwarves, even as "Sua Altezza" laughed at this overworked staging.

[116] ASMn, AG 1086, July 10, 1535: "Altre volta racoomandai a V.Ecca quell presento Francesco nano, incarcerato per la sua gran poverta e Io feci moso da Compassione come per essermi el poveretto affetionato, e raccomandatomi da persona a ch'io desidero far cosa grata per le qual cose di nuovo, son forzato raccomandarlo a V.Ec, promettendomi che cosi com'io son volonta coso che la si degni mostrarmi I quell ch'io possi server questo mio officio habbi I qualche parte aprofitarvi al Francesco et alle sue miserie. Baccio le man a V.E. raccomandomi sempre sella sua bona gra. Di Fi."

[117] ASF, MP 4, 297, June 13, 1541. Notably, Pagni mentions the affront made to Lorenzo di Galeotto de'Medici and the offense perpetrated on the dwarf in the exact same manner and using the same tone: "Mi son meravigliato assaj che Sua Eccellenza habbi hauto tanta patientia con questo signore et che habbi indugiato tanto a risentirsi delle insulentie sue, la una delle qualj fu non molti mesi doppo la arrivata di Sua Signoria qui, che hebbe ardire di dar di mano addosso a Lorenzo di Galeotto de'Medicj, che era sul terrazzino che è dinanzi alla camera dove Sua Eccellenza dava audientia nel Palazzo de'Medici, alla presentia d'una copia grande di cittadinj et di cortigianj et con superbissime parole cacciarlo di quell palazzo, minacciando di mettergli la spada ne'fianchi se non s'andava con Dio [...]. Detto Signore [Pirro Colonna] [...] disse queste o similj parole verso il Nano di S. Ex.a che li era allato a veder' giocare, cioè: 'Egli è questo porcho del Nano che mi fa malo augurio', comandandadolj se li levasse dapresso [...] et multiplicando le parole tra l'uno et l'altro, il Signor Pyrro senza alcun rispetto di questo Ex.tie, le qualj, V.S. sa, quanto amino questo Nano, li dette un gran straffo [...]."

[118] ASF, Pratica Segreta 186, ca. 126v, *Cosmus Medicus Dei gratia Florentie dux*: "et cum animadveremus ad debilem patrimonium tuum tueque parenne et quod ni tibi a nos sucurratur semper in pauvertate viveres et post vitam tuam parum vel nihil filis tuis relinqueres [...]."

[119] Christiane Klapisch-Zuber, "Nobles or Pariahs: The Exclusion of Florentine Magnates from the Thirteenth to the Fifteenth Centuries," *Society for Comparative Study of Society and History* 39, no. 2 (1997): 218.

[120] ASF, MP 241, 94, March 6, 1573: "Ufitiali, Provveditore et Ministri del Monte della Pietà di Fiorenza. In virtù di questo mandato vi commettiamo che paghiate a ms. Thomaso de'Medici nostro tesoriere scudi [...] per più conti come appresso, cioè: [...] Scudi X per darli a Morgante Nano [...]."

[121] Lorenzo Legati, *Museo Cospiano: Annesso a quello del famoso Ulisse Aldrovandi E donato alla sua Patria dall'Illustrissimo Signor Ferdinando Cospi Patrizio di Bologna e Senator, ecc.* (Bologna, 1677), 7, as cited in Zakiya Hanafi, *The Monster in the Machine: Magic, Medicine, and the Marvelous in the Time of the Scientific Revolution* (Durham and London: Duke University Press, 2000), 86.

[122] Pauli Zacchiae Romani, totius status ecclesiastici proto-medici generalis. *Quaestionum medico-legalium, tomi tres. Editio prima Veneta, Lugdunensi & Noribergensi, quae passim soedis scatebant erroribus multò emendiator: Accedunt Interpolationes, & Auctaria ex novis Inventis & Observationibus Recentiorum Auctorum. Curà Joannis Danielis Horstii, Diversorum S.R.I. Principum Archiatri, & Collegii Medici Moeno-Francofurtani Senioris. Opus omnibus medicinae et juris utriusque peritis, Necnon Tribunalium (Ecclesiastici, Civilis) Assessoribus maximè necessarium* (Venice: Bonifacii Viezzeri, Superiorum Permissu, 1737).

[123] Charles Avery and Anthony Radcliffe, *Giambologna: Sculptor to the Medici* (Edinburgh and London: The Arts Council of Great Britain, the Westerham Press, 1978), 101. It is interesting that this fountain was meant for Francesco I, thus attesting that Morgante's fame did not wane immediately after Cosimo I's reign but held for several years before it faded.

[124] Ibid., 103.

[125] Holderbaum, "A Bronze," 440–42.

[126] *Ragionamenti del Signor Cavaliere Giorgio Vasari pittore e architetto aretino sopra le invenzioni da lui dipinte in Firenze nel Palazzo di loro altezze serenissime con lo illustriss. Ed eccellentiss. Signore D. Francesco Medici allure Principe di Firenze insieme con la invenzione della pittura da lui cominciata nella cupola. Con due tavole, une delle cose più notabili, e l'altra degli Uomini Illustri che sone ritratti, e nominate un quest'opera* (Arezzo: Michele Bellotti, 1762), particularly 134–49.

[127] Stephen Mennell and Johan Goudsblom, eds., *Norbert Elias: On Civilization, Power, and Knowledge. Selected Writings* (Chicago and London: University of Chicago Press, 1998), 55.

[128] Paolo L. Rossi, "*Sprezzatura*, Patronage, and Fate: Benvenuto Cellini and the World of Words," in *Vasari's Florence: Artists and Literati at the Medicean Court*, ed. Philip Jacks (Cambridge: Cambridge University Press, 1998), 61.

[129] *Ragionamenti* (1762), 134–40: "V.E. sia la ben venuta [...]"; "V.E. dice il vero [...]"; "come V.E. può avvertire, l'ho divisato in tre invenzioni [...]"; "Quando piaccia a V.E., io comincierò da questi quartieri della Città di Firenze [...]."

[130] It is interesting to note that Vasari's effort were not commonplace and not every artist attempting to forge a courtier identity for himself through the adoption of intellectual written endeavors and/or acquisition of distinguished manners at court was rewarded with the same success as Vasari. Benvenuto Cellini, for instance, remained banned from the Medici court, in spite of his numerous attempts at *civiltà*. See Rossi, "Sprezzatura."

[131] Janet Cox-Rearick, "Art at the Court of Duke Cosimo I de'Medici (1537–74)," in *The Medici, Michelangelo, and the Art of Late Renaissance Florence* (New Haven and London: Yale University Press, 2003), 35.

[132] Janet Cox-Rearick, *Bronzino's Chapel for Eleonora di Toledo in the Palazzo Vecchio* (Berkeley and London: Berkeley University Press, 1993), 37.

[133] Janet Cox-Rearick's entry for *Agnolo Bronzino: Eleonora di Toledo and Her Son Giovanni*, in *The Medici, Michelangelo, and the Art of Late Renaissance Florence*, 145.

[134] Jonathan Nelson, "Creative Patronage: Luca Martini and the Renaissance Portrait," *Mitteilungen des Kunsthistorisches Institutes in Florenz* 39 (1995): 285–93.

[135] Caroline Murphy, *Lavinia Fontana: A Painter and Her Patrons in Sixteenth-century Bologna* (New Haven: Yale University Press, 2003), 161.

[136] For a larger discussion on portraits of children in Renaissance Italy, see Marian M. Methenitis, *More than Mirrors: Portraits of Children in Renaissance Italy*, unpublished dissertation (University of Dallas, 1995).

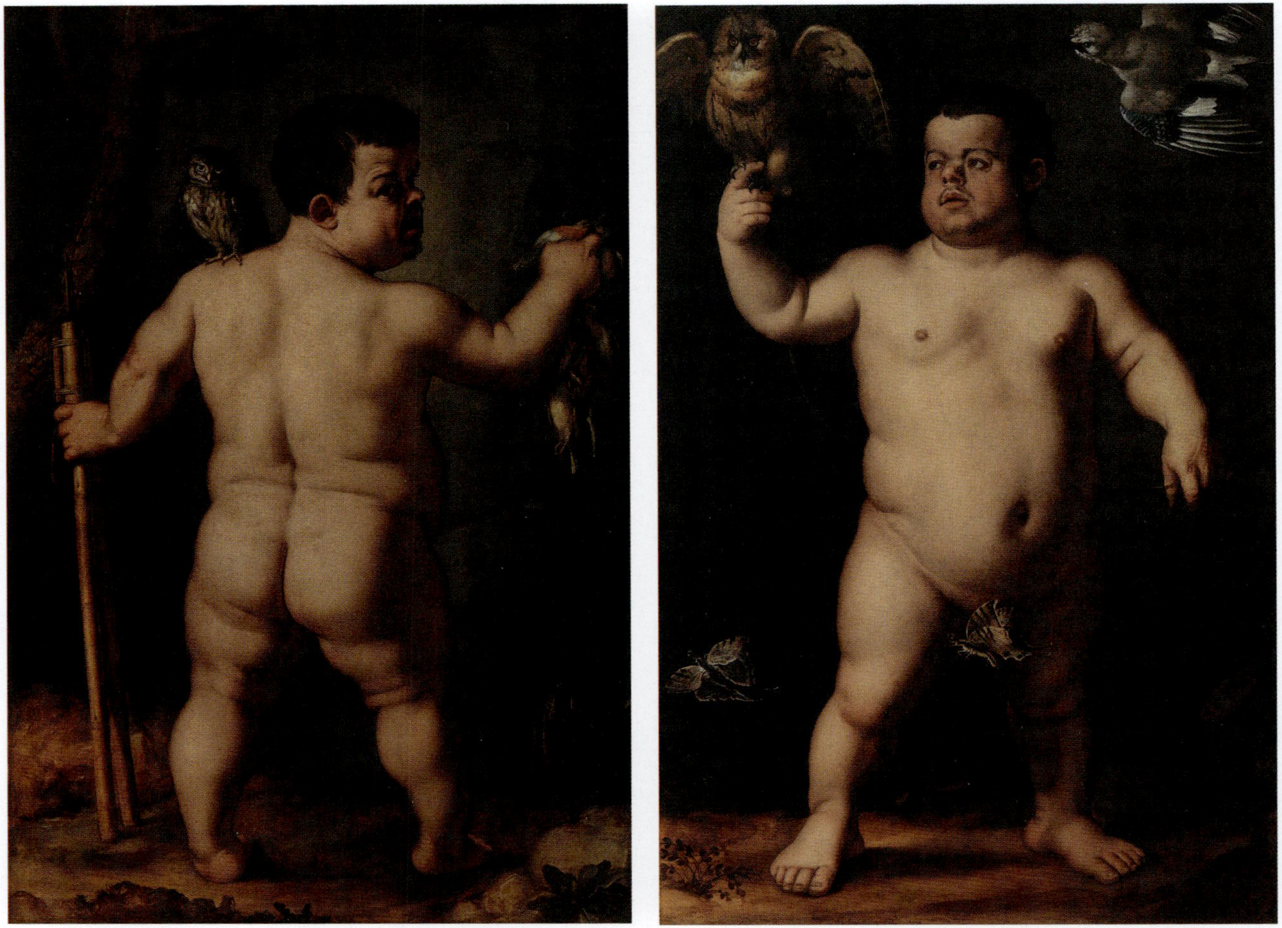

Plate 1 (*verso and recto*). Agnolo Bronzino, *Portrait of Morgante*, ca. 1547, Galleria degli Uffizi, Florence

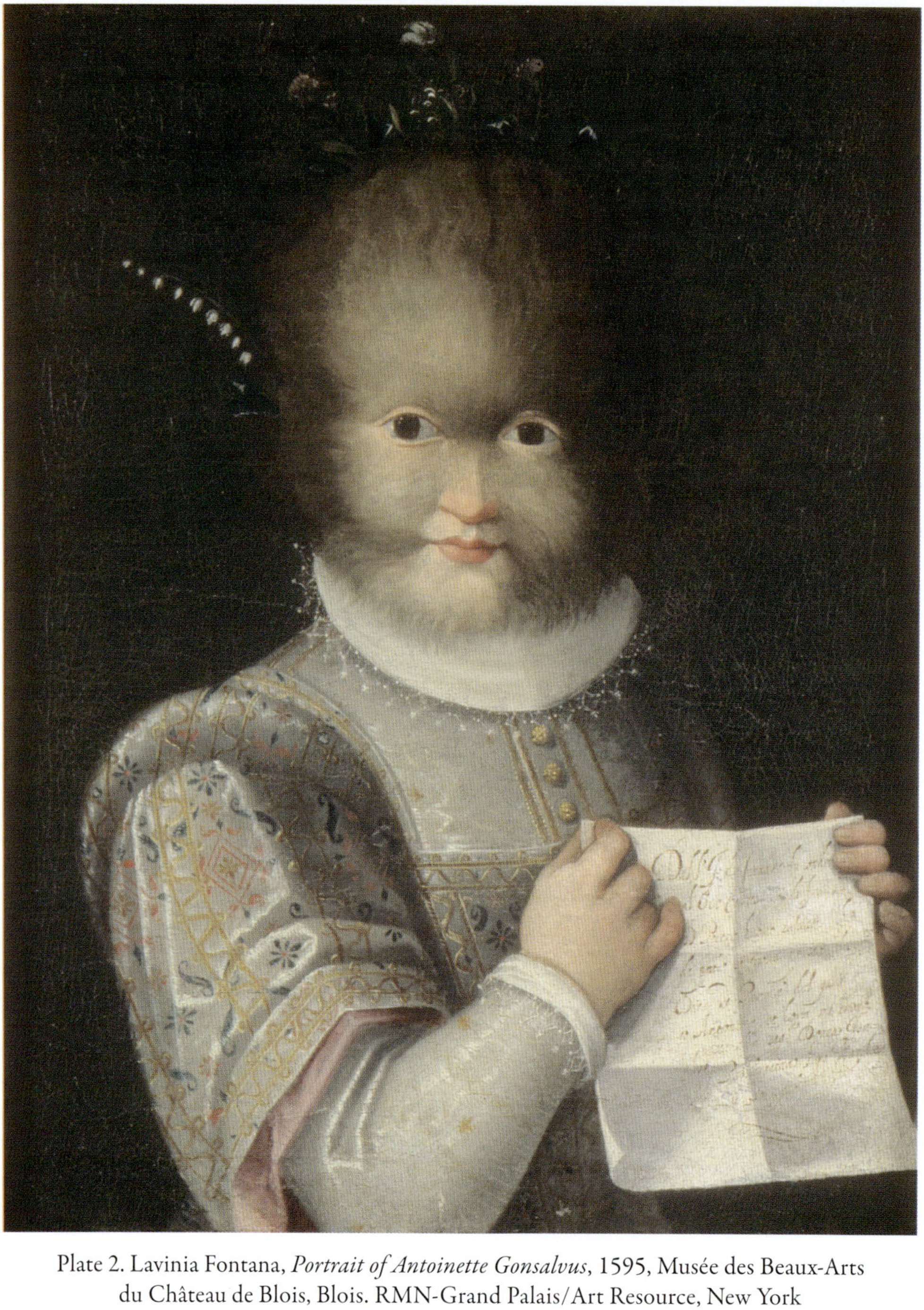

Plate 2. Lavinia Fontana, *Portrait of Antoinette Gonsalvus*, 1595, Musée des Beaux-Arts du Château de Blois, Blois. RMN-Grand Palais/Art Resource, New York

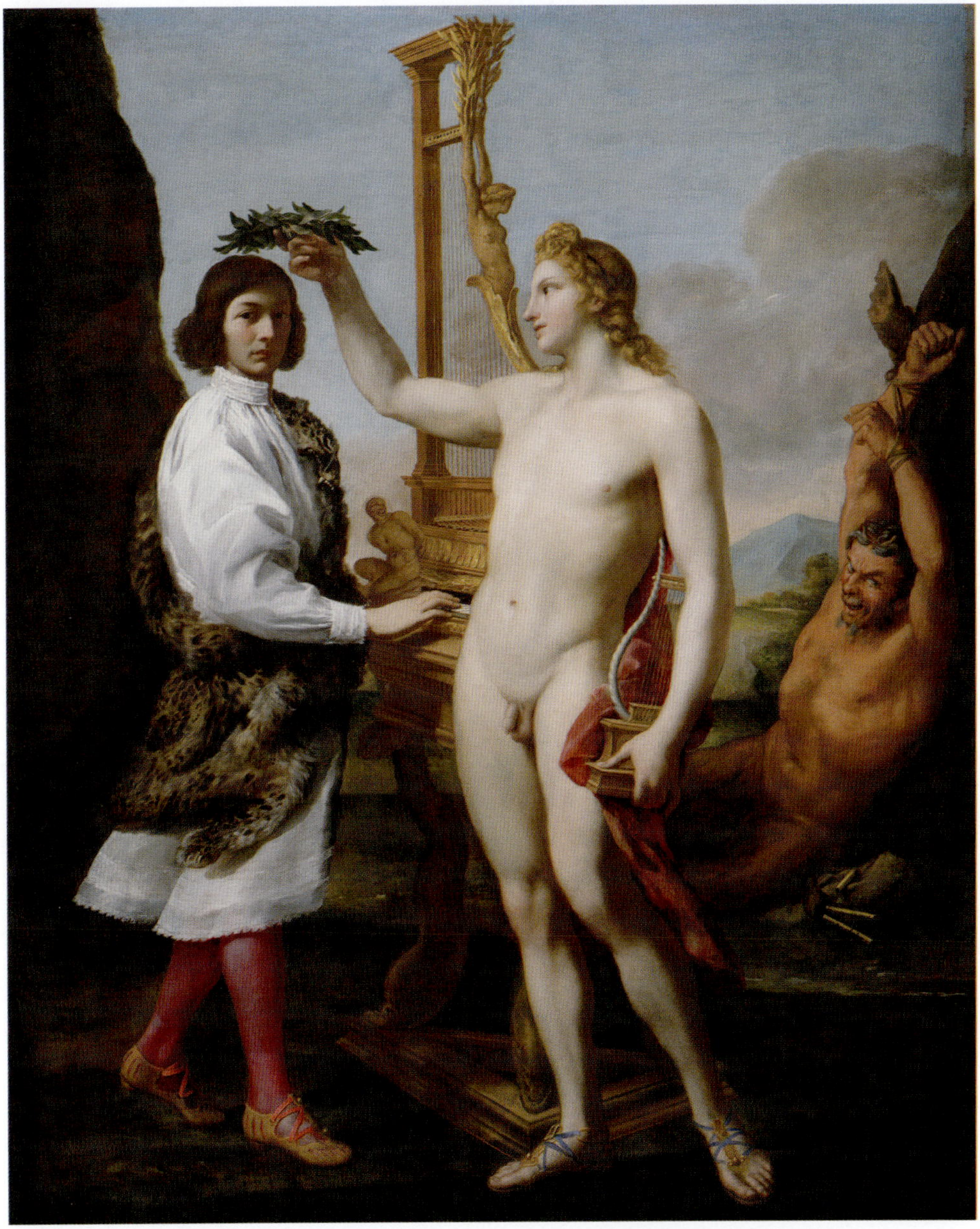

Plate 3. Andrea Sacchi, *Portrait of Marc'Antonio Pasqualini*, 1640, Metropolitan Museum of Art, New York

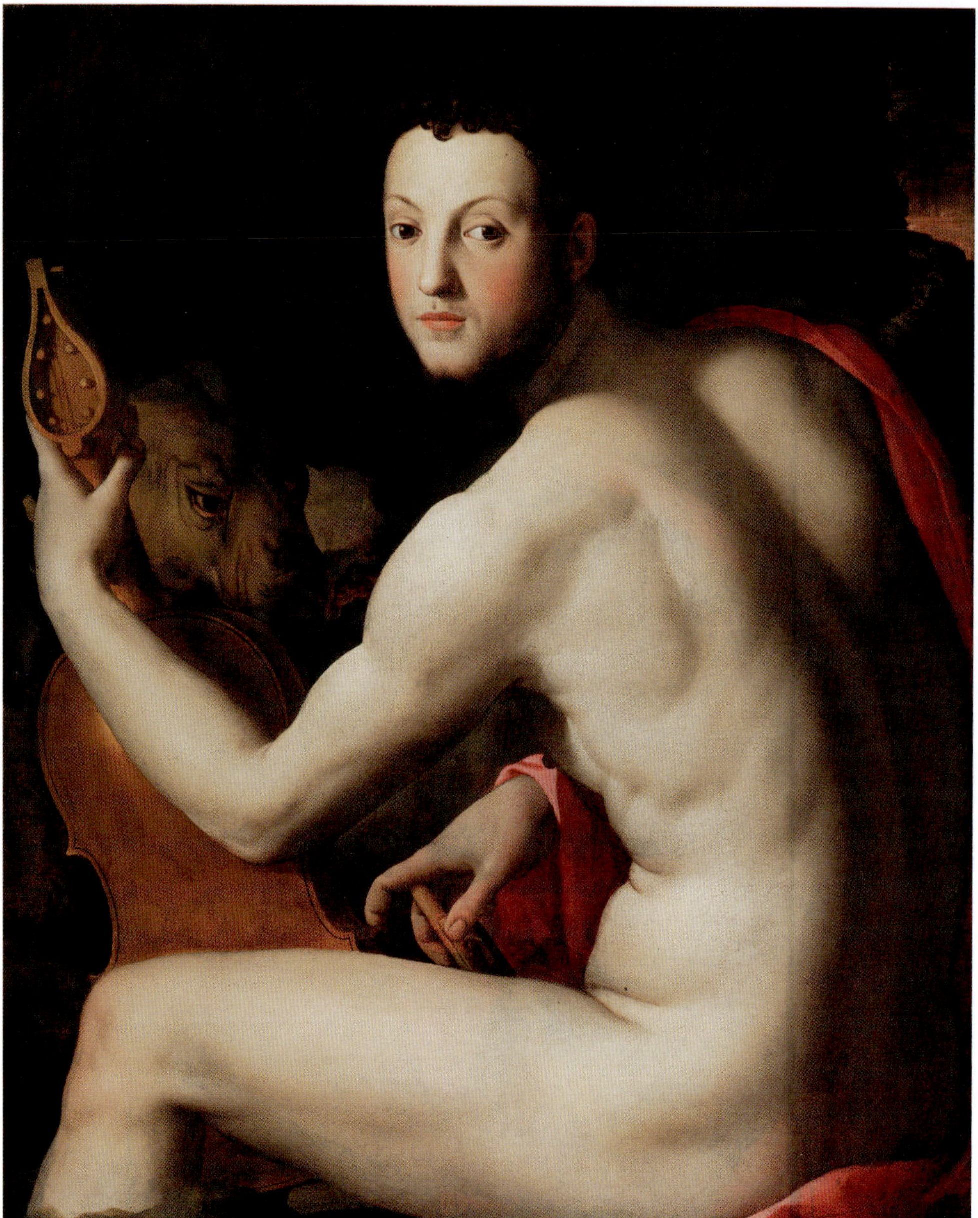

Plate 4. Agnolo Bronzino, *Cosimo I de'Medici as Orpheus*, ca. 1539, Philadelphia Museum of Art, Philadelphia

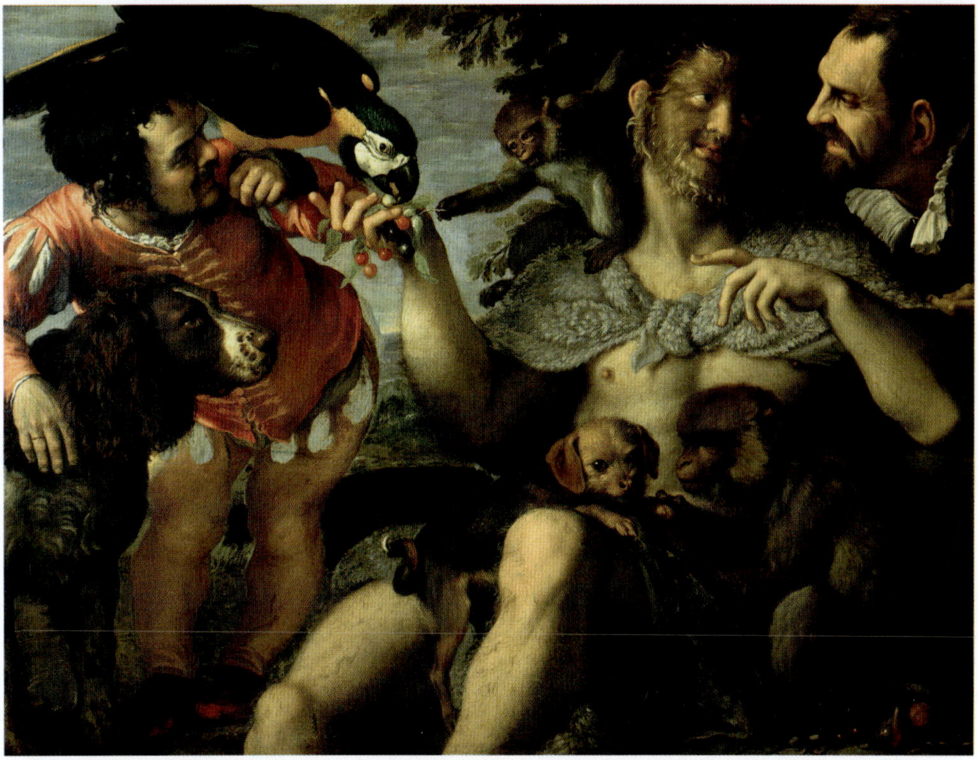

Plate 5. Agostino Carracci, *Composition with Figures and Animals*: *Hairy Harry, Mad Peter and Tiny Amon*, 1598, Museo di Capodimonte, Naples. Scala/Ministero per i Bene e le Attività culturali/Art Resource, New York

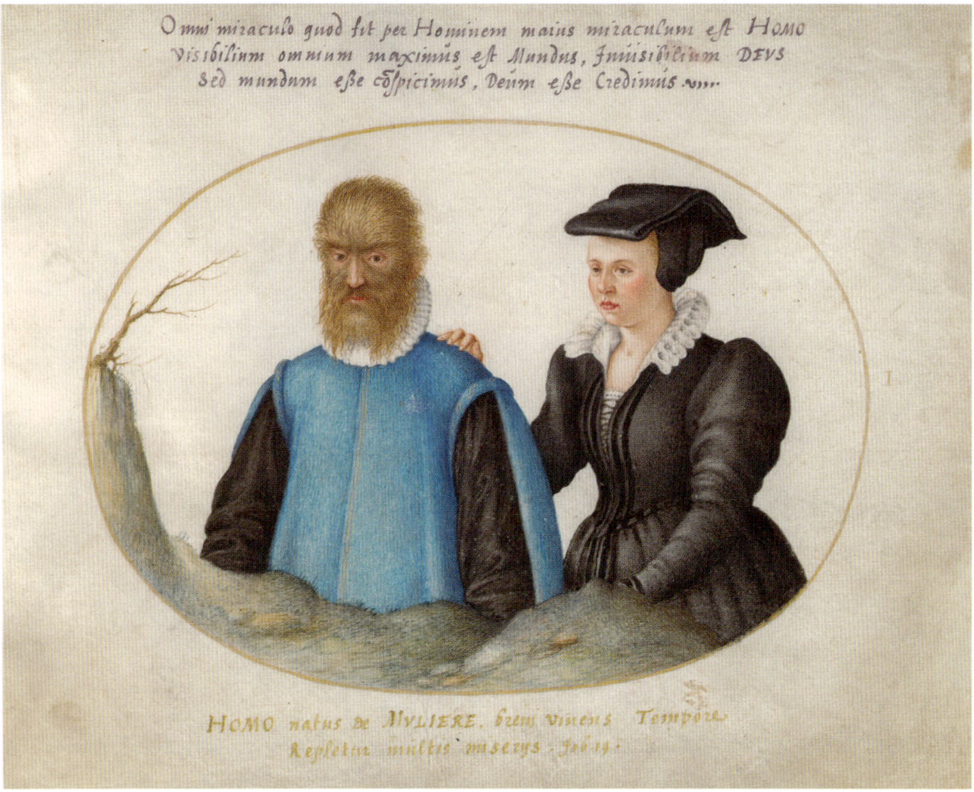
Omni miraculo quod fit per Hominem maius miraculum est HOMO
Visibilium omnium maximus est Mundus, Inuisibilium DEUS
Sed mundum esse cōspicimus, Deum esse Credimus
HOMO natus de MULIERE, breui viuens Tempore
Repletur multis miserijs. Job 14.

Plate 6. Joris Hoefnagel, *Plate I* from *Animalia Rationalia et Insecta (Ignis)*, ca. 1575–80, National Gallery of Art, Washington, D.C.

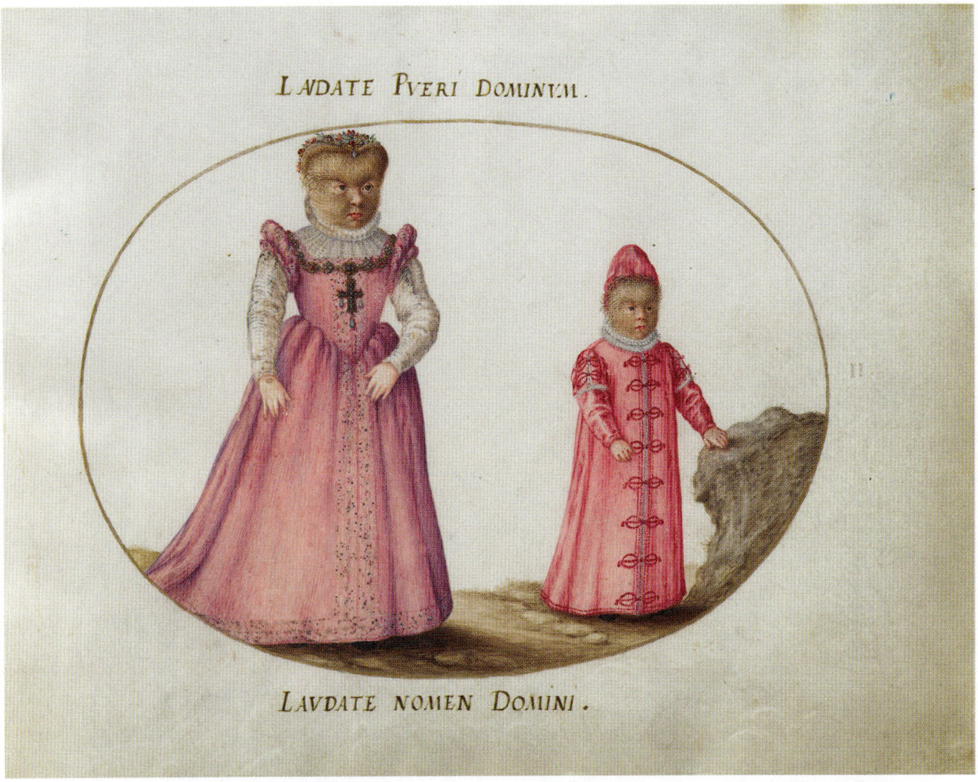

Plate 7. Joris Hoefnagel, *Plate II* from *Animalia Rationalia et Insecta (Ignis)*, ca. 1575–80, National Gallery of Art, Washington, D.C.

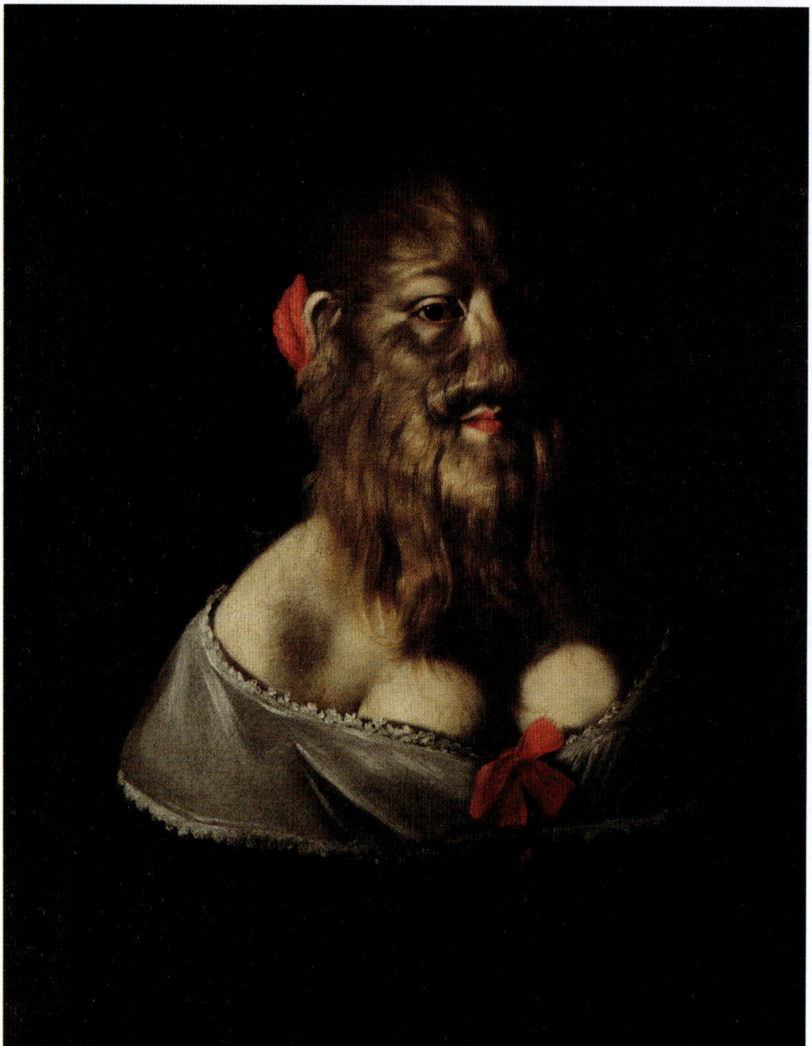

Plate 8. Jusepe de Ribera(?), *Portrait of Madeleine Gonsalvus*(?), ca. 1615, Thomas Agnew & Sons, London

Chapter 4

A Civilized Savage: The Hirsute's Conquest

ALTHOUGH MEN AND WOMEN WITH hypertrichosis—the excess growth of hair over most of the body—did not hold a status as commonly valued as that of dwarves, their presence at court followed the same channels. The combination of their unusual appearance and their ability to match their patrons intellectually guaranteed them positions as court companions. As a result, they were a valuable presence at court and, like dwarves, they sat for portraits. One such family was the Gonsalvus family, who became the most painted hirsute family in Europe.[1] The visual record left by patrons who commissioned these paintings is immensely valuable, as it allows for an investigation of the position held by the Gonsalvus family in various courts and to determine how their medical condition transformed them into marvels. In turn, the Gonsalvus family's proximity to ruling authority questioned the notion of monstrousness by framing power in relation—and in opposition—to otherness. It is in their visualizations that we see the tension between *ritrarre* and *imitare* take unsettling and unsettled forms. Unlike dwarves who did not often come to court and generate families who looked like them, the Gonsalvuses held a unique position because they were a family of beings with extraordinary bodies. The human ties that connected them together and the education they received made them closer in kin to courtiers than dwarves were. Therefore, artists struggled to use artistic rhetoric to depict a family—a decidedly human concept—of hairy monsters. Ultimately, it is in these unresolved vacillations that we see the conflicted position held by the Gonsalvuses as courtly participants, objects of scientific explorations, sentient beings, and fascinating visual subjects.

In 1595, Ranuccio Farnese, Margaret of Parma's grandson, presented Henri Gonsalvus—the son of a hirsute man found in the Canary Islands, Pierre Gonsalvus—as a gift to his brother, Cardinal Odoardo Farnese. Following his adoption by the cardinal, Henri was depicted in a group portrait by Agostino Carracci (1557–1602) painted between 1598 and 1599 (Plate 5).[2] I have discussed this group portrait in chapter 3 in terms of its commission details, the importance of the animals on a metaphorical and literal level, as well as the commentary this painting makes about possessing monsters in courtly circles. However, one notable point is that by the time Carracci painted the portrait, Rodomonte (Amon) had been dead more than four years and Pietro Matto (the buffoon) had already left Rome.[3] Henri Gonsalvus was thus the only live model accessible to Carracci. Interestingly, Carracci does not accentuate the hairiness of the hirsute man, but rather inserts external indices that point to the hirsute's personal history and social position. Henri is shown wearing a goatskin garb called a *tamarco* and typical of the inhabitants of the Canary Islands—where Henri's father, Pierre, was found. Additionally, both Amon and Pietro turn toward Henri who grounds the entire composition of this painting. Henri turns to Pietro, while his left hand and index finger point to Amon, implying the connection occurring between the buffoon and the dwarf through him. If, as Roberto Zapperi has suggested, this painting was not commissioned by Cardinal Farnese, but rather by one of the sitters, Henri was most likely the patron of this work. Not only is his wild nature not visually emphasized through the depiction of his excessive growth of hair, but Carracci also shows him as the one gathering others in what seems to be a civil conversation. The ability to converse becomes a supplementary civilizing index in a painting that speaks to humanity's potential for peace. And it is through Henri that all of these elements acquire visible manifestations. Because Henri was legally adopted by Cardinal Farnese and given almost full juridical status, his agency may have been greater than some of the physically different individuals discussed in the previous chapter (and, in fact, even greater than that of his sisters).[4] What this portrait does emphasize unequivocally, however, is the sustained interest in not only dwarves, but in hirsutes as well. Henri Gonsalvus and his family became famous not only because of their congenital condition, but also and mostly because courtiers were drawn to their physical appearance that artists, then, immortalized.

As the first documented family with visible hypertrichosis, the Gonsalvuses set a precedent for this disease. They also attached their name to the congenital condition called Ambras syndrome because of the numerous portraits of the Gonsalvus family that were held in Schloss Ambras, in present day Austria. In a study published in 1993, F.A.M. Baumeister, along with three colleagues, states the main visible characteristics associated with Ambras syndrome:

> The whole body is covered with fine, long hair, except areas in which ordinarily no hair grows: the palms, the soles, the dorsal terminal phalanges and the mucosa. The accentuation of the hypertrichosis on the shoulders, the face and the ears is characteristic. The forehead, eyelids, nose, cheeks and preauricular region are uniformly covered with hair, reaching a length of several decimeters if not shaved. The hair is light coloured, silky or golden. Only the scalp hair, the eyebrows, the eyelashes and the axillary hair are darker. The hypertrichosis of the external ears is typical: if not cut, long curls protrude from the external auditory canal. The eyelashes may become very long; in one case [...] the eyelashes were reported to be absent.[5]

This syndrome is also called congenital hypertrichosis lanuginosa and is the result of an inherited autosomal dominant trait.[6] Although the endocrine system controlling the growth of hair may be affected by various intrinsic and extrinsic factors, the genetic factors are the most important in the transmission of hypertrichosis.[7] As an autosomal trait, the gene causing hypertrichosis is found on one of the non-sexual chromosome pairs and its occurrence is therefore not dependent on the sex of the parent transmitting the gene. Because of the meiotic genetic recombination, the children acquire half the genetic material from each parent. If, in the case of the Gonsalvus family, one parent possessed the dominant gene located on the eighth chromosome, the children had a 50 percent chance of inheriting the disease.[8]

Visually, Lavinia Fontana's (1552–1614) 1595 portrait of Antoinette Gonsalvus (Plate 2) matches perfectly the phenotype associated with the Ambras syndrome. In accordance with Françoise Launay, research engineer at the CNRS in Paris, the distribution of the hair on the little Gonsalvus girl, her glabrous—smooth-skinned, hairless—hands, and the coloration of her facial hair all indicate that indeed, Antoinette Gonsalvus suffered from hypertrichosis lanuginosa universalis.[9] Consequently, we can assume that if she did in fact marry a man who was not a carrier of the Ambras gene, her children may have been glabrous and thus lost for history, since they would have been of no scientific or visual interest. As opposed to her brother Henri, who fathered hairy children, Antoinette and her children may have disappeared from public life thanks to the gamble of genetic recombination. Her portrait is therefore the last remnant of her actual existence.

Fontana's portrait of Antoinette is the most puzzling portrait of the Gonsalvus family, and one that gives an instructive glimpse into the discourse that framed their presence in early modern European courts. Although this painting was executed after the Gonsalvus family left the court of France, the details and the history embedded in this portrait reveal the convoluted social path that the Gonsalvuses took from the arrival of Antoinette's father Pierre to the court of Henri II of France, to the disappearance of the family from most historical records. Whereas rigid societal rules might have suppressed the identity of Antoinette as a sentient individual, evidence suggests that, in fact, that which made her exotic and collectible also guaranteed her a safe position as a courtier, companion, and educated young woman. Antoinette's different body signified a flawed human form, yet unlike a generic curiosity, she acquired a social mobility that transcended her body and allowed her to be educated, benefit from full juridical personhood, and pursue an—almost—independent life. Fontana knew the strong cultural references associated with hirsutes—wildness, savagery, violence, illiteracy—and combined them with the personal history of the Gonsalvuses, all the while subtly pointing to the tenuous position of a little girl/monster whose family grew up in one of the most rigid courts of early modern Europe.

A life-size, three-quarter-length portrait measuring 57 cm by 46 cm, the portrait of Antoinette Gonsalvus appears to be an accurate and highly detailed visual representation of the daughter of the most famous hirsute of the Renaissance, Pierre Gonsalvus. Completed in 1595, this painting came to be ascribed to Lavinia Fontana only recently.

Until 1990, this painting was attributed to a follower of Veronese, making the identification of the subject next to impossible. Indeed, without the knowledge of Fontana's connection to Ulisse Aldrovandi (1522–1605), and her previous drawing of the hirsute girl, the anonymity of the portrait's sitter would have persisted. The provenance of this painting is as important for the identification of the subject, as it is essential to understanding the impetus behind its commission. The portrait traveled from Mantua, where it belonged to Vincenzo Gonzaga to end up eventually with the Gordon family in Aberdeen in the nineteenth century. Most likely, Archie Gordon, Fifth Marquess of Aberdeen bought the portrait in an auction around 1834, and Sotheby's London sold it for David Gordon to R.E.A. Wilson in 1947. Bought by the Haskell family, the portrait was sold to Phillips in London in 1990, then moved to the Galleria Pietro Scarpa in Venice, and was finally acquired by the Musée des Beaux-Arts du Château de Blois in 1997. Along the way, the portrait gained in value, particularly when it became associated with Lavinia Fontana.[10]

Adopting the courtly three-quarter-length pose, the subject of this painting gazes directly at the viewer. Her eyes look forward, while her mouth faintly hints at a smile. Antoinette is wearing a lavish dress, complete with gold embroideries, lace, elaborate collar and sleeves. Her costume is typical of the dress worn by young female courtiers. In her hair, two sets of flowers are visible against the dark, indeterminate background: behind her right ear, a sprig of lilies of the valley, and on top of her head a crown of clovers, snow drops, and carnation. Her face is covered with hairs of various lengths and color gradations, while both her hands are glabrous. Fontana painted every strand of hair on the face of the sitter with great attention, akin to a scientific exploration of a unique specimen. The face is not darkened to imply hairiness, neither is the pilosity exaggerated. The texture of the hair Fontana rendered on the canvas bears a soft, delicate, and almost sensuous quality. Most visibly, Antoinette's hair, extending to her white collar seems to imply a fluid movement that serves as a rich transition between the wildness of the hair and the luxurious civility of the costume worn by the sitter. In this intentional pictorial language, Fontana is combining an aesthetic vocabulary that idealizes the sitter but that remains truthful to her appearance—a difficult balance to achieve, but one that speaks to the *invenzione* of Fontana in combining *ritrarre* to accomplish *imitare*. Antoinette holds a letter that reads

> Don Pietro, wild man, was brought from the Canary Islands to his most serene Highness the King of France, Henry. At the present time, he is at the court of the most serene Duke of Parma, where I, Antoinette, used to be, and now I am nearby with Lady Isabella Pallavicina, the Marchioness of Soragna.[11]

By following the text of this letter, the chronological elements of Antoinette's life unfold. It is by detangling them that we can follow and understand the life of Antoinette and the complexities that lay in the portrait Fontana painted of the hirsute subject.

Sold in 1947 under the title "The Wild Boy," this painting is now recognized as part of Lavinia Fontana's oeuvre. Known as one of the foremost Renaissance artists of Bologna, Fontana painted many religious altarpieces and a significant number of secular works.[12] Her subject, Antoinette Gonsalvus (ca. 1588–?), exemplifies the vexed issue of physically anomalous bodies in the context of highly normative court settings; indeed, even the portrait's 1947 catalogue description attests to the confusion it inspires for the uninitiated viewer: Sotheby's London described the work as "a dwarf with a monkey-like head, holding a letter in both hands which states him to be in the service of Donna Isabella Pallavicini."[13]

As the daughter of a hirsute, Antoinette should at best have been a courtly wonder. But her father Pierre, who came to the court of Henri II as a marvel, received extensive education and married under the auspices of the French king. Antoinette benefited indirectly from the education her father received, and the circles in which the family moved; also, due to courtly exchanges, she was better traveled than most young women her age. Years after the death of his benefactor Henri II, and shortly after the death of his widow Catherine de'Medici Valois, Pierre and his family traveled to various places, including the court of Margaret of Austria, Rome between 1594 and 1595, and eventually they settled in Parma.

Fontana's portrait was original in its form and composition, yet still followed a typical court format. It was not copied from one of the many representations of the famous Gonsalvus family; in fact a preliminary drawing of Antoinette attests to the originality of Fontana's composition and study from nature (Fig. 4.1).[14]

Fontana met the Gonsalvus family when they came to Bologna, and she had the chance to see the family again after that original meeting, leading to her drawing and, eventually, finished portrait of Antoinette. The portrait found its way to the collection of Vincenzo Gonzaga (Duke of Mantua, 1562–1612), but it was originally commissioned by Isabella Pallavicini (ca. 1545–1623) from Parma, Marchesa di Soragna. During a trip to Bologna, Isabella saw the senator Mario Casali—a close friend of the Fontana family—and she may have asked the famous Bolognese naturalist Ulisse Aldrovandi to contact Fontana, who then created the portrait of Antoinette. Though this complicated series of negotiations have been addressed by the scholarship on the Gonsalvus family, the collaboration between Aldrovandi and the artist is often regarded as the primary reason behind this portrait's commission.[15] Aldrovandi was interested in exceptions to the rules of nature, and the Gonsalvus family provided him with a perfect and rare example; therefore, scholars have interpreted this portrait as an illustration of Aldrovandi's scientific ethos.[16] The congenital condition that turned a little girl into a monster, however, also secured her a place at court and in the collective scientific memory. Indeed, Fontana's representation of Antoinette Gonsalvus exemplifies the tension between the external appearance of the subject and her place at court. Rhetorically, Fontana's portrait of

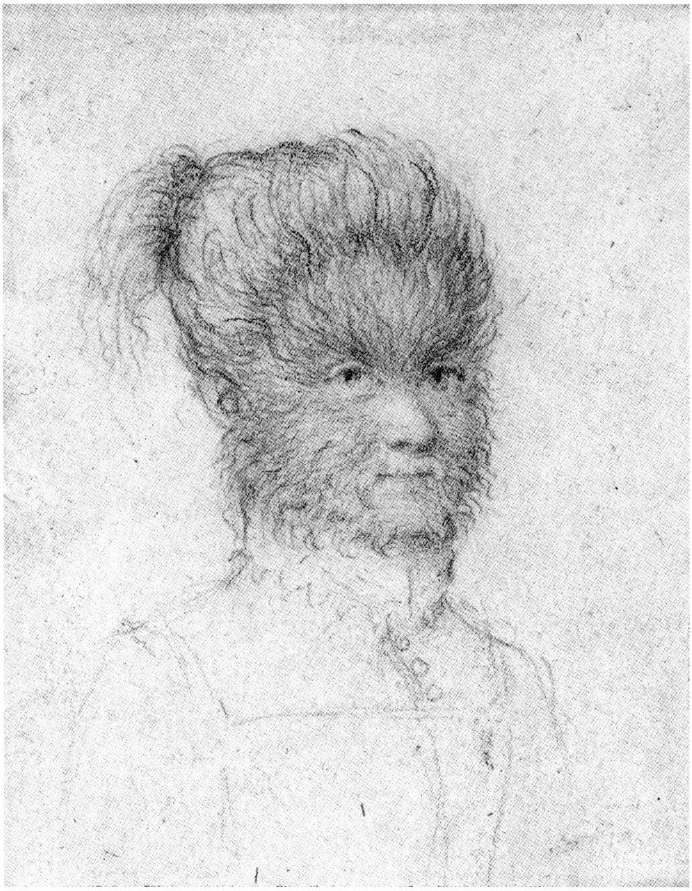

Figure 4.1. Lavinia Fontana, *Portrait of Antoinette Gonsalvus*, 1595, The J. Pierpont Morgan Library, New York

Antoinette challenged a seemingly homogeneous courtly vocabulary of forms and modes of presentation, while visually tracing the encounter between a female artist, an educated but non-normative individual, enthralled patrons, and a puzzled scientific community.

Explanations for the existence of hirsutes did not lack for originality in the Renaissance and the Middles Ages. Believed to have been born from the imagination of perverse women during conception, or to be faithful descendants of mythological satyrs, or savage giant creatures living in the woods, hirsutes deeply puzzled those who encountered them in actuality or in written and imaged works. The ambiguous appearance of the "wild man" made his characterization all the more troubling. Neither civilized enough to be part of human society, nor beastly enough to be entirely relegated to the animal world, hirsutes occupied a liminal position between the two categories. From the margins of illuminated manuscripts to popular engravings, the visual presence of people who had hypertrichosis challenged the fragile, porous layers of cultural associations that defined society. Lavinia Fontana's portrait, which contributed to this evolving pictorial conversation, is no exception.

Although manuscripts such as *Marvels of the East* (ca. 1040) included illuminations depicting hairy men involved in wild activities as early as the eleventh century, these works did not systematically classify wild men within a defined category.[17] The rise in the number of representations of wild men in the twelfth and thirteenth centuries coincided with the satyr's loss of pagan divinity in the mind of an increasingly rigid Christian society.[18] Therefore, the wild man became more of an outcast savage, than a supernatural being possessing mystical powers. In the collective imaginary, however, the wild man's feral qualities were conflated with his great power and immense knowledge of nature. Some traditions, still enacted today in folkloric festivals in eastern and southern Switzerland, speak to the contradiction inherent in both fearing and invoking a being whose powers were deemed super-human. While not Italian, this example demonstrates beliefs that seeped throughout most of Europe and affected the ways in which the Gonsalvus family was viewed in France and in the courts they entered subsequently. The Swiss belief held in the early modern period maintained that in order for the wild man to share his wisdom about nature, he had to be captured with copious amounts of alcohol.[19] In the town of Evolène, for instance, male Carnival celebrants wear beastly masks and straw-stuffed bags around their bodies and jump out to frighten passers-by. At night, it is customary to catch these men and drink with them.[20]

Literature reinforced the untamed notion of the wild man who lived in the woods and possessed supernatural strength. In the first 1483 edition of Matteo Boiardo's epic poem *Orlando Innamorato*, the description of a hirsute leaves no doubt to his appearance; he is described as having a long beard, much hair, and hairy all over from head to toe.[21] *L'omo bestiale inumano* is described as a dangerous and solitary being, who captures women in the woods. Eventually killed by Brandimarte, the wild man in this narrative is finally tamed, and his violent and monstrous qualities disappear with him at his death. Then with *Orlando furioso* (1516), Ludovico Ariosto included the figure of the wild man in his epic *canti*. This time, however, Brandimarte does not physically kill the *omo bestiale inumano*. The wild man in *Orlando furioso* is Orlando himself, having gone mad—a behavioral wilderness—after discovering Angelica's betrothal; Brandimarte kills the wild man *in* Orlando, bringing him back to his civilized self.[22]

As European societies moved toward defining themselves as early modern states, they became more rigid in their structures and the wild man acquired an iconic status. Civilized minds associated him with the longing for a simpler and untainted way of life.[23] Although this shift did not allow hirsutes to completely evade the connection made between their condition and the mythology of the wild man, by the sixteenth century hirsutes were simply understood within a range of naturally occurring monsters.[24]

As such, they appealed to the early modern classifying impulse. In 1566, for example, Pierre Boaistuau (1517–1566) in his *Histoires prodigieuses* included hirsutes among his catalogue of stories from Greek and Latin ancient authors, imaginary biblical occurrences, fantastic animals, and congenital diseases.[25] In his fifth chapter, titled *Prodigieuses des enfantemens monstrueux, & de la cause de leur generation*, Boaistuau illustrated an image of a hirsute woman standing in front of a king. Behind her, a child, with completely black skin, is walking (Fig. 4.2). The text reads:

> It is certain that most often these creatures preceded the judgment, justice, punishment and curse of God, who allows fathers and mothers to generate such abominations, testifying to the horror of their sin, because they rush indifferently, like wild animals, or their greed guides them without allowing them to respect old age, time, place, or other Laws given by nature.[26]

Boaistuau suggested it was the parents' greed and bestial instincts that has led to such monstrous offspring. Because the parents' strayed from the laws of nature, their children were punished and carried the visible signs of their parents' moral deviations.

Though he adopted the generative approach proposed by Boaistuau, Ambroise Paré (1510–1590) did not see sin and punishment as the reason for hirsute children. Of the thirteen causes that were believed to produce monsters, Paré indicated the fifth one, imagination, as the source of hirsutes.[27] In his book on surgery, first published in 1573, Paré included a section on monsters and marvels. In this section, he often appropriated stories and images from earlier authors, including Boaistuau from whom he borrowed the illustration for his hirsute woman. Appearing in chapter IX under the title *Exemple des Monstres qui se font par imagination*, and placed once again next to a black child, the hirsute woman served as an example of what happened when a mother's imagination was fertilized by concrete visual aids. The hirsute woman, for Paré was thus the result of her own mother's overactive mind, just as the black child was the result of the imagination of his mother:

> Damascenus, grave author, testifies that he saw a girl who was hairy like a Bear, and she had been born deformed and hideous because the mother had looked too intently at the figure of Saint John wearing a fur skin, an image that was tied at the bottom of her bed while she was conceiving the child.[28]

Pierre Gonsalvus's and his hirsute children's appearance was therefore a visible mark that recalled many imaginary, literary, and folkloric stories that stamped their human presence and therefore their visual representations.

As extraordinary beings, hirsutes' legal rights were controlled by restricted juridical status. We can assume that the Gonsalvus family paved the way for other persons with hypertrichosis, as there is a specific mention of their case in Paolo Zacchia's (1584–1659) medico-legal questions. Personal physician to the popes and legal advisor to the

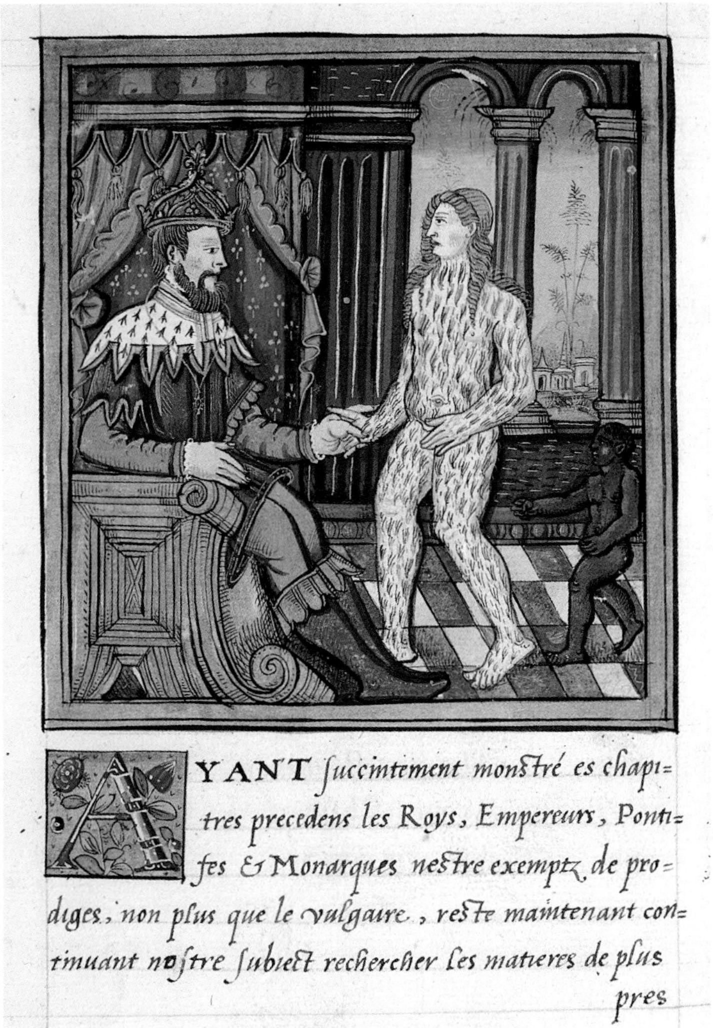

Figure 4.2. Pierre Boaistuau, *Hairy Woman and Black Child*, illustration from *Les Histoires Prodigieuses*, 1559, Wellcome Library, London

Rota Romana, Zacchia explored questions that combined current medical knowledge with ethical and legal issues. In his seventh book, beneath the entry *Homo pilosus & hujusmodi hominum ortus quails*, Zacchia describes the case of the Gonsalvus family, their travels from court to court, and his correspondence with the Swiss physician Felix Platter (1536–1614) about his observation of Pierre Gonsalvus.[29] By establishing the Gonsalvuses as legal precedents, Zacchia *de facto* gave hirsutes juridical personhood—a conclusion he justified through medical examinations and biblical quotes. Though he did not establish their ability to possess material goods or marry—his treatise appeared years after these precedents had already taken place—Zacchia nevertheless confirmed the fully human and independent status of hirsutes.

Another indication related to the independence of the Gonsalvus family is the fact that they were assigned a servant upon arriving in Parma in May of 1591. Not only was the family given a personal attendant, but they were also given a subvention of 11 scudi and 32 soldi, which later increased to 14 scudi and 20 soldi.[30] At a more personal and significant level, the marriage of Henri to Girolama di Giacomo Cintura, which occurred on June 15, 1602 in the church of Capodimonte, provides a relevant example of juridical independence of hirsute men. Not only was Henri's ties to the Farnese family materialized through the dowry that Odoardo Farnese gave to the man's glabrous bride, but he was also allotted a piece of land bordering the Farnese estate in Capodimonte.[31] These instances do not, however, confirm the consistency of human status for hirsutes. Indeed, a Medici Christmas inventory dated 1546 lists a box of fruit and animals made of sugar, two savage men, masks, glass animals, and cloth for a dwarf's socks and undergarment.[32] As inventories were records of ducal and regal possessions, they offer glimpses into the politics of display associated with the households that produced them. In this case, the liminal position of these *homini salvatichi* is particularly legible—even if they were not actual hirsutes, they were "wild men" and, as such, monsters on the margins of civilized codes. Because no rhetorical difference is noted between the ways in which the objects and the live beings are listed, this inventory thus registers the savage men as objects akin to glass animals given to Medici children. The only potentially humanizing difference here is found in the way in which another type of non-normative individual, the dwarf, is clearly referred to as a subject since he needs garments. The status of the Gonsalvus family was not one that erased the construction of hirsutes and their association with wildness; it only provided a distinct category for them as paradigmatic human abnormalities.[33]

As an identifiable family, the Gonsalvus members have left documented traces. In an account book related to the expenses of the court of Parma during the rule of Ranuccio Farnese, an entry from May 1591 reads: Don Pietro Gonzales Selvaggio.[34] This entry marks the first official record of the title and name given to the Tenerife-born man whose family became the most painted hirsutes in Europe. At least a decade before, in his four-volume study of natural history (published between 1575 and 1582), Joris Hoefnagel (1542–1601) had included illustrations of Pierre Gonsalvus and his wife—the only representations, indeed, of any humans found in all four volumes (Plate 6 and Plate 7). In the folio preceding the illustration of the couple, Hoefnagel inscribed a text that not only identified Pierre, but also traced his journey from the Canary Islands to France, where he had married and fathered hirsute children.[35] (The text held by Antoinette in Lavinia Fontana's depiction refers to her origins in the Canary Islands, as well.) The conquest of Tenerife in 1495 marked the end of the Canary Islands' independence and the beginning of their political and territorial attachment to the Spanish kingdom. Just like many native

Guanches, Pierre Gonsalvus's fate was to become a slave.[36] Paradoxically, however, his odd appearance, which would have ostracized him in an independent society, saved his life in an enslaved one. Indeed, he was offered not as a common slave, but rather as a precious gift upon the conquerors' return to the mainland.[37] A couple of years after these presents were brought back, the Venetian ambassador to Spain, Francesco Cappello, returned to the *Serenissima* with gifts from the Iberian peninsula. Those gifts included colorful parrots and a strange savage boy—Pierre Gonsalvus—who could not speak any comprehensible language.[38] The arrival of Pierre Gonsalvus at the age of ten to the court of Henri II of France therefore did not occur because of a direct Franco-Spanish connection, but via Venice. He was transported from Venice to the French court in connection with other courtly diplomatic gifts bestowed upon the future Henri II on the death of his father, François I, on March 31, 1547.[39] For forty-two years, Petrus Gonsalvus lived in Paris as part of Henri II's court, where he received military training and a literary education including Latin—an accomplishment that made him unusual, even among French courtiers.[40] During those years, Pierre Gonsalvus married a glabrous woman named Catherine, with whom he eventually had seven children.[41]

Following the crowning of former Huguenot Henri de Navarre as Henri IV, King of France, many religious disputes and armed conflicts arose. After the death of Henri II in 1559, Pierre Gonsalvus stayed in court under the auspices of François II, Charles IX, and Henri III, though it is probably the Queen Mother Catherine de'Medici Valois (1519–1589) who pushed for the continuum in the life of the Gonsalvuses at the court of France. However, once Catherine de'Medici Valois died in 1589 and her Catholic son Henri III was assassinated, the Gonsalvus family found itself without protection. Because he was the nephew of the King of Spain Felipe II, Alessandro Farnese (1545–1592), Duke of Parma, was sent to Paris to help the Catholic Legion headed by the Duke of Mayenne, Charles de Lorraine. Feeling tired and sick, Alessandro Farnese decided to return to Parma and, having taken an interest to the Gonsalvus family while in Paris, opted to send them to Parma as well. Even though Alessandro Farnese died in Arras before reaching Parma, the Gonsalvus family's fate was sealed.[42] Pierre Gonsalvus, his wife Catherine, their son Henri, and daughters Madeleine, Françoise, and Antoinette were sent to Parma. These tumultuous times crystallize the moment when Catherine de'Medici Valois's protection of this hirsute family becomes particularly relevant. When Henri II died, it was Catherine de'Medici Valois who offered her protection as Regent of France to the family of monsters. Owning the Gonsalvus family did not afford Catherine the same status as owning dwarves; whereas dwarves served as social indicators of status, hirsutes were seen by most people as neither civilized enough to be part of a human society, nor beastly enough to be entirely relegated to the animal world. Indeed, while Henri II and Catherine may have viewed the Gonsalvuses as having acquired civilized manners, succeeding monarchs and courts may not have shared in this opinion. Catherine's gesture to protect the Gonsalvus family referred to her husband's desire to educate and shelter the hirsute family, and to her own desire to protect them and salvage the family her husband had supported. Through the kingships of her sons Charles IX and Henri III, and eventually through that of her son-in-law Henri IV, Catherine did not falter in her pledge to the Gonsalvus family, and by extension, to her late husband, in spite of the implication of savagery and foreignness associated with hirsutes in the collective imaginary. After the death of her husband, Catherine needed to establish herself as an essential instrument of rulership, to maintain what she had fought to establish. Through her visible role as Regent, she tightly controlled the politics of her adopted country and attempted to assure the continuity of the Valois dynasty. Through her private protection and adoption of monsters, she transcended her foreignness and established a dual type of legitimacy: that of a courtier linked to the strongest ruling families of Europe, and that of a caring widow, safeguarding her husband's emotional legacy.

Interestingly, Catherine's 1589 testament is silent on what is to be left to the Gonsalvus family; whereas it states that 2,000 *écus* be given to each of the dwarves, no entry appears for any of the Gonsalvuses.[43] This omission complicates the juridical personhood attributed to the hirsute family. Dwarves' positions oscillated between that of subject/object, as is demonstrated in inventories where dwarves appear as either objects of curiosity or attendants; because of their rarity, however, the legal position of the hirsutes was neither well-defined nor, as in the case of Catherine's testament, defined at all. Legal documents attesting to the details of the life of Pierre Gonsalvus at the court of Henri II only press the issue further. For instance François de la Vacherie, who was the *gouverneur* in 1552, had the "charge and governing authority of the Savage of the King our Lord" and authorized to give fifty *sous* per day for the "food, governing, and expenses of the Savage."[44] However, the title of the de la Vacherie as *gouverneur* problematizes the position of the hirsute at court, for one could be a *gouverneur* to either animals or humans. This unresolved dichotomy becomes even more complex after the death of Catherine de'Medici Valois. Until 1589, the Gonsalvuses remained with her—one assumes under her more or less distant protection—in Paris. It is only following her death that records of their travels to Bologna, Parma, Ferrara, and Rome appear. Whereas loss of patronage does not necessarily mean loss of protection, in this case and because of the many political turmoils that occurred in and around the court of France, it is very likely that until the Queen Mother was alive, protection was guaranteed to the hairy family; when she died, their wellbeing was no longer guaranteed. They had to use their wondrous qualities as human-beasts to be shown, adopted, or accepted in various courts, as their only means of survival. Once the different Gonsalvuses found their ways into suitably protective courts, their human qualities could resurface. One could infer that it is precisely this situation which Catherine sought to avoid for the Gonsalvuses. By allowing them to remain in Paris, she allowed them to remain human. Whereas Catherine's public presentation as a widow guaranteed her position as Regent of France, her protection of the Gonsalvus family signaled her loyalty to Henri II. The dwarves visualized her courtly status, while the hirsutes provided her with a radical alterity beyond her own. Their presence at court might have provided a physical presence that was even more foreign than that of Catherine, but they also stood as reminders of Henri's human generosity.

Interestingly, although Catherine was occasionally depicted with court dwarves, there are no known images that associate her with the Gonsalvus family. This absence echoes the carefully-constructed public choices made by this exiled Italian ruler. Depicting herself alongside "wild men" in the French collective imaginary would not have supported her ruling ambitions. Mimicking the ruler-dwarf pairing found in other powerful European courts, on the other hand, did promote her objectives—even if this required that her compassionate private behavior be eclipsed by a publicly calculating performance. Indeed, hirsutes did not function as imperfect mirrors of perfect royal bodies in the same way that dwarves did. The bodies of the Gonsalvuses were so distant from the civilized normative self promoted at court that their wildness could only, remotely, serve to mitigate Catherine's foreignness. A close visual and recorded association may have been equivalent to admitting records of social ties to these uncivilized monsters.

After they left the court of France, the Gonsalvuses need to travel to the various courts where patrons could offer them a decent standard of living, one to which they had grown accustomed. On their way to the Farnese state, the Gonsalvuses stopped in Basel in 1591. While there, the Swiss physician Felix Platter examined Pierre Gonsalvus and noted his observations *post facto* in a medical treatise written between 1612 and 1614.[45] Though he did not distinguish Pierre by name, the Helvetic doctor identified him as an exceptionally hairy man who was very dear to Henri II. Platter did not attribute any monstrous qualities to the hirsute man and kept his examination within the realm of the medical, including his observations in the third volume of his treatise, which dealt entirely with deformities.[46] Under the title *Pilosi et Hirsuti admodum hominess quidam*, Platter devoted two full pages to explicating the details of the visual appearance of this hairy family.[47] Platter wrote about a distinct family and during a specific time in order to look at them under a purely objective medical lens. In this way, he dissociated himself from previous writings loosely based on the idea of hirsutism, rather than on a series of case studies illustrating a congenital disease and not the symptom of a moral failure. Platter, and later Aldrovandi, had no understanding of the causes for the unusual corporeal pilosity of the Gonsalvuses. However, the written and visual accounts they left have helped identify the genetic causes that affected Pierre, his three daughters, and two of his four sons.

Lavinia Fontana's portrait also leaves a visual trace of the phenotypical articulation of the Ambras syndrome. In addition to her portrait of Antoinette, many other paintings and prints of the Gonsalvus family were created in the sixteenth century and survive today. For instance, four paintings, each representing a different member of the Gonsalvus family, were produced around 1582 (Figs. 4.3, 4.4, 4.5, and 4.6).

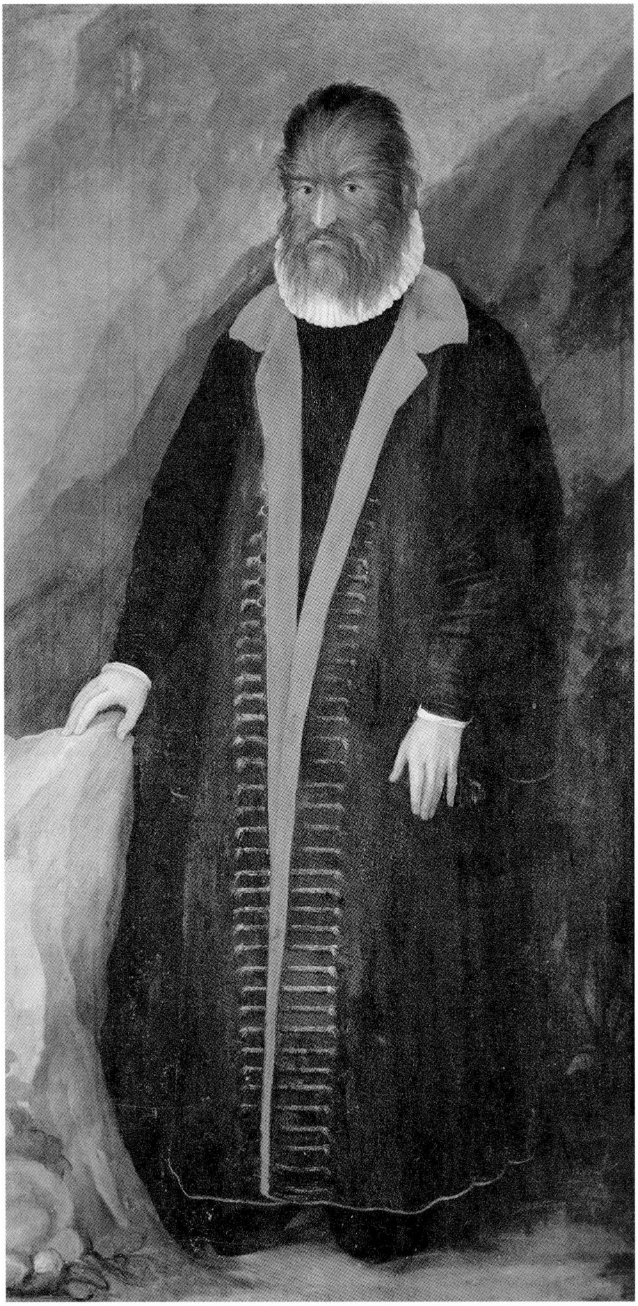

Figure 4.3. Anonymous, *Portrait of Pierre Gonsalvus*, ca. 1585, Schloss Ambras, Innsbruck. Erich Lessing/Art Resource, New York

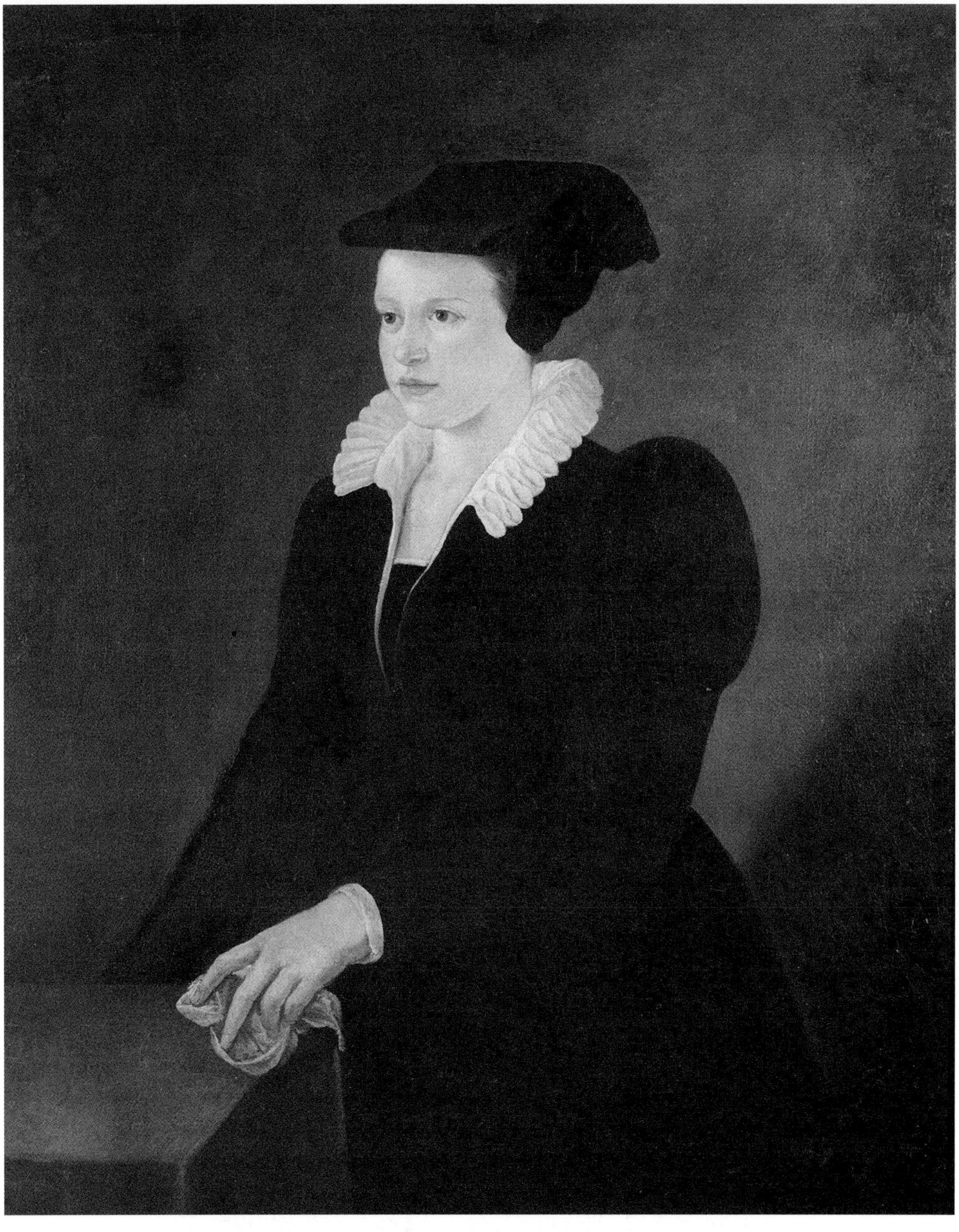

Figure 4.4. Anonymous, *Portrait of the Wife of Pierre Gonsalvus*, ca. 1585, Kunsthistorisches Museum, Vienna

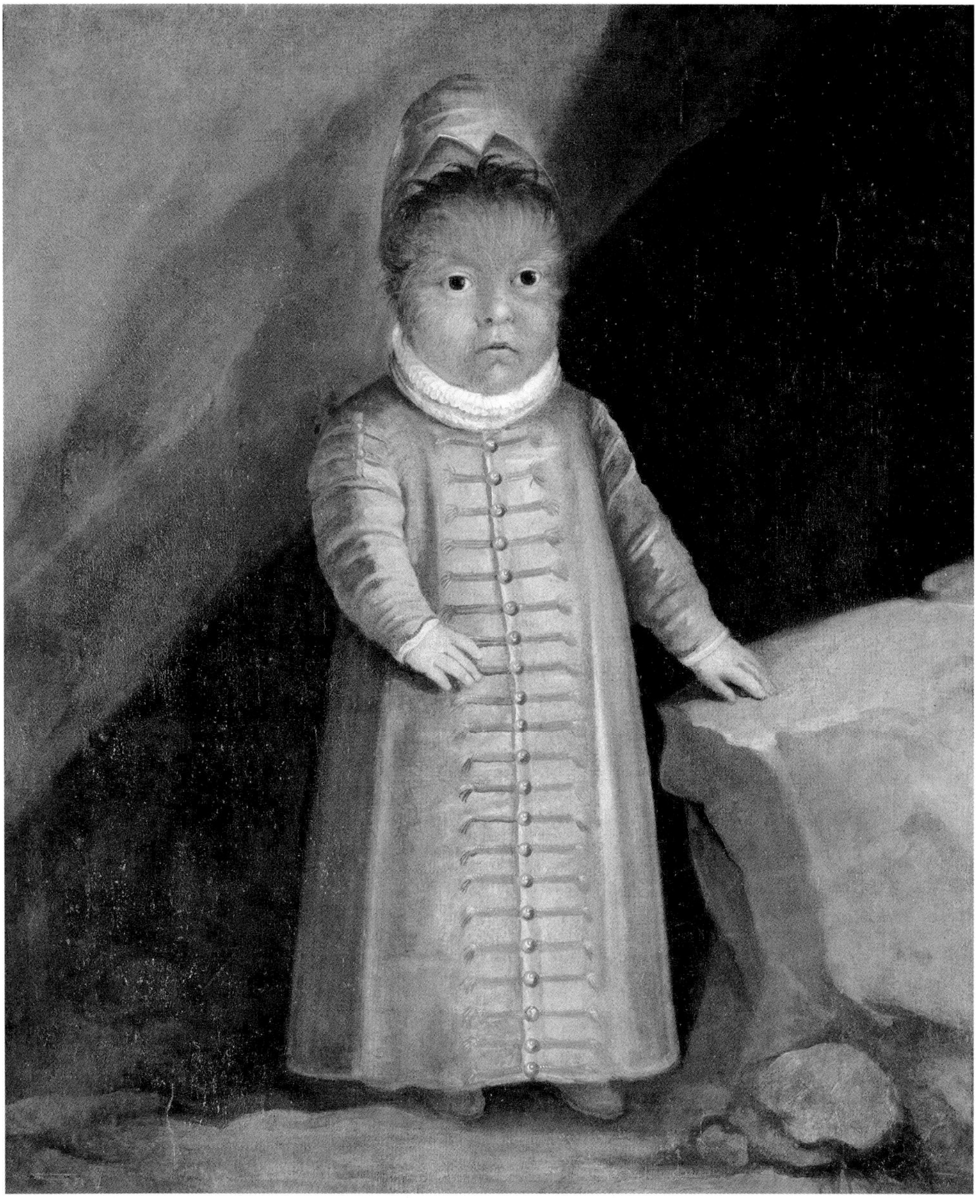

Figure 4.5. Anonymous, *Portrait of the Son of Pierre Gonsalvus*, ca. 1585, Schloss Ambras, Innsbruck. Erich Lessing/Art Resource, New York

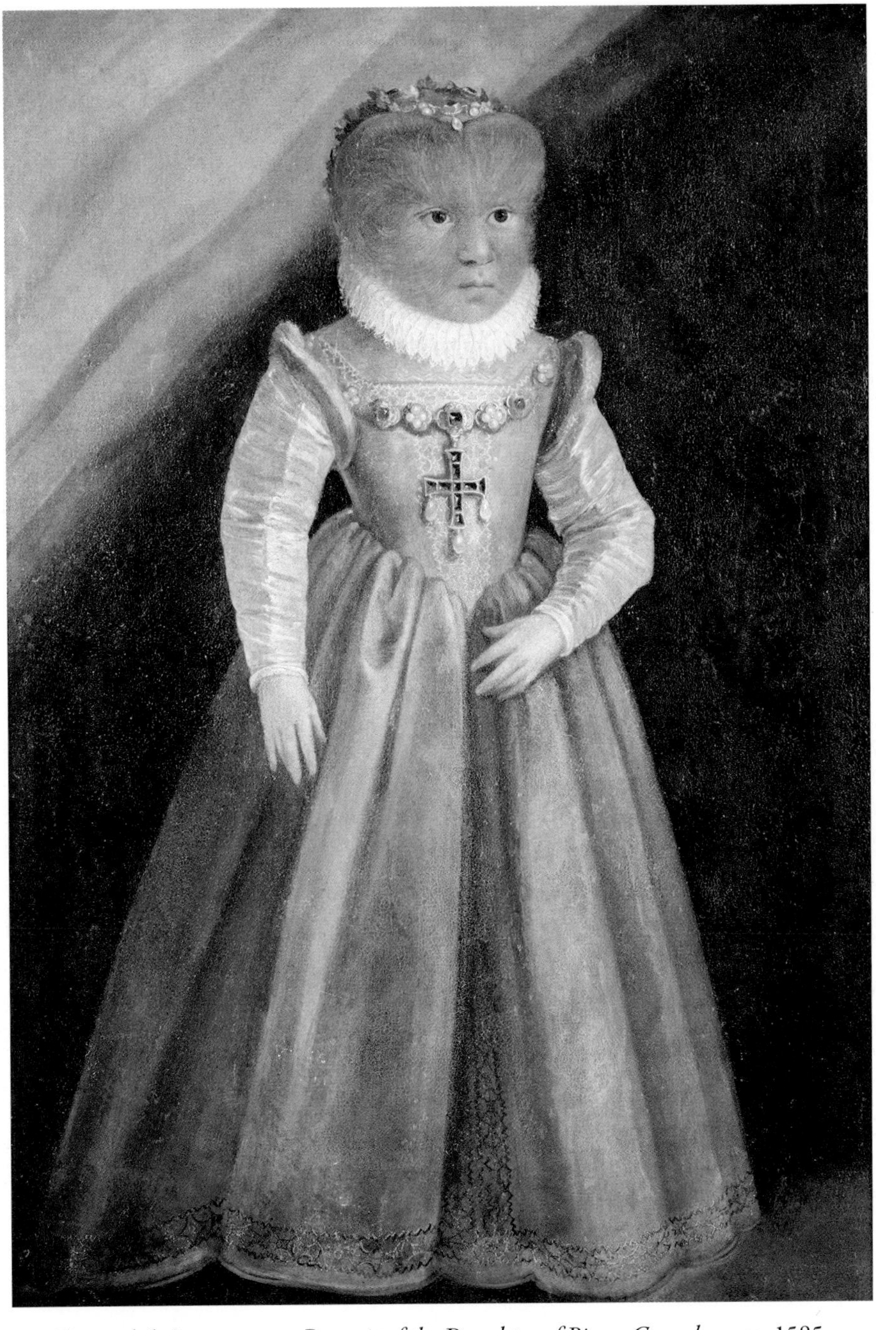

Figure 4.6. Anonymous, *Portrait of the Daughter of Pierre Gonsalvus*, ca. 1585, Schloss Ambras, Innsbruck. Erich Lessing/Art Resource, New York

Pierre Gonsalvus, his daughter Madeleine, his son Henri, and his wife Catherine are the lone subjects of the series. Pierre, Madeleine, and Henri all wear clothes that identify them as potential civilized human beings; however, they are all painted in front of cave-like backgrounds. Christiane Hertel has argued that these settings, in contrast to the courtly clothing that the Gonsalvus family wears in these images, link them to a "primitive" and "hidden" place in nature.[48] Though the dress of the Gonsalvuses—and of Antoinette in particular—played a crucial role in the projection of their characters, the cave setting was also reference to their foreignness, as well as a wild one. Indeed, many Guanches were troglodytes—cave dwellers—and the conquering Spaniards would have been able to witness the private dwellings of the people they were enslaving. The subsequent association of the Gonsalvus family with caves therefore likely referred to their origins in the Canary Islands.[49] Furthermore, only Catherine is painted in an interior scene, whereas the rest of her family is evidently outside, closer to nature. The juxtaposition of the courtly garb with a coarse external setting serves to highlight the unsettling tension found in representing anatomically unusual individuals as part of a courtly discourse and thus in framing monstrous visual subjects with an artistic rhetoric meant to idealize aesthetic qualities. Aside from Catherine who was glabrous, the detail on the face and hands of the Gonsalvus family are similar to those found later in Fontana's portrait of Antoinette. Hoefnagel's *Ignis* illustration does not stray from this standard, since it presents the Gonsalvus family as possessing all characteristics associated with hypertrichosis lanuginosa universalis. Hoefnagel also places the elegantly dressed Gonsalvus family in a nature scene, indicated by branches to the right of Petrus and by rocks, on which Henri leans. Unlike the Austrian depiction, however, Hoefnagel does not isolate Catherine in an interior scene and in fact emphasizes her connection to her husband: her right hand rests on the back of Pierre's left shoulder, intimating the relationship between them. Dirck de Quade van Ravesteyn's portrait of the Gonsalvus family painted between 1600 and 1612 also emphasizes their external qualities (Fig. 4.7). In particular, the painter pays great attention to showing the hair on the face of the subjects, while emphasizing the smoothness of the hands of the hirsute family. Yet, unlike Hoefnagel or the Austrian portraits' artist, Ravesteyn paints classical columns behind the family. His portrait bears the most resemblance to that of Fontana because of the tension found in juxtaposing deformed individuals to indices of civility. Not only do their clothes speak to their human qualities, and the columns to their cultural access, but the composition also echoes typical family portraits where the position of each member speaks to his or her place in the nuclear social realm. To the right, Catherine is seated, both her hands placed on her son Henri's shoulder. He leans on her lap while his sister Madeleine stands to his right, holding his hand. Standing taller than anyone in the painting is Pierre, gazing directly at the viewer and thus presenting his family.

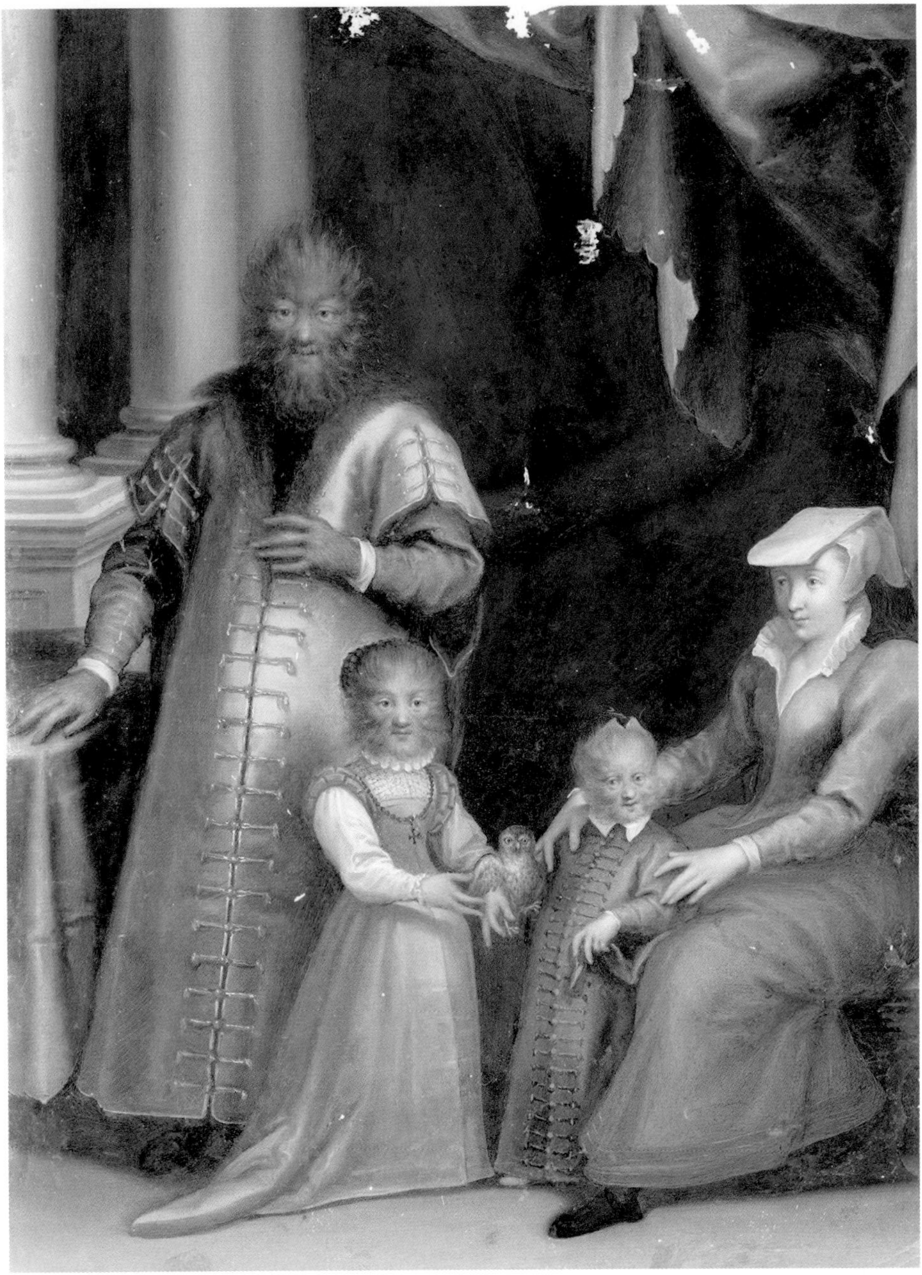

Figure 4.7. Dirck (de Quade) van Ravesteyn, *Petrus Gonsalvus and His Family*, ca. 1600–12, Österreichische Nationalbibliothek, Vienna

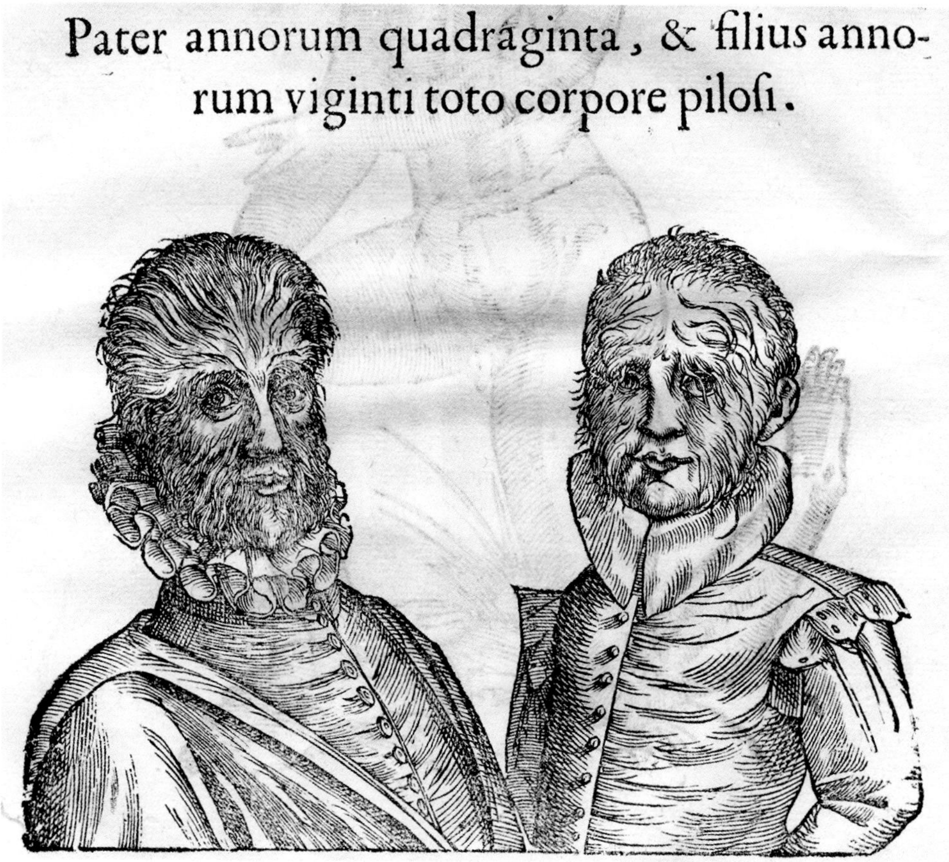

Figure 4.8. Ulisse Aldrovandi, prints of the Gonsalvus family from *Monstrorum Historia*, 1642, Wheaton College Permanent Collection, Newell Bequest Fund, Norton, Massachusetts

Using a different visual vocabulary, Ulisse Aldrovandi's prints, produced in the 1590s, and published posthumously in 1642, assert the medical syndrome of the Gonsalvus family members by omitting such human narrative and by presenting the viewer mostly with the unusual facial characteristics of the family (Fig. 4.8). In fact, Catherine is not depicted at all, since she held no anatomically intriguing qualities. Unlike previously mentioned artists, Aldrovandi's connection to the Gonsalvuses was not primarily guided by visual curiosity, but rather by a scientific inquiry, one that led to fruitful productions and interesting collaborations.

Ulisse Aldrovandi had a particular interest in anatomical and pathological rarities, since monstrous individuals allowed curious scientists to apply at once their medical, natural, and sensory knowledge. Within this conceptual framework, the Gonsalvus family provided an ideal subject of inquiry for the Bolognese naturalist. However, while condoning the study of monstrous objects or entities who aroused wonder, Aldrovandi condemned excessive representations of such *mirabilia* that strayed away from the truth and added marvelous qualities to increase the stimulation of the senses.[50] Therefore, not only did he need to experience first-hand the marvelous qualities of the Gonsalvus family, but he also needed an artist who would stay true to *imitare* while maintaining a semblance of *ritrarre*; displacing the balance toward the latter would only tilt the truth. The idea of the artist as a visual witness was essential to Aldrovandi.[51] The negotiations that occurred between Lavinia Fontana and Ulisse Aldrovandi are not entirely clear, however we do know how the two came into contact. Prospero Fontana (1512–1597), Lavinia Fontana's father, entertained a close friendship with Bologna's most famous naturalist; among the elite intellectual network that revolved around Aldrovandi, Gabriele Paleotti (1522–1597), his brother the senator Camillo Paleotti, and the historian Carlo Sigonio (1523–1584) were all friends of the Fontanas and commissioned works from Lavinia Fontana.[52] It is no surprise that Aldrovandi's relation with Lavinia Fontana developed during the life of her father and lasted after Prospero died. The naturalist mentioned her, as well as Prospero, in his *manoscritti* in 1577 where he refers to Lavinia Fontana as *Lavinia pictrix*.[53] Meeting the Gonsalvuses, and having their likeness recorded, involved another series of planned choices. Lavinia Fontana and Antoinette Gonsalvus's acquaintance was not accidental. The inscription held by Antoinette in her portrait indicates not only the location and provenance of the painting, but also those of the hirsute girl. At the court of Ranuccio Farnese beginning in 1591, the Gonsalvus family had become almost well known in the city of Parma as they were among the Farnese family. In 1593, the Marchioness of Soragna, Isabella Pallavicini moved to a palazzo in Parma. There, she met little Antoinette and requested the girl as a gift; her wish was granted.[54] During a trip to Bologna in April of 1594 to see the senator Mario Casali, Isabella Pallavicini took Antoinette with her—and thus, at Casali's suggestion, she introduced the hirsute girl to Aldrovandi.[55] Following Aldrovandi's examination of the hirsute girl, the Marchioness of Soragna asked Fontana to create a picture of Antoinette (in fact, Mario Casali himself may have contacted Lavinia Fontana independently, since his brother became Lavinia's son's godfather and they were all well acquainted with each other).[56] Although it is known that the Marchioness commissioned the painting, the recipient of the painting—if other than herself—remains unknown. It could have been someone who did not have the opportunity to see Antoinette often or at all, as the portrait would have served as a replacement for direct observation. In a 1626–1627 inventory for the Duke of Mantua, Vincenzo I Gonzaga (1562–1612), a portrait of a hairy girl is recorded, most likely Antoinette's portrait.[57] It is known, therefore, that the portrait eventually ended up with the Gonzaga family before it was bought and sent to England. However, from 1595, when it was commissioned, to 1626–1627 when a source places it in the Gonzaga family collection, its whereabouts remain unknown.

The chance to observe the hairy girl *ad vivum* did not elude Aldrovandi, who also took advantage of Antoinette's presence to have her depicted. A man named Brumanno recorded the little girl's features, and the images he produced were later used for the woodprints that populated the posthumous 1642 *Monstrorum Historia* (Fig. 4.9).[58]

Interestingly, Aldrovandi chose to display images of the Gonsalvus family in his villa in San Antonio di Savena; he did so by framing the portraits of himself and his wife Francesca Fontana with the Medici grand dukes—Francesco I (1541–1587) and Ferdinando I (1549–1609)—on one side and the Gonsalvuses on the other.[59] The elaborate iconographies that were used to decorate Aldrovandi's villa were based on the myth of Ulysses, but were developed in more complex ways so as to tie the naturalist's biography with his theories on nature and his social stance. It was also an expansion of the concepts elaborated in his museum, but one that could find a more personal articulation and more discrete audience. Paula Findlen aptly states that the visual program of Aldrovandi's villa was an extension of his unfinished autobiography.[60] The *imprese* and the portraits found there were thus intricate statements on the naturalist's identity.[61] Between the portraits of highly civilized patrons—the Medici grand dukes—and those of "wild" creatures, we find Aldrovandi and his wife, linking nature and civilization, allowing them to communicate. Lina Bolzoni suggests that the presence of the Gonsalvuses so close to the Medici and the Aldrovandi also holds a moral component difficult to disregard: Aldrovandi is able to observe and gather the principled teachings that nature can offer to humans.[62] In this regard, Aldrovandi's enterprise joins Agostino Carraci's in the presentation of Amon, Henri, and Pietro: men learn from nature, but monsters who are closer to animals understand these teachings more immediately than men who have to gather that knowledge less instinctively. Fredrika Jacobs has convincingly argued that the costumes of the Medici, thus juxtaposed with those of the Gonsalvuses, established equivalences rather than differences.[63] However, removed from the villa, the portraits of Aldrovandi's treatise lost their meaning. They fell, instead, within the realm of the scientific and left little room for humanization since the Gonsalvus family was presented among monsters and, thus, lost this complex and rich contextual explanation.

Lavinia Fontana may have observed Antoinette by permission of Aldrovandi and probably in his presence. Yet her depiction of the hirsute girl and her understanding of Antoinette as part of a human family with a complex personal history differed greatly from that of the Bolognese naturalist. Most of the scholarship dealing with the Blois painting establishes that Antoinette's portrait was the direct result of a collaboration between Fontana and Aldrovandi, with Aldrovandi holding the pivotal role in the relationship. However, aside from Caroline Murphy, no scholar mentions the crucial relation between Fontana and Senator Mario Casali. In fact, since the Marchioness of Soragna was staying with Casali in Bologna, it is more than likely that Fontana might have been contacted at the same time, if not *before* Aldrovandi.[64] Her interaction with Antoinette might thus have been less scientifically oriented than has been previously assumed. For her portrait

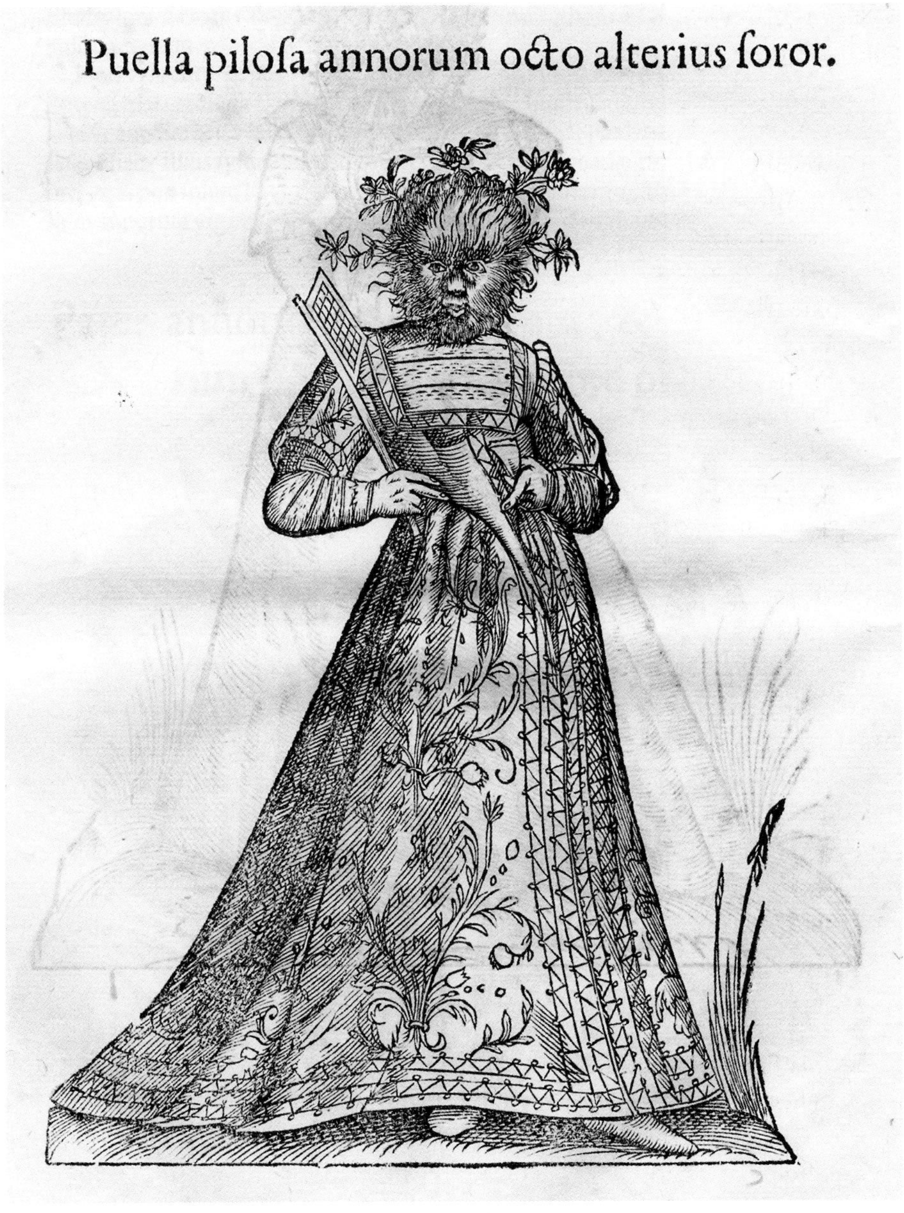

Figure 4.9. Ulisse Aldrovandi, print of Antoinette Gonsalvus's family from *Monstrorum Historia*, 1642, Wheaton College Permanent Collection, Newell Bequest Fund, Norton, Massachusetts

of Antoinette Gonsalvus, Fontana's preliminary drawing confirms the originality of her composition and study from nature (Fig. 4.1). The J.P. Morgan Library owns nineteen drawings by Lavinia Fontana gathered in an album designed specifically to hold them: the album, which is bound in dark blue goatskin and is tooled in gold, measures 334 mm by 284 mm and has only nineteen pages, enough to accommodate all nineteen drawings. In addition, the various drawings look as if they have been cut out from their original support and glued onto the pages of this album. Each has a drawn squared frame, added after the collage was completed. On most of the drawings, it is possible to see an original ruling separation, delineating the future location of each mini-portrait.[65] The portrait of Antoinette Gonsalvus appears on the eighth folio. The use of red and black chalk gives the drawing delicate lines and defined hues. Even though the outline of Antoinette's shirt is visible, most of the details stop at her neck; the ruffles of her shirt are outlined, but the chalk traces fade and eventually disappear below her shoulder. Visually, Lavinia Fontana treated the hirsute girl in the exact same fashion as she treated all of her preliminary portrait drawings. That is to say, the artist mainly emphasized the facial features of her subject and did not pay much attention to her garb. In a sense, the drawing of Antoinette is just another generic portrait in red and black chalk, just like those of Aldrovandi or Fontana in the same series. Unlike Aldrovandi's scientifically guided endeavor however, Fontana's seems to have been, from the onset, more personal and humanizing.

Antoinette's position was a complex one. Whereas her mother was a "normal" glabrous French woman, her father was a foreigner who carried the burden of his physical appearance. However, it is precisely because of her father's education and noble contacts, gained through his condition as a hirsute, that the whole family found protection and livelihood in courtly spheres. This central dichotomy in Antoinette's life is echoed in Fontana's representation of the girl. The main unresolved dichotomy of Antoinette's life was the seemingly impossible reconciliation of her physical appearance with a "normal" and civilized life. Her father's success at court opened many social and legal doors for the little hirsute girl, yet when Fontana painted her, Antoinette was too young to grasp the unique nature of her station in life (she was around seven years old when the portrait was painted). She was also at the end of a tumultuous period in which her family's fate was dictated by political alliances and wars of religion. Fontana's iconographical insertions thus served as markers of what the artist saw in her subject's life and her turbulent family history. Antoinette was born in the court of Henri II. Though she was born with physical deformities, she was the daughter of a respected man whose title had been recorded officially as "Don" only three years after her birth. Consequently, Antoinette grew up in several court circles and, probably like her father, benefited from the educational opportunities there. The inherent tension in showing a monstrous-looking individual holding a written letter did not escape Lavinia Fontana. Antoinette's delicate gesture and knowing gaze establish her literacy, paralleling the first-person account found in the inscription. Furthermore, the text of the letter stands in for the girl's noble lineage. Fontana's brush established for her both a voice and a dignified family tree.[66] The flowers in Antoinette's hair emphasize her dual nature in another way. Behind her right ear we see a sprig of lilies of the valley, and on top of her head rests a crown of flowers made of clovers, snowdrops, and a carnation.[67] The lily of the valley was recognized as a symbol of humility, because it blooms face down; purity, because of its white color and light crisp scent; and wilderness, because it grows without needing care.[68] The crown of flowers is an obvious attempt to show her gentility yet even this symbol is ambiguous. The flowers here are carefully chosen to emphasize humility and femininity—particularly the small rose—yet all are common native species that grow in the wild. This vacillation between wild and delicate, humble and savage, speaks to the social conflicts Fontana may have foreseen in little Antoinette's future struggles. Though the flowers do not have any specific association in Cesare Ripa's *Iconologia*, the crown in which they are arranged looks very similar to flowers seen on the heads of young maidens in other portraits done by Lavinia Fontana. For instance, we see a comparable display in the hair of two women in the retinue of the Duke and Duchess of Mantua, depicted in Fontana's *Visit of the Queen of Sheba to Solomon* (ca. 1600) (Fig. 4.10).

In her *Portrait of a Noblewoman*, painted in the early 1590s and depicting a young woman to be married (Fig. 4.11), Fontana carefully painted a crown of flowers on the head of the betrothed.[69] The association of crowns of flowers with young women, or women to be married, is a notable one as it places Antoinette within the same realm as other Bolognese women fashioning themselves as feminine and graceful assets for a future family. Cesare Ripa notes that the crown of gold surmounting a virgin's head stands for purity; this unbroken circle is paralleled in the one Fontana places on Antoinette's head.

One of the most telling visual tensions in this portrait is Fontana's juxtaposition of a monstrous face with luxurious garments. Most viewers would have easily assessed the worth of the cloth worn by Antoinette.[70] Fontana took care to paint the sheen on the cloth, thus indicating silk, and she also paid great attention to the embroideries on the sleeves of Antoinette's dress. Both of these elements would have represented a significant outlay of labor and material for the little girl's clothes. Silk, a specialty of Bolognese weavers, was expensive in the sixteenth century—whereas the workmanship put into the embroidered sleeves of Antoinette's garment further accentuates the lavishness of her costume.[71] This luxurious choice reflected the social status of the patron who commissioned the portrait, of course, but it also lent Antoinette herself a sense of prestige. Indeed, the type of cloth represented in Antoinette's portrait is akin to that of many other Bolognese noblewomen. The length of the portrait and its dark undifferentiated background serve only to highlight the precious clothing of the hirsute girl.[72] The costume in Antoinette's portrait is telling in its difference from Carracci's painting of Henri where the hirsute man is presented wearing a *tamarco*, thus linking him to the Guanches. Furthermore, because the *tamarco* is in fact made of animal skin, the visual association of Henri with

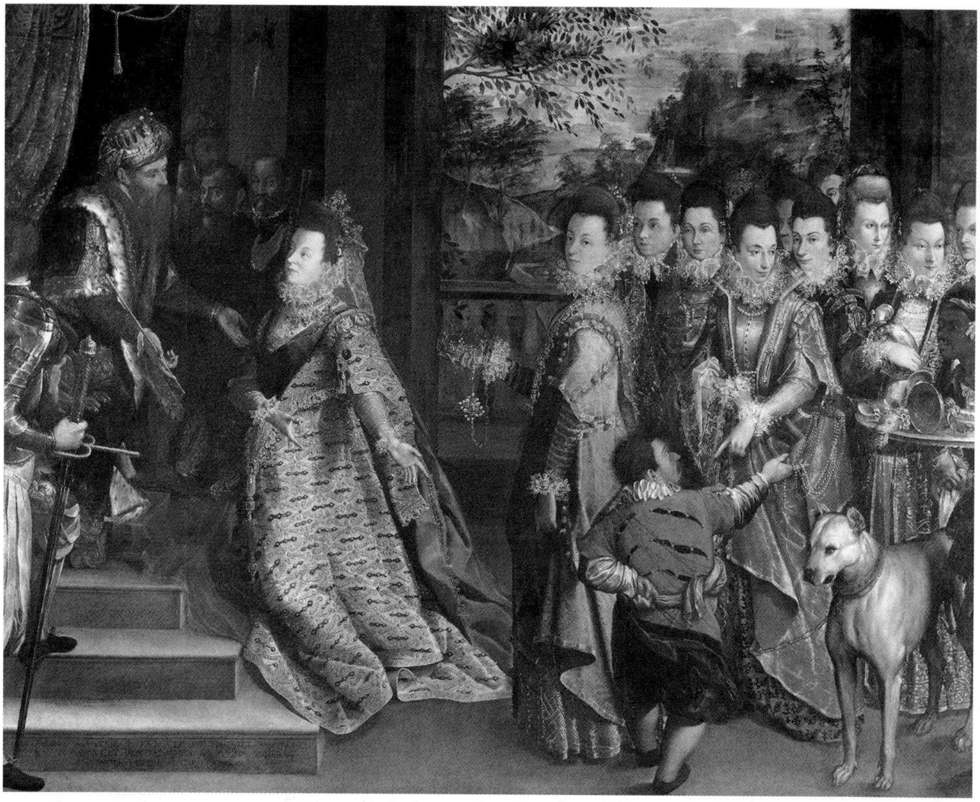

Figure 4.10. Lavinia Fontana, *Visit of the Queen of Sheba to Solomon*, ca. 1600, National Gallery of Ireland, Dublin

the animal kingdom is undeniable. In opposition, Fontana ascribed decidedly human qualities to Antoinette.[73] Antoinette did embody the wondrous qualities sought in a collectible monster, but she did not come to court as an entertainer or earn her life through grotesque displays. Therefore, while she was also a collectible monster, her status differed from that of Morgante since she was born in a court of a courtly educated father, and benefited directly from the pecuniary and educational advantages of the social sphere in which she lived. The active intervention of her portrait in the discourse on Renaissance portraiture thus does not lie in the reversal of *imitare* and *ritrarre*, but rather in the expansion of *imitare* to equate the purpose of *ritrarre* in deciphering the noble character of the sitter. Far from masking the hypertrichosis condition of Antoinette Gonsalvus, Lavinia Fontana used it to emphasize the position of a human being whose position oscillated between that of a curious object and that of a dignified subject. Like Fredrika Jacobs, I believe Antoinette was not depicted as an "anomaly" but rather as an "asperity," a being filled with unequal qualities.[74] In spite of the careful attention paid to Antoinette's

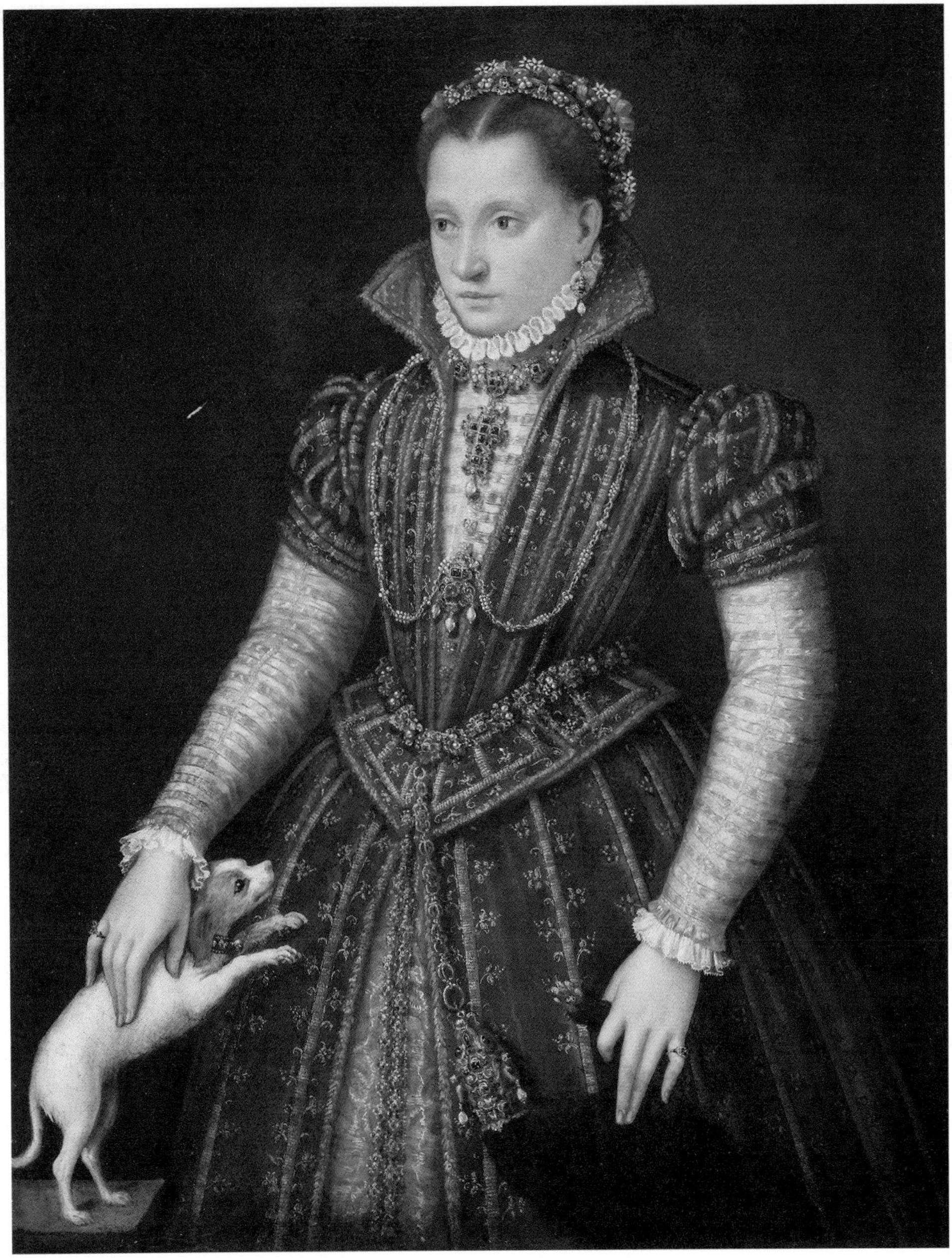

Figure 4.11. Lavinia Fontana, *Portrait of a Noblewoman*, early 1590s, National Museum of Women in The Arts, Washington, D.C.

condition, the rest of the details in this portrait almost obliterate the little girl's monstrous attributes. The combination of her epigram with those flowers and the silk brocade of her garment turn this "monstrous" girl into a marriageable member of the retinue of Isabella Pallavicini. Indeed, as with the portrait of any courtier, it is the character of Antoinette that emerges as the strongest subtext of this painting—not her ties to wild men, their feral qualities, or her status as a collectible object.

Lavinia Fontana's visual choices transformed Antoinette from a savage being to a civilized young girl, expunging the stigma of wilderness attached to her genetic condition. Fontana purposefully depicted Antoinette as a courtier able to master *civiltà* and consequently, as a civilized member of a court retinue. Fontana allowed Antoinette to play against the viewer's expectation by depicting her civilized *behavior* rather than by pointing to the predictable indices of savagery viewers would anticipate. Paolo Zacchia's use of the Gonsalvus family as legal precedents for the establishment of hirsutes' juridical personhood joined, rhetorically at least, Lavinia Fontana's effort by adding a sense of agency to the objectified subject. Fontana's portrait of Antoinette re-inscribed the curious within an early modern framework, ultimately adapting the precepts of Renaissance court portraiture to express not the monstrosity of her subject but her civility. The artist expanded the fixed meaning attributed to a court portrait, however, precisely by choosing the ways in which she depicted such an unusual subject. By means of this portrait, both Fontana and her subject created unstable and expandable boundaries for the representation of physical difference, as well as for early modern aesthetic sensibilities.

Notes

[1] The Gonsalvus name has many different forms, from Gonzales to Gonsalvez and to Gonsalus. For the sake of clarity, I use the more neutral and commonly used surname Gonsalvus. However, I use the French version of the given names for consistency and because most of the Gonsalvus children were born in France and their parents were educated in France.

[2] Henri is known as Arrigo Peloso in Carracci's painting. For general discussions on the Gonsalvus family, see Giovanna Galli, "Strano è bello," *Stile Arte* 63 (November 2002); Christiane Hertel, "Hairy Issues: Portraits of Petrus Gonsalvus and His Family in Archduke Ferdinand II's *Kunstkammer* and Their Contexts," *Journal of the History of Collections* 13, no. 1 (2001): 1–22; Alberto Manguel, "Lavinia Fontana: The Image as Understanding," in *Reading Pictures: A History of Love and Hate* (New York: Random House, 2000); and Merry Wiesner-Hanks, *The Marvelous Hairy Girls: The Gonzales Sisters and Their World* (New Haven and London: Yale University Press, 2009); and Roberto Zapperi, *Il selvaggio gentiluomo: L'incredibile storia di Pedro Gonzalez e dei suoi figli* (Rome: Donzelli Editore, 2005).

[3] Roberto Zapperi, *Un buffone e un nano fra due cardinali: Aspetti della comicità a Roma nell'ultimo Cinquencento* (Rome: Fondazione Camillo Caetani, 1995).

[4] The life of Henri is the most recorded of that of the Gonsalvus children. His four marriages and six children are all documented.

[5] F.A.M. Baumeister et al., "Ambras Syndrome: Delineation of a Unique Hypertrichosis Universalis Congenital and Association with a Balanced Pericentric Inversion (8)(p11.2;q22)," *Clinical Genetics* 44 (1993): 126.

[6] Daniel S. Wendelin, David N. Pope and Susan B. Mallory, "Hypertrichosis," *Journal of the American Academy of Dermatology* 48, no. 2 (February 2003): 164.

[7] Sigfrid A. Muller, "Hirsutism," *The American Journal of Medicine* 46, no. 5 (May 1969): 803–17.

[8] While this information is ahistorical in its detailing of balanced structural chromosomal aberration, it is important for the modern scholar as it allows for a more thorough understanding of the Gonsalvus's family condition and its phenotypical manifestation (visible). Information compiled from Gerald Karp, *Cell and Molecular Biology: Concepts and Experiments* (New York: John Wiley & Sons, 1996), 520 and 636–37 in particular. The ratio of genetic transmission is easily verifiable through a simple karyotype. Though the stability of the gene located on the eighth chromosome is debatable, it does not affect the inheritance ratio. Dr. Esther Guevara-Sanguinés suggests the possibility of a gene attached to an X chromosome in the case of a Mexican family in which males were more affected than females. However, the ratio of two sons/three daughters in the case of the Gonsalvus family eliminates this option. In addition, the genetic heterogeneity of the hypertrichosis trait does not affect its transmittal ratio, only its phenotypic expression. See Esther Guevara-Sanguinés et al., "Congenital Generalized Terminal Hypyertrichosis with Gingival Hyperplasia," *Pediatric Dermatology* 19, no. 2 (2002): 116.

[9] Personal letter from Françoise Launay to Sylvain Bellanger, May 12, 1997. Dr. Launay mentions two articles referring to the Ambras syndrome prior to public knowledge of this portrait. The articles in question are: James G. Ravin and Gerard P. Hodge, "Hypertrichosis Portrayed in Art," *JAMA* 207, no. 3 (1969): 533–35 and W. Felgenhauer, "Hypertrichosis Lanuginosa Universalis," *Journal de Génétique Humaine* 17 (1969): 1–44.

[10] Information gathered from Archie Gordon, *A Wild Flight of Gordons: Odd and Able Members of the Gordon Families* (London: Weidenfeld and Nicolson, 1985); Fiche recapitulative pour la demande de subvention présentée au fonds regional d'acquisition des musées, March 3, 1997; *Bulletin de la Société des amis du Château et des Musées de Blois*, 25 (June 1997): 8–9; and Francis Haskell, Personal letter to Sylvain Bellanger, August 18, 1998. While the portrait was sold for only 32 pounds in 1947, the Musée des Beaux-Arts du Château de Blois acquired it for 287,300 francs, the equivalent of approximately 26,000 pounds, more than 800 times its estimated value fifty years earlier.

[11] "Dall'I(s)ole Cannare fu condotto / al Ser.o Enrico re di Francia / D.Pietro huomo salvatico / de presente si trova presso / il ser.mo Duca di Parma del quale [fui] / io Antoinette, et hora mi trovo a presso alla Sig.ra Donn Isab[e]ll[a] / Pallavicina Sig.ra Marchesa / Di Soragna."

[12] Vera Fortunati, *Lavinia Fontana of Bologna 1552–1614* (Milan: Electa, 1998).

[13] Francis Haskell, Personal letter to Sylvain Bellanger, August 18, 1998, archives du Musée des Beaux-Arts du Château de Blois.

[14] Some relevant examples of portraits of the Gonsalvus family or members of the Gonsalvus family are: Anonymous artist, *Portrait of Petrus Gonsalvus* and *Portrait of Antoinette Gonsalvus*, 1580, Kunsthistorisches Museum, Vienna; Dirk de Quade van Ravestyn, *The Gonsalvus Family*, 1582, Osterreichische Nationalbibliothek, Vienna; Joris Hoefnagel, *Antoinette and Her Brother*, 1582, National Gallery of Art, Washington, D.C.

[15] This is indeed the main argument used by Giovanna Galli, Christiane Hertel, and Alberto Manguel.

[16] Joy Kenseth, ed., *The Age of the Marvelous* (Hanover: Hood Museum of Art, Dartmouth College, 1991), 329.

[17] Timothy Husband, *The Wild Man: Medieval Myth and Symbolism* (New York: The Metropolitan Museum of Art Press, 1980), 22. The manuscript in question is *Marvels of the East*, from England, eleventh century, Cotton Ms. Tiberius B. v., vol. i, fol. 81v., found in the British Library of London.

[18] Richard Bernheimer, *Wild Men in the Middle Ages: A Study in Art, Sentiment, and Demonology* (New York: Octagon Books, 1970), 22.

[19] Lynn Frier Kaufmann, *The Noble Savage: Satyr and Satyr Families in Renaissance Art* (Ann Arbor: UMI Research Press, 1984), 33.

[20] Ibid., 35. The author confirms Kauffmann's assessment since she participated in this tradition during the winter of 1988. *À bon entendeur* [...].

[21] Matteo Maria Boiardo, *Orlando Innamorato*, ed. Giuseppe Anceschi (Milan: Garzanti, 1978), 1:XXII, 7–8; 1:XXIII, 2–18: "Con lunga barba e gran capigliatura, / tutto peloso dal capo alle piante."

[22] Ludovico Ariosto, *Orlando furioso*, ed. Emilio Bigi (Milan: Rusconi, 1982), XXIII, 133: "E poi si squarciò i panni, e mostrò ignudo / l'ispido ventre e tutto 'l petto e 'l tergo."

[23] Kaufmann, *The Noble Savage*, 36–41. Additionally, Jean Bourdichon's early sixteenth-century depiction of the wild family fits into that schema. His image was accompanied by a text on the Four Conditions of Society and associated the wild state with a pure one, void of the fake and superficial riches of society. See Debra Higgs Strickland, *Saracens, Demons, and Jews: Making Monsters in Medieval Art* (New Jersey: Princeton University Press, 2003), 247.

[24] There is, nevertheless, an overlapping of the "wild" and magical qualities of hirsutes that never fully disappeared from the collective imaginary.

[25] Pierre Boaistuau, *Histoires prodigieuses* (Paris: Robert le Mangnier, 1566).

[26] Ibid., chapter 5, 14: "Il est tout certain que le plus souvent ces creatures monstrueuses precedent du iugement, Iustice, chastiement & malediction de Dieu, lequel permet que les pere & meres produisent telles abominations, en l'horreur de leur péché, par ce qu'ils se precipitent indiferemment, comme bestes brutes ou leur appetit les guide, sans respect ou observation d'age, de lieu, de temps, ou autres Loix ordonées de nature [...]."

[27] Ambroise Paré, *Les Oeuvres d'Ambroise Paré, conseiller et premier chirurgien du roy. Divisées en vingt huict Livres, Avec les figures & portraicts, tant de l'Anatomie, que des instruments de Chirurgie, & de plusieurs Monstres. Revueuës & augmentees par l'Autheur*, 4th edition (Paris: Gabriel Buon, 1585), chapter 1, 2010, Des Causes de monstres.

[28] Ibid., chapter 9, 2037: "Damascene, autheur grave, atteste avoir veu une fille velue comme un Ours, laquelle la mere avoit enfantee ainsi difforme & hideuse, pour avoir trop ententivement regardé la figure d'un sainct Jean, vestu de peau avec son poil, laquelle estoit attachée aux pieds de son lict, pendant qu'elle concevoit."

[29] Pauli Zacchiae Romani, totius status ecclesiastici proto-medici generalis, *Quaestionum medico-legalium, tomi tres, Editio prima Veneta, Lugdunensi & Noribergensi, quae passim soedis scatebant erroribus multò emendiator: Accedunt Interpolationes, & Auctaria ex novis Inventis & Observationibus Recentiorum Auctorum, Curà Joannis Danielis Horstii, Diversorum S.R.I. Principum Archiatri, & Collegii Medici Moeno-Francofurtani Senioris, Opus omnibus medicinae et juris utriusque peritis, Necnon Tribunalium (Ecclesiastici, Civilis) Assessoribus maximè necessarium* (Venice: Bonifacii Viezzeri, 1737), 107.

[30] Information gathered by Roberto Zapperi from the Archivio di Stato di Parma, Mastri Farnesiani, vols. 11–16. As cited in Zapperi, *Il selvaggio gentiluomo*, 167.

[31] Letter dated December 9, 1605 from Henri Gonsalvus to Cardinal Odoardo Farnese regarding the future construction of a house on the terrain given to him by the Cardinal: "Questa settimana proscima coprirò la mia casa si piace a iDio," and a letter dated to May 11, 1608 where Enrico Gonsalvus tells the Cardinal he now lives in his new home; "quattro giorni sono ho cominciato a mangiare nella casa nova." Archivio di Stato di Napoli, Archivio Farnesiano, 613 (II), cc. 932r and 936r; 614 (II), ca. 1004. Cited in Zapperi, *Il selvaggio gentiluomo*, 172 and 124.

[32] ASF, MP 1172, 1, 27. The list reads: "Scatola di frutte e animali di zuccero. 2 homini salvatichi. Maschere. Animaletti di vetro. La drappa per calze e gippone, al nano." Caroline Murphy generously shared this document with me and I am thankful to her.

[33] While examples of wild men and women do not abound in literature from the early modern period, later examples provide a notable contrast to the highly principled way in which the Gonsalvus family was treated. The bafflement of societies toward inhabitants of the wild did not diminish with the legal establishment of hirsutes as full juridical entities. The eighteenth century saw numerous episodes related to the conundrum posed by a being whose appearance was fully human, but whose behavior was incomprehensibly savage. The story of two boys found in the woods of the Aveyron region of France perplexed the inhabitants of the county, as well as the legal and medical authorities. Peter and Victor were found in 1724 and captured. Though visibly humans, accounts of their lives post-capture do not leave room for an assessment of the boys as fully human. These feral children provided an interesting counterpoint to the case of hirsutes. Indeed, physical appearance did not always matter as much as social skills in the determination of monstrousness or legal personhood. For more about eighteenth-century discourse conflating hirsutes and children raised in the wild, please see Julia V. Douthwaite, *The Wild Girl, Natural Man, and the Monster: Dangerous Experiments in the Age of Enlightenment* (Chicago and London: University of Chicago Press, 2002).

[34] Archivio di Stato di Parma, Mastri farnesiani 11, 250.

[35] The inscription reads: "GONSALVUS Alumnis REGIS GALLORUM / Ex Insulis Canariae ortus / Me teneriffa tulit: villos sed Corpore toto / Sparsit opus mirum naturae: Gallia, mater / Altera, me puerum nutrivit adusque virilem / Aetatem: docuitque feros deponere mores / Ingenuasq. Artes, linguamque sonare Latinam / Contingit et forma praestant; munere Divum / Coniunx et Thalami charissima pignora nostri / Cernere naturae licet hinc tibi munera: nati / Quod referunt alii matrem formaq. Colore / Ast alii patrem vestiti crine sequuntur / Conparvit Monachii boiorum Ao:1582."

[36] It is worth noting that the enslavement of Guanches was problematic: because they were Christians, Church officials did not condone the acquisition of, in this case, Catholic slaves.

[37] Felipe Fernández-Armesto, *The Canary Islands after the Conquest: The Making of a Colonial Society in the Early Sixteenth Century* (Oxford: Oxford University Press, 1982), 6, 37, and 40.

[38] Geoffrey Symcox, Giovanna Rabitti, and Peter D. Diehl, eds., *Italian Reports on America 1493–1522: Letters, Dispatches, and Papal Bulls. Repertorium Colombianum X* (Turnhout: Brepols Publishers, 2001), 91, 105, 107, 109–110, 111–112, 115–116.

[39] In a letter dated April 18, 1547 to the Duke of Ferrara, Ercole II d'Este (1508–1559), his ambassador Giulio Alvarotto described the gifts given to the future Henri II, including a ten-year-old boy covered in hair. Archivio di Stato di Modena, Archivio segreto estense, Cancelleria ducale,

Sezione estero, Carteggio ambasciatori, Francia, b. 24: "È stato donato al re un putto de circa X anni portato dalle Indie, molto bello, ma tutto piloso il volto et tutta la vita, come appunto si dipingono gl'humani silvatici. I pelli sonno longhi circa cinque dita. Sonna rari molto, tanto che si vedeno tutti i lineamenti deall fazza. Sonno di colore tané chiaro et molto sottili et fini più che'l pello di zebelino, et sanno de buon. Lui parla spagnuolo et va vestito come è l'ordinario d'ognuno. Però su per la vita ha il pello frusto. Non si chi l'habbi donato a Sua Maestà." Roberto Zapperi's transcription corrects the previously published one by C. Occhipinti, which contained several mistakes. See Zapperi, *Il selvaggio gentiluomo*, 158.

[40] Françoise Waquet, *Le latin ou l'empire d'un signe: XVIe–XXe siècle* (Paris: Albin Michel, 1998), 273.

[41] Zapperi, *Il selvaggio gentiluomo*, 65. The names of the children were: Madeleine (born ca. 1575, hirsute), Paul, Henri (born ca. 1580, hirsute), Françoise (born ca. 1582, hirsute), Antoinette (born ca. 1588, hirsute), Horace (born 1592, hirsute), Hercule (born 1595).

[42] Historical information gathered from André Alba et al., eds., *Malet et Isaac: L'Histoire Tome 2: L'Age classique: 1497–1789* (Paris: Hachette, 2002) and Zapperi, *Il selvaggio gentiluomo*, 71–76.

[43] MF 3952, Testament de Catherine de Médicis, 294r.

[44] Archives Nationales de Paris, Minutier Central, XIX, 184 and 187: "charge et gouvernement du saulvaige du roy nostre sire" and "nourriture, gouvernement, and despence du saulvaige."

[45] In his writings, Felix Platter dates his encounter with the Gonsalvus family to 1583. However, evidence regarding the age of the children he mentions, as well as the travel route of the Gonsalvus family would make such an encounter impossible in 1583. In addition, Platter also misdates several other events: for instance, he records the 1568 wedding of the Duke of Bavaria Wilhelm von Wittelsbach with Renata de Lorraine to 1574. This mistake is very telling since Platter actually attended the event. For details on Felix Platter's writings and his chronological inaccuracies, see Katharina Huber, *Felix Platters "Observationes": Studien zum Frühneuzeitlichen Gesundheitswesen in Basel*, Basel Beiträge zur Geschichtswissenschaft 177 (Basel: Schwabe, 2003).

[46] Felix Platter, *Observationum in Hominis Affectibus plerisa corporie animo, functionum laesione, dolore, aliave molestia et vitio intommodantibus* (Basel: Ludovici König and Conradi Waldkirchii, 1614).

[47] Ibid., 553–54. Platter detailed the bodily parts that did have hair and those that did not. He also gave a historical trace of the Gonsalvuses by linking them to the court of Henri II and that of Parma.

[48] Hertel, "Hairy Issues," 5.

[49] To Hertel's defense, she did not have knowledge of the Blois portrait before publishing her 2001 article and thus could not use the portrait as comparison material. For instance, the lack of cave-like setting in Antoinette's portrait may be due to her holding a letter that speaks to her father's origins. Personal letter from Christiane Hertel to Thierry Crépin-Leblond, April 30, 2002.

[50] Biblioteca Universitaria di Bologna (BUB), Aldrovandi Manoscritti, MS 83, 335r: "Altri mostri sono [...] nella qualita dell'uno et dell'altro [... pero] qui alla mostruosita di natura il pittori vi n'aggiungere un'altra per la sua imaginationi facendo la cosa piu mostruosa."

[51] For the idea of artists as witnesses to truth in science, please see Andrea Carlino, "Fatti contraffatti tra curiosità e scienza," *Arte + Architettura in Svizzera* 57, no. 1 (2006): 37–44.

[52] Caroline Murphy, *Lavinia Fontana: A Painter and Her Patrons in Sixteenth-century Bologna* (New Haven and London: Yale University Press, 2003), 52.

[53] BUB, Aldrovandi Manoscritti, MS 136, XXIV, 21–35.

[54] Zapperi, *Il selvaggio gentiluomo*, 82.

[55] This trip is recorded by Antonio Francesco Ghiselli, chronicler of the city of Bologna and is found in BUB, Memorie antiche manuscritte di Bologna, MS 770, XIX, 645: "Ritrovandosi certa gran signora alloggiata con Mario Cavalier Casali figliuolo del già Andrea ambi senatori, era con essa lei fanciulla di circa dieci anni tutta nella faccia pellosa fuori che la punta del naso e punta del mento, e parimente pellosa la coppa, le spalle, le braccia, le gambe, ma non il resto."

[56] Murphy, *Lavinia Fontana*, 163.

[57] Raffaella Morselli, ed., *La celeste Galeria: Le raccolte* (Milan: Electa, 2002), 200–201.

[58] BUB, Aldrovandi manoscritti, MS 136, XVI, 271v–272v under the title "De muliere Sylvania ex litteris Brumanni Brumanni": "Co che V.S. forze savera dubitato che non mi sia riuscito de mantenere la promessa ch'io le feci del ritratto di quella femina salvatrica che l'Alt. del Sig. Duca di Parma mandò adonare alla Sign.ra Marchesa di Soragnia. Et per quello ch'io intendo il padre madre et fratelli di q.ta salvaticha il detto Sig.ra Duca li tiene nel Castello di Parma. Mi pensava di poter far copiar detto ritratto qui in Milano, per mane di quello Giovane tant va lente, ma quando ni [...] io di gra era stato mandato altrone. Dove investigando ne ho ritrovato un altro in Parma dove ora residdo se ben al presente mi ritrovo qui in Milano et questo è stato la causa della tardanza che so fatto à mandarlo. Credero anco in breve di mandarle il ritratto d'un serpente bizarre et stravagante di grossezza d'un Colombo di sano, longo cureba duo palmi compresso la coda, era do colori stravaganti prima che seccassio creddo c'habbia Quattro piedi et a le trapate. In soma non sò d'haver piu mai visto un simile fu ammazato nel navigho vicino a Milano a tre miglia quattro anni sono da un contadine [...] et l'ebbe un prese che lo dom al Sig.r Co. Antonio della lo maglia m. mio Sig.r. qual se lo tiene fre le suo cose piu case in uno suo studio. Creddo me ne serrura da farlo ritrare , il che faro quanto prime per mandarlo ritratto a V.S. la qual fra tanto goderia il rittratto della salvatica ch'io li mando qui mi chiusa [...]."

[59] Findlen, *Possessing Nature*, 306–11.

[60] Ibid., 307.

[61] In this vein, we are reminded of the ways in which collectors determined their *Kunst- und Wunderkammern* as extensions of themselves and as self-fashioning tools.

[62] Lina Bolzoni, "Parole e immagini per il ritratto di un nuovo Ulisse: L' 'invenzione' dell'Aldrovandi per la sua villa di campagna," in *Documentary Culture: Florence and Rome from Grand-Duke Ferdinand I to Pope Alexander VII*, ed. Elizabeth Cropper, Giovanna Perini, and Francesco Solinas (Bologna: Nuova Alfa Editoriale, 1992), 346–47. Bolzoni also points to the importance of the script found below the images, they are as follows: "in effigiem puellae hirsutae, viri sylvestris ex Europoea filiae" and "Forte videns bardus similem quandoque colonus // effigiem, subito simia dixit, ave": then between the verse "in effigiem hominis sylvestris, puellae iam dictae patris, toto corpore hirsuti" and "Hirsutum faciem atque manus me monstrat imago, // at sub veste rigent caetera membra pilis." She cites BUB, Aldrovandi Manoscritti, MS 99, c. 40v.

[63] Fredrika H. Jacobs, *The Living Image in Renaissance Art* (Cambridge: Cambridge University Press, 2005), 143.

[64] Murphy, *Lavinia Fontana*, 181 for the detail regarding the fact that Casali contacted *both* Aldrovandi and Fontana to view the little hirsute girl.

[65] All physical observations of the album and the drawings it contains are the author's, based on a November 2006 visit to the Pierpont Morgan Library.

[66] It is not too much of a stretch to assume familial ties between Antoinette and the Marchioness of Soragna since we know Odoardo Farnese actually adopted Henri after the boy was sent to him as a gift.

[67] I am indebted to Meghan Pennisi for identifying those flowers during a trip to the Musée du Château de Blois when we both had a chance to look closely at the portrait of Antoinette Gonsalvus. I am grateful to her for sharing her knowledge of flora and its iconography with me.

[68] Lucia Impelluso, *Nature and Its Symbols*, trans. Stephen Sartarelli (Los Angeles: The J. Paul Getty Museum, 2003), 78–81, also for visual precedents.

[69] Murphy, *Lavinia Fontana*, 106–14.

[70] Carole Collier Frick, *Dressing Renaissance Florence: Families, Fortunes, and Fine Clothing* (Baltimore and London: The Johns Hopkins University Press, 2002), 3: "everyone, from *sottoposti* (laborer) to magnate, knew cloth and could easily evaluate the worth of its wearer."

[71] Roberta Orsi Landini and Mary Westerman Bulgarella, "Costume in Fifteenth-century Florentine Portraits of Women," in *Virtue and Beauty: Leonardo's* Ginevra de'Benci *and Renaissance Portraits of Women*, ed. David Alan Brown (Princeton and Oxford: Princeton University Press, 2001), 90–91.

[72] Murphy, *Lavinia Fontana*, 98.

[73] To add to this sibling comparison: a recently discovered portrait (Plate 8) of someone presumed to be Madeleine Gonsalvus has been acquired by Thomas Agnew & Sons in London. Around 1610, when both Jusepe de Ribera (1591–1652) and Madeleine were at the court of Ranuccio Farnese, she was married to the Duke of Parma's "keeper of dogs." In this portrait, the sitter is older than Antoinette was in Fontana's painting and her facial hair is greatly emphasized, as are the red feather in her hair, her red lips, and the red bow on the décolletage of her dress. The dark background allows for the hair and the sanguine iconography to emerge strongly, thus presenting the viewer with a much more sensuous portrayal than Fontana's. I am greatly indebted to Cliff Schorer for bringing this portrait to my attention.

[74] Jacobs, *The Living Image*, 146.

Chapter 5

Audible Absence: The Castrato's Voice

THE PHYSICAL ABNORMALITY OF THE castrati was different from that of dwarves or hirsutes. But the living conditions of castrati joined those of dwarves and hirsutes as court attributes meant to arouse interest through difference. Using Andrea Sacchi's (1599–1661) portrait of Marc'Antonio Pasqualini (1614–1691) (Plate 3) as its point of entry, this chapter elaborates on the particular anatomical anomaly that constructed castrati. It also explores the ways in which the physical mutilation that resulted in an audible manifestation could be made visible. Castrati began life as normal, healthy, intact males. Most of them came from poor families who were promised fame and glory through their sons' musical destinies. Before they reached adolescence and if they showed talent in their musical training, these boys underwent castration and, following the removal of their testes, undertook an even more intensive musical training. Because these boys came from families with little to no connections with the patrons who would one day hire them as singers, the stigmas on the families were almost inexistent—they simply did not live in the same social spheres. The connection among castrati, dwarves, and hirsutes lies in the medical approach to their anatomical anomalies. Indeed, looking at Realdo Colombo's 1559 *De re anatomica libri XV*, Andrea Carlino states that the understanding of monsters as omens and products of the imagination was overruled by the *anatomical* definition of their physical abnormalities.[1] Carlino suggests that anatomical inquiry initiated a change in the perception of monsters; although they were still seen as omens and as marvels, Colombo began to redefine them through their anatomical abnormalities.

This significant shift in the history of monsters is precisely the one my book traces. If monsters could fall under the domain of medicine, rather than only under the domain of the supernatural or the wonderful, according to Carlino, then castrati fall into the same category as dwarves and hirsutes. They, too, demonstrated anatomical distinction of medical interest. In addition, just like dwarves and hirsutes, castrati's legal status and ability to define their personhood juridically was entirely dictated by their physical difference—regardless of the fact that their extraordinary bodies were manmade. It is this anatomical absence, of course, that led them to a courtly setting in the first place; there, they became audible court monsters, collected for their musical abilities. Though recordings of castrati would make for an appropriate complement to their visual representations, very few of these recordings still exist. The simple fact that there are no more castrati today greatly hinders any exhaustive study, as a first hand experience of their vocal performances is impossible.[2] Portraits and written accounts of castrati stand virtually alone, then, as evidence for their presence and influence at court. Although this part of the book centers around Sacchi's portrait of Pasqualini, in order to understand the composite position of castrati in court and church, and their resulting presence in official portraiture and unofficial caricatures, this chapter turns first to the body of the castrato and the ways in which it was understood socially and visually.

The allegorical characteristics of Sacchi's portrait have been addressed by the scholarship on seventeenth-century Roman painting and the concepts behind the *idea del bello*, yet most authors have remained silent on the implications of castration in relation to the sitter. The inclusion of Marsyas in the background of this painting, the presence of Daphne, as well as the centrality of Apollo's genitals, all covertly reference physicality throughout the composition. Although the theme of Marsyas is intended to simultaneously reflect and deflect the mutilation of the artistic body, Apollo's genitals assert Pasqualini's virility, in the absence of his own physical testimony to it. In addition, the juxtaposition of Apollo and Marsyas reinforces the unresolved tension between tamed and unbridled sexuality, and the castrato's accepted and forbidden social and legal rights.[3] This chapter examines Andrea Sacchi's painting of MarcAntonio Pasqualini, considering how the work's iconographical, compositional, and contextual dimensions reveal the contested nature of the castrato's body, gender, sexuality, and social position. To this end, this part of the book considers the evolving social status of castrati in seventeenth-century Italy and their juridical and legal difference from eunuchs. In addition, this chapter examines anatomical inquiries into hermaphroditism, and explores how the castrato's ambiguous physical persona was translated visually into images. By assessing the social, cultural, and artistic context that surrounded the castrated male singer, we eventually see that his body shaped patrons' and audiences' perceptions; he was considered both a monstrous individual—if an artificially created one—and a musical prodigy. The castrato's musical abilities allowed him to become a cherished participant in courtly life, and to find artistic glory in elite realms. It is because of his mutilated body, and the subsequent musical talent that stemmed from it, that he was able to enter these spheres. The tension between musical splendor and a mutilated body remains unresolved in most depictions of the castrato, who, like dwarves or hirsutes, paradoxically used his non-normative body as a vehicle for social acceptance and as the only commodity valuable enough to allow him entry into courtly circles. But this tension was particularly dissonant in Sacchi's portrait, where the myth of Apollo and Marsyas—and that of Apollo and Daphne—centered the anxiety surrounding the body of the castrato in multiple ways.

The story of Apollo and Marsays provides one of the most graphic narratives of Ovid's *Metamorphoses*. The satyr Marsyas found the discarded flute that Athena had thrown away, and being very pleased with his own musical skills, declared himself the greatest of musicians. This displeased Apollo, master of the lyre and god of the arts. Apollo subsequently challenged Marsyas to a competition and promised that the winner could do as he pleased to the vanquished. While Apollo could play the lyre and sing at the same time, Marsyas could only play his flute *or* sing. He therefore lost the challenge and was skinned as punishment.[4] Ovid only presents the scene that confronts his reader with the sentence of Marsyas, his painful flaying, and the tears that turned into a stream in Phrygia.[5] Less gruesome, but no less tragic is the story of Apollo and Daphne. Told in its entirety by Ovid, the tale explains Cupid's role in making Daphne impermeable to love. Apollo, however, felt the reverse sentiment and seeing Daphne's beauty pursued her. In order to elude the god's advances, Daphne asked to be turned into a tree and as Apollo's chase came to a close, she turned into a laurel and escaped him.[6]

Andrea Sacchi used both myths in his depiction of Pasqualini. On a large 243.8 cm by 194.3 cm canvas, Sacchi paints a crowning scene involving three main protagonists: Pasqualini to the left, Apollo in the center, and Marsyas in the right background, tied to a tree, his pipe instrument on the ground to his left, and about to be flayed. As a fully clad Pasqualini plays a clavicytherium (a type of harpsichord, an upright spinet) and stares directly at the viewer, a nude Apollo, holding a lyre in his left hand, is turning toward Pasqualini and placing a crown of laurel atop his head. Framed to the left by a rock formation and to the right by the tree to which Marsyas is tied, the entirety of the scene takes place in an idealized exterior landscape, an unusual placement for an instrument generally found in lavish interiors. On this clavicytherium, we see sculptures that reinforce the central narrative, while adding strident elements to it: a kneeling and tied Marsyas is sculpted on top of the key block by the lower end of the keyboard. He is looking up toward Daphne and is closest to Pasqualini. Daphne is part of the soundboard holding the strings together vertically. The base for her sculpted body is at the top rail of the clavicytherium, but because Apollo's body masks her point of origin, she is visually closest to Apollo's right shoulder from which she seems to emerge. In the process of transforming into a tree, her legs have disappeared into the bark and, from her fingers, laurel leaves grow. In fact, the gold color of the instrument—including that of Daphne's sculpture—mirrors the blonde hair color of Apollo. It is in the covert, but strong, dialogue occurring between these various characters that the castrato's physical abnormality and his position as a castrato become evident, as is developed further in this chapter. But in order to enter these realms productively, an explanation of castrati's lives is necessary.

At the time of his death in 1922, Alessandro Moreschi was the director of the Sistine Chapel Choir and also the last living castrato.[7] The practice of creating and training castrati had ended many years before, yet Moreschi belonged to a line of male soprano singers who had kept this tradition alive for almost four hundred years. A set of documents in the Sistine Chapel dates the first appearance of a castrato—a man, castrated before puberty, and trained to sing in the range of a soprano, mezzo, or contralto—in

Italy to 1562; their steady decline started in the mid-eighteenth century and led to their eventual disappearance by the early twentieth century.[8] Reaching their apogee in the seventeenth and eighteenth centuries, castrati were simultaneously admired and ridiculed. Their performances, however, were unequivocally praised. The outstanding quality of the castrati's vocal production was the primary reason for their fame, as well as the *leitmotif* for the mutilation they suffered between the ages of six and thirteen.[9] Whereas musicological scholarship has amply addressed the castrati phenomenon in regard to musical compositions and the development of opera, the social and physical contexts that affected castrati and dictated their visual presentation have scarcely been explored. The rise of opera coincided with the rise of castrati, yet the taste for their voices preceded the musical form that would define their careers.[10] Well before the castrato's integration into seventeenth- and eighteenth-century operatic compositions, he formed a prominent role as court singer. Gugliemo Gonzaga, third Duke of Mantua and an important patron of music, supported numerous castrati at his court; similarly, Cardinal Montalto, grandnephew of Pope Sixtus V, included castrati among the numerous musicians whom he patronized.[11] In fact, even when castrati served as opera singers, they still depended on patrons who either controlled opera houses or wielded sufficient influence to impose their musical taste and thereby determine the artists' fates.[12] To belong to the court or entourage of a powerful ruler brought the castrato financial benefits and glory, but it also meant that his fate was bound to that of his patron; wars or political and religious changes could directly affect the status of the singer, just as it affected that of his patron. In the same vein, because a castrato was entirely reliant upon the graces of his patron, he relinquished any pretense of autonomy.[13] Church choirs provided a somewhat more secure and stable environment for the castrato, for they assured a steady income and a lifelong position (though a more anonymous one).[14] These choirs were very possessive of their castrati, however, and attempted to prevent them from leaving for more glorious, if less reliable, milieux.[15]

The presence of castrati in church choirs raises important questions about the position the Catholic Church adopted regarding castrati and castration in early modern Europe. Most scholars situate the origins of castration for explicit musical purposes in ecclesiastical decrees and interpretations. In accordance with Saint Paul's teachings, and reinforced by Clement VIII, women were not allowed to speak in church—nor were they even allowed to appear on stage in any of the Papal States, following an edict by Innocent XI.[16] It therefore became necessary for church choirs to employ boys and men who artificially sang female parts—falsetto singers, today known as counter-tenors—in order to reach the higher soprano notes.[17] However, young boys' voices changed at puberty and the voices of adult artificial *falsetti* were not always deemed pleasant. The castrato voice offered a solution to this problem. Not only was the castrato's voice as beautiful as, yet more powerful than, a young boy's, but it also had the advantage of being a permanent attribute of a grown man.[18] The castrati had the perfect male "white voice" sought by the Church and the public alike. The white voice of the castrato could hold soprano notes (without the vibrato found in female voices), had the purity found in children's singing, and could perform at stronger levels than either. The castrato was thus inherently the perfect *created* combination of male power and female range, delivered in a sound package meant to remind audiences of the innocence of children. Castrati became favored human musical instruments, though highly fraught ones since they straddled several spheres—including those of gender boundaries—which made their status completely blurred and liminal.[19]

Employment by the Church alone does not explain why, in the seventeenth century, hundreds of Italian boys suffered castration. To gamble with a son's virility was risky, and the increase in castration in the 1620s has been seen as a response to the economic crisis faced by most of the Italian peninsula.[20] As wars and plagues struck most Italian cities, landholding became the main source of income for the upper classes—an option not as readily available to others struggling. The plague of 1630–1631 cost cities such as Milan 30 to 60 percent of their population, while proto-industrialization in rural areas destabilized employment and urban work settings, affecting the economies of both rural and urban areas.[21] Whereas marrying a son and providing him with an official career was extremely costly, placing him into monastic orders was much less expensive and could even bring the family benefits such as tax concessions.[22] Children recruited as choristers within these orders were more often than not from disadvantaged families; by allowing their sons to be castrated, families could prolong their steady income and provide a remedy to their financial needs.[23] The position of the castrato, therefore, provides one of the rarest instances of the pairing of emasculation and material gain.

Against the backdrop of religious rituals, musical taste, and financial need, castration may have appeared to those who performed or sanctioned it to be a simple, if painful solution to a pressing problem. The physical act of castration, however, had strong corporeal and social repercussions for the boys on whom the operation was performed. It is difficult today to fully assess these effects because not even does the contemporary medical literature offer a comprehensive study of human castration.[24] The production of castrati was not regarded as a scientific experiment, and therefore no records were kept that trace its evolution or its effects; only inferences from portraits, caricatures, and contemporaneous written accounts allow us to reconstruct this vanished practice (a reconstruction made all the more difficult as classical myths about eunuchs often became intertwined with the reality of human castrati).[25] Furthermore, as a rule, castration was performed clandestinely, and often by the parents themselves. A graphic description given by Charles d'Ancillon in 1707 provides gruesome details about a homemade castration and offers a glimpse into the suffering—much downplayed in this description—of a hapless young boy:

> the boy five to seven years of age was placed in a hot bath to soften and make supple the parts, making them more tractable. He was given a potent drink, the jugular veins were compressed, and when he became groggy, the organs were snipped out with a knife with scarcely any pain. In the very young, constant compression and rubbing of the tiny gonads were done until they were no longer palpable.[26]

One of the main reasons the procedure remained secretive was its official condemnation by the Church.[27] Paradoxically, the Church was also the greatest employer of castrati; in order to rationalize this inconsistency, the Church stated that those who had been mutilated by accident were allowed to join the Church and sing to the glory of God. Ecclesiastical authorities thus maintained that while they did not condone castration for artistic purposes, they were willing to help those who, by accident had suffered such a loss. Because therapeutic reasons were often offered as to why the removal of the testicles might help a young boy's health—to prevent gout, elephantiasis, leprosy, or hernias—it is therefore no surprise that among the hundreds of boys who underwent such an operation, very few knew the actual intention of their parents or guardians.[28] Most believed they were the victims of unfortunate, and sometimes fantastic, accidents such as falling from a horse or being bitten by a pig.[29] After the decree of Benedict XIV, castration as a practice was tolerated but never authorized or officially encouraged.[30] Despite the absence of comprehensive scholarship on the history of castration, there is some historical evidence for when and why castrations were performed.[31] Notarial contracts between young Italians and music teachers stipulate the need for castration prior to the engagement of a student, and thus provide evidence for the widespread nature of the practice in seventeenth-century Italy.[32] For instance, the parents and uncle of a young boy named Paolo Nannini of Viterbo agreed to have him castrated for the sake of learning music (interestingly, the expense for this operation fell on his teacher).[33] Similarly, in 1697, an eight-year-old was to be castrated before receiving musical instruction from brother Bonaventura Tricarico—an arrangement that clearly benefitted the boy's parents.[34]

Orchiectomy—the removal of testicles—kept the larynx from growing and dropping, thus preserving the sound of the prepubescent voice.[35] Other effects of orchiectomy stem from its disruption to the endocrine system. Testosterone, responsible for the growth of the larynx and secreted in the testes, also stimulates male sexual characteristics. Its absence causes visible changes, some of which were witnessed in the appearance of castrati: increased height, long limbs, disproportionately large thorax, accumulation and feminine distribution of fat, beardlessness, smooth skin, and droopy eyelids.[36] The overall feminization of the castrato depended on his own physiological endocrine system, and the degree to which his lack of testosterone was overwhelmed by the production of the female hormones that promoted the growth of breasts.[37] Depending on the age at which the castration was performed, the degree of sexual maturation of the castrato would differ—yet regardless of the extent to which his secondary sexual characteristics were visually manifested, an adult castrato would often find himself to be caricatured for being too effeminate, for lacking sexual power, and for possessing a weak intellectual authority.[38] Popular perceptions of castrati depended largely upon their stereotypically odd physical appearances. Even though some castrati did not fit these commonly held stereotypes, they nevertheless belonged to a specific category marginalized from dominant groups of society. Their careers could be framed in superhuman glory if they were talented, fortunate, and patronized in propitious social spheres; but they could also be viewed with repugnance and disgust, relegating them to the lower depths of the same Italian society that adulated them—in his travels through France and Italy in 1770, Charles Burney noted that Italians were ashamed of castrati and denied that they were produced locally.[39] Indeed, the labeling of castrati as physically different and abnormal never ceased even at the height of their fame. The castrato, those who taught him music, those who listened to him, and those who employed him in a church choir all maneuvered in a murky arena, where the castrato was unambiguously cast as "other."[40] This otherness, of course, directly derived from the stigma attached to the act of castration. Disavowed in their creation by the authorities that condoned their mutilation, exploited for art's sake, often the product of poverty, and yet artistically and religiously valuable, the castrato embodied a peculiar social and economic space defined by the oscillating responses they received—admiration and aversion. Their unresolved condition, and the subsequent inconsistent public reaction to their bodies, made them not only others, but monsters, with all its subsequent implications. Like dwarves or hirsutes they were produced to be shown, even if their mutilated bodies held a different kind of monstrosity due to the value placed on their audible abnormality. Because it was uniformly produced, their monstrousness was almost tamed—a taming that was completely dependent on the elite culture that appreciated and indirectly created them.

The mutilated bodies of castrati pointed to centuries of historical and mythological violence associated with the act of castration. Used as a sign of punishment or as means of torture, castration was always conceived as an act of mutilation—one that theological rules and seventeenth-century penal codes permitted only for the punishment of criminals.[41] The punitive association with castration pervaded the social interactions castrati faced, since their mutilation was an audible and visible mark left for all to hear. Furthermore, the removal of the testes signified the removal of sacred symbols of divine and masculine power; indeed, etymologically, the word "testify" finds its origins in the Latin word *testis*, or "witness," referring to the act of placing one's hand on one's testes while taking an oath—a requirement that consequently excluded women and eunuchs from testifying.[42] Thus prohibited from testifying, eunuchs lost their juridical status as fully independent and whole human beings. The remnants of this legal stripping certainly influenced how castrati were perceived within a structured legal and societal system, yet it is relevant to note that there were differences in juridical personhood between castrati, eunuchs, and hermaphrodites depending on their reproductive powers. It comes as no surprise that castration was rarely seen as an innocent procedure; as Meyer Melicow has indicated, the practice was most often associated with punishment, revenge, or forced exclusion.[43] Because of these associations, castrati became an embarrassment for early modern Christendom—and yet, ironically, castrati who failed to become remotely accomplished singers were allowed to become priests.[44] The popular distaste for the bodies of castrati persisted up until the twentieth century, a reticence that explains the general rejection castrati felt in the social, legal, and artistic discourse framing their lives. These forms of prejudice both constructed the monstrosity of castrati, and also shaped their peculiar appreciation by the Church and the public. The unique, man-made talent was as much a curse as it was a blessing.

The social and psychological impact of the castration stigma found its way into visual representations of castrati. Caricatures are perhaps the most telling instances of the ways in which castrati were perceived in the collective imaginary, as very few examples of seventeenth-century portraits of castrati exist (most illustrations date to the eighteenth century, when castrati and their representations became more popular). The scarcity of castrati portraits in the seventeenth century makes Sacchi's work an intriguing exception. As neither this painter nor his subject had access to a large corpus of work on which to build this composition, Sacchi's choices are thus inherently personal and rich with

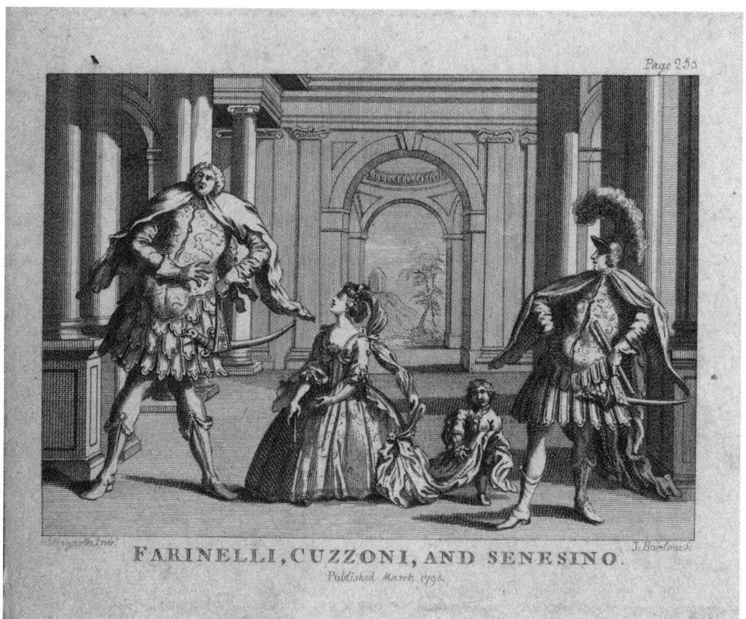

Figure 5.1. After William Hogarth, engraved by John Berlow, *Farinelli, Cuzzoni, and Senesino*, performance in 1723, published in 1798, The Victoria and Albert Museum, London

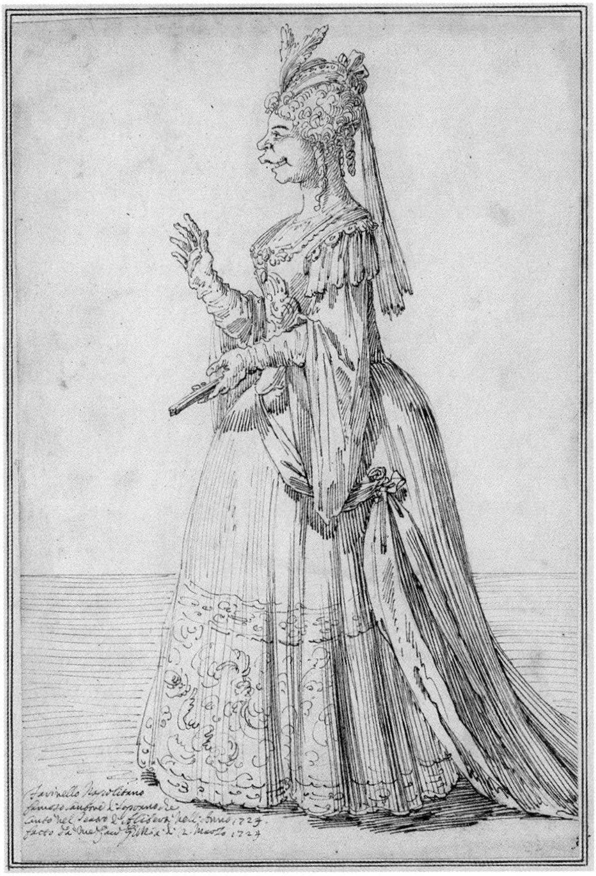

Figure 5.2. Pier Leone Ghezzi, *Caricature of Farinelli in a Female Role*, ca. 1740, The J. Pierpont Morgan Library, New York

information. The very absence of earlier castrati portraits makes Sacchi's statement in Marc'Antonio Pasqualini's portrait all the stronger. Eighteenth-century caricatures offer a hint of the place castrati held in this earlier period. Several sketches by William Hogarth (1697–1764) and Pier-Leone Ghezzi (1674–1755) depict the castrato Farinelli (a.k.a. Carlo Broschi, 1705–1782) in various operatic roles (Figs. 5.1 and 5.2).[45]

Letters and odes written at the height of Farinelli's fame, or shortly after his death, testify to his attractive physical appearance; back from his travels through France and Italy in 1794, John Courtenay wrote, in verse, to Robert Jephson, telling him about his various opinions about politics and the arts there. By the time Courtenay published his odes, including one about the famed castrato, Farinelli had been dead twelve years, yet Farinelli's fame had not dwindled and his beauty was still actively remembered in most musical circles. Courtenay, in his writings, presented the glory of the castrato and the admiration the singer inspired and he was no exception.[46] But in spite of Farinelli's renowned beauty, Hogarth and Ghezzi's caricatures highly deform and exaggerate the awkwardness of his body. Whereas the costumes refer to the theatricality of the scene being represented, the physical features of the castrato unmistakably suggest an uncomfortable relation between the body of the castrato and its public perception. Ghezzi's drawing of Farinelli in a female role is particularly telling of the uneasy gender position occupied by castrati. The artist does not refrain from depicting the elaborate female costume, but does so while inscribing the awkward and unattractive face that accompanies such a lavish and feminine costume. Mirroring the ways in which castrati's white voices disturbed a gendered binary, their caricatured physical depictions heightened this discordance. The juxtaposition of Farinelli's odd face and the elegant female dress certainly contributes to a sense of discomfort in the artist's—and viewer's—mind. It is worth noting that, at the time these caricatures were produced castrati were flourishing and Farinelli was arguably the most famous among them. It would therefore seem natural for eighteenth-century castrati to have relinquished their status as oddities. These caricatures problematize the issue of the castrato's body, however, revealing that it remained an inherently challenging part of his persona. In spite of the acclaim castrati like Farinelli received, his body and the history attached to it did not allow him to relinquish his status as a marvelous oddity, playing with his audience's senses as they watched and listened to him. Whereas a castrato's vocal ability made him musically superior to his contemporaries, a castrato's body cast him as physically anomalous. Even when "musical castration" had become more commonplace, its victims were still perceived as curiosities—men whose otherwise invisible mutilation became immediately apparent the moment they opened their mouths.[47] Indeed, the castrato existed *because* of a physical mutilation. Like a dwarf, a castrato acquired his social mobility precisely because he was physically out of the norm—and yet the degree of his popularity still depended on his artistic talent, just as a dwarf's wit might confer upon him the title of favored companion. The difference here lies in the invisibility of the castrato's anatomical irregularity. Just like dwarves were the foils to perfect courtly bodies and hirsutes were the foils to perfect courtly behaviors, castrati became the foils to perfect courtly masculinity. It is via complex iconographies that the androgyny—or hypersexuality, in the case of Pasqualini—of the castrato was made visible rather than audible only. The castrato's otherness needed to transcend his voice in order to be captured.

Eighteenth-century official portraits of Farinelli, notably, do not emphasize the potential peculiarity of his physical appearance and here we can see a continuation of discourses tied to idealization in representations meant to enhance the status of the sitter. It is also very possible that Farinelli's actual physical appearance did not immediately betray the consequences of his body's absence. These portraits emphasize the high social status of the singer, Farinelli's attractiveness, as well as his musical penchant and talent. Farinelli himself commissioned Amigoni—thus giving Farinelli his own voice, so to speak—for

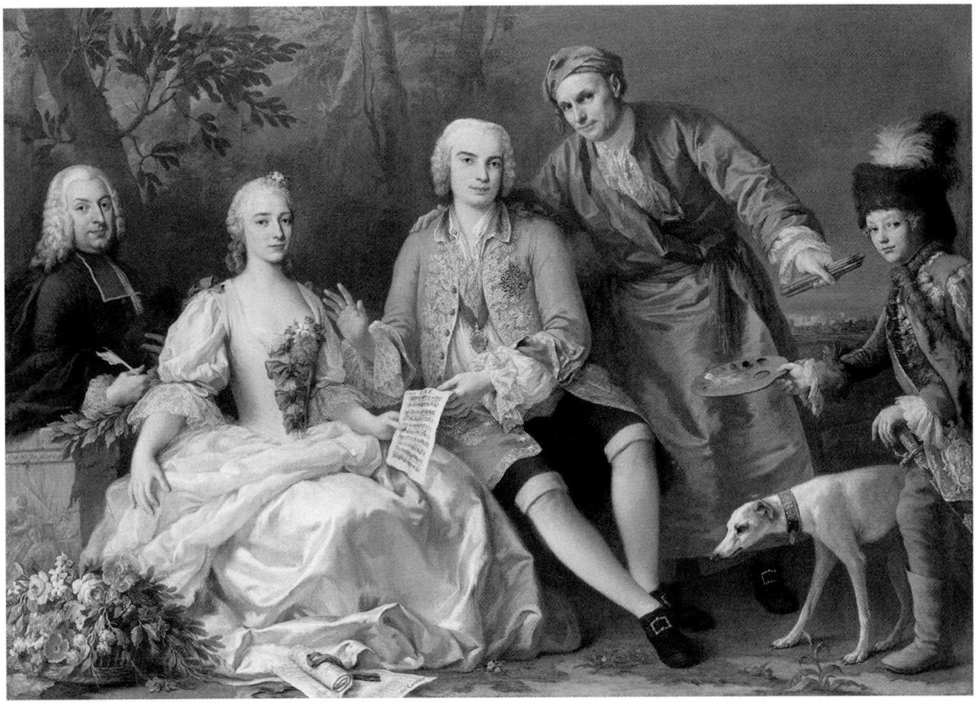

Figure 5.3. Jacopo Amigoni, *Musical Portrait Group: The Singer Farinelli and Friends*, ca. 1750–52, Felton Bequest 1950 (2226–4), National Gallery of Victoria, Melbourne

his 1750 *Musical Portrait Group: The Singer Farinelli and Friends* (Fig. 5.3) a work that hangs today in the National Gallery of Victoria in Melbourne.

In this singular group portrait, Farinelli is shown centrally, wearing the insignia of the Order of Calatrava, an honorary military and religious order bestowed by the King of Spain.[48] In addition to including himself in the painting, Amigoni also represented the Milanese soprano Teresa Castellini, the abbot and writer Pietro Metastasio holding a quill, and a Hungarian hussar who might be the young imperial Prince Joseph holding a dog bearing Farinelli's initials.[49] The emphasis on the knightly order and Farinelli's various other social connections removes stigma of his castration and diverts the viewer's attention instead to the relationships implied by the painting. Castellini and Farinelli hold a musical score that is based on a poem written by Metastasio and that Farinelli himself set to music. The poem speaks of the departure of a lover and it is certainly tied to the narrative that Farinelli wants the viewer to read in his relationship to Castellini. Amigoni has emphasized the closeness of Castellini and Farinelli not only in their placement alongside each other, but also in their sharing of a sheet of music—one that speaks to their story since Castellini was about to leave Madrid and thus Farinelli—and in Farinelli's hand gesture toward the soprano: he is about to touch her with his right hand. All of the protagonists were Italians who found themselves in Madrid, therefore the painting may speak to the imminent dissolution of their expatriate gatherings since Metastasio had already left and Castellini was preparing her departure.[50] More importantly, however, Amigoni uses typical visual decorum to emphasize Farinelli's masculinity in his clothing and particularly in his implied romantic ties to Castellini. It comes as no surprise that Farinelli would not want to emphasize the—perceived—liminal gender qualities resulting from his mutilation, but rather underline his high artistic and social standing. Other portraits of Farinelli follow suit. The painters emphasize the castrato's wealth as much as his artistic abilities and highlight the currency of Farinelli as an artist, convincing audiences that the castrato would be an invaluable presence in operatic productions. Once again, there are no physical insinuations regarding Farinelli's mutilation.

Among the few additional portraits of castrati that represent them sympathetically, rather than as caricatures of themselves, only one drawing, of Antonio Paccini by Antoine Watteau (Fig. 5.4) somewhat hints at the unusual physical appearance of castrati: in this drawing the hormonal effects of castration are seen in the additional fatty deposit on the face, as well as in the droopy eyelids, which were common symptoms. On the whole, sanctioned portraits of castrati did not contain overt or covert iconographical references to castration; rather, they used visual language to convey social prestige and artistic prowess.

The physical traits that characterized castrati went largely unrepresented, a situation that highlights the pointed dynamic between oral and visual media. Indeed, the only way for the viewer to know about the corporeal anomaly of the subject could occur most effectively through the direct experience of the voice of the sitter, who in these images is able to safely hide behind the social and visual conventions on the canvas.

Andrea Sacchi's portrait of the castrato Marc'Antonio Pasqualini differs from such conventions while still integrating recognizable elements of art and music.[51] The portrait depicts Marc'Antonio Pasqualini playing a musical instrument while being crowned by Apollo. In the right background, the satyr Marsyas is tied to a tree and about to be flayed. Pasqualini is wearing the white robe of the pontifical singers, as well as an animal skin—an allusion to his theatrical and dramatic abilities.[52] Gianpietro Bellori (1615–1690) interpreted Pasqualini's animal skin as a shepherd's costume, which would have evoked one of Pasqualini's roles in a production designed by Andrea Sacchi in the Palazzo Falconieri in 1634.[53] Pasqualini is shown playing a clavicytherium, which is identifiable as an instrument belonging to cardinal Antonio Barberini, his patron.[54] Indeed, an examination of the Barberini inventories shows an entry for one of Antonio Barberini's instruments, which matches the one painted by Sacchi.[55] The table on which the clavicytherium rests provides additional signs that this instrument was in fact part of the Barberini family possessions; its three legs, classical illustrations of dolphins,

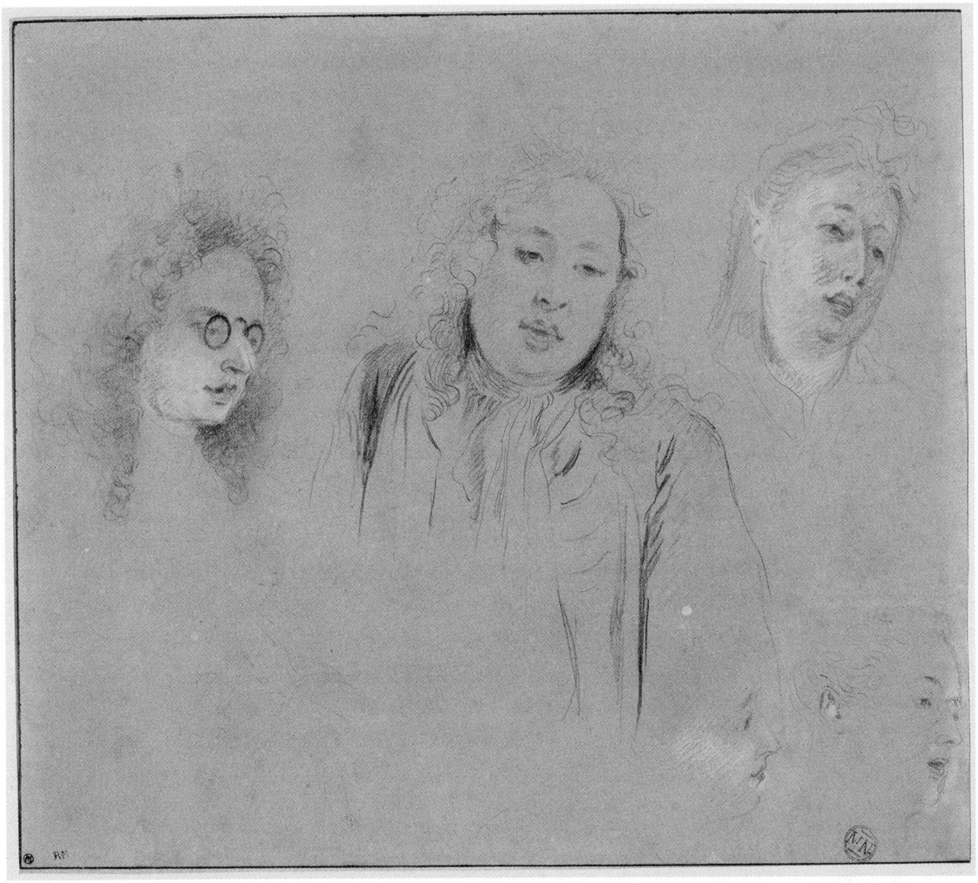

Figure 5.4. Jean Antoine Watteau, *Antonio Paccini*, 1720, Musée du Louvre, Paris. RMN-Grand Palais/Art Resource, New York

represented the quality of princely benefaction that was particularly associated with the Barberinis, and seen in Gianlorenzo Bernini's (1598–1680) 1642 Triton fountain, only steps away from the Palazzo Barberini in Rome, an emblem common to the family.[56]

The most overt allegory in the painting refers not only to the musical abilities of Pasqualini, but also to his poetic talents and social prominence.[57] Born in 1614 in an impoverished family of eight children, Marc'Antonio Pasqualini entered the choir of San Luigi de'Francesi in 1623, where he also attended school.[58] In 1630, one month after the school of San Luigi dei Francesi was suppressed, Pasqualini was taken under the protection of Cardinal Antonio Barberini and made *cantore pontificio*. He remained in the chapel until 1659, but this appointment did not keep him from singing secular works or from being a part of the Barberini household.[59] Pasqualini soon became cardinal Antonio

Barberini's favorite artist in residence, and by 1641 was widely known for his insolence.[60] Circulating in the aristocratic circles of Rome, Pasqualini achieved what only a select number of artists accomplished: he reached the highest social spheres through his talent and fortunate connections. His impertinence eventually led cardinal Antonio Barberini to distance himself from his protégé, for whom he found a position in the church of Santa Maria Maggiore.[61] Pasqualini's life, though rare in its level of success, was no exception for the famous castrati who found recognition in spite (and because) of, their mutilation. Discovered and protected by a powerful patron, the castrato would depend on his patron, perform for him in the operas he commissioned, and then either teach, compose, or direct a church choir in his later years.[62] The fact that Pasqualini moved in intellectual and aristocratic circles has been used to explain this portrait's allegorical content; indeed, by representing Apollo crowning the castrato, Sacchi referred to the art of *poesia*, as found in Cesare Ripa's *Iconologia*.[63] Franca Trinchieri Camiz has convincingly argued that this portrait illustrates the musical, intellectual, and poetical aspirations of Pasqualini, as opposed to an informal portrait of a castrato such as Caravaggio's 1595 *Musicians* (Fig. 5.5).[64]

This insistence upon the castrato's artistic and intellectual dimensions seems to have remained quite popular, since other extant portraits of castrati discussed previously in this chapter but produced later than Sacchi's work also and mainly emphasized the social and intellectual aspect of the castrato's life. Nicoletta Guidobaldi has taken the argument further and introduced the figure of Marsyas within this iconographical analysis. For Guidobaldi, Apollo crowns Pasqualini not only because of his artistic abilities, but also because of his artistic *supremacy*; the figure of Marsyas in the background serves as a reminder of the musical contest lost by the satyr and won by Apollo, who in fact may even be giving his own crown of victory to Pasqualini.[65] This chain of artistic transmission finds resonance in the body of the castrato as the perfect vehicle for art, since his body was created for the sole purpose of serving the musical arts. Todd Olson also provides an impressive reading of Sacchi's painting and an excellent analysis of the role of Marsyas in the painter's composition. Olson argues that the correlation of violence and mutilation associated with the torture of Marsyas speaks to the castration endured by Pasqualini; he also offers an interesting psychoanalytical reading of the castrato's gender performance and its visual expression by Sacchi.[66] However, we can push this argument further by looking at the fact that Pasqualini himself commissioned this portrait and was well versed in the implications of including such complex iconography.

Two figures fracture the mere allusion made to a musical contest or to the uncontested artistic supremacy of the castrato: Marsyas and, on a different register, Daphne. The figure of Marsyas speaks to the tension that exists in glorifying an artist whose skills were the result of physical mutilation: the flayed Marsyas serves as a reminder of the latent imperfection of Pasqualini's damaged body. Yet, the fact that the work was commissioned by Pasqualini himself makes the allegorical allusions even more complicated.[67] The figure

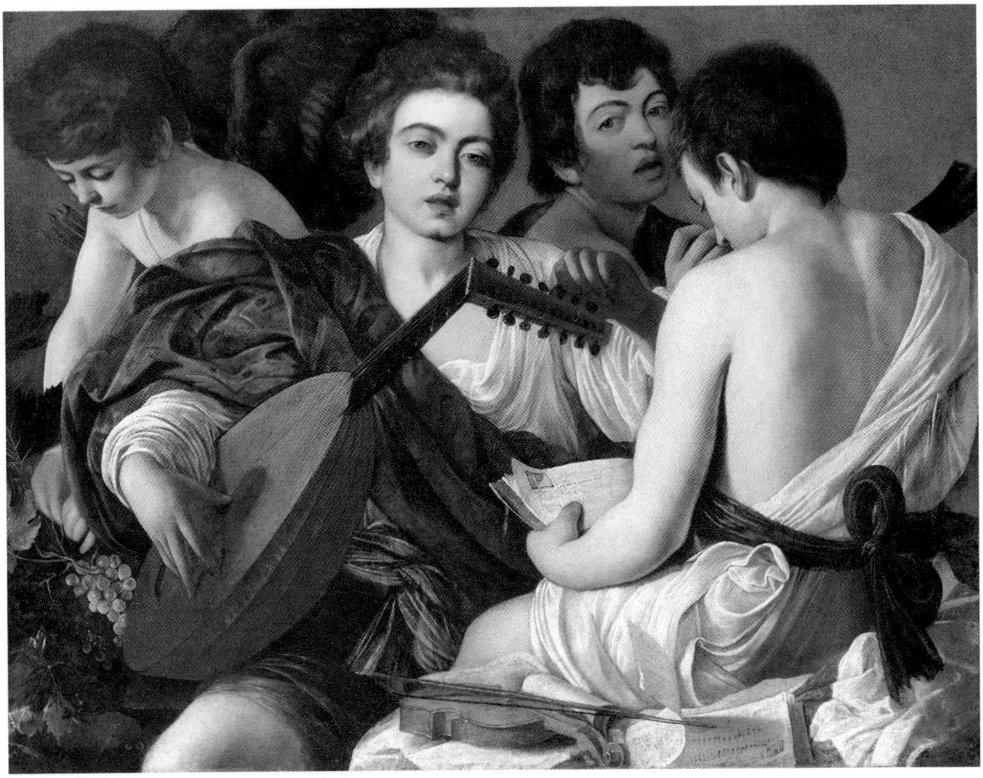

Figure 5.5. Michelangelo Merisi da Caravaggio, *The Musicians*, ca. 1595, Metropolitan Museum of Art, New York

of Daphne, on the other hand seems inescapable since the sculpture is an inherent part of the Barberini clavicytherium painted by Sacchi; yet, Sacchi's placement of Daphne and the subsequent bridge she provides between Apollo and Pasqualini was an intentional supplement to a composite visual program. The complex triad of Pasqualini, cardinal Antonio Barberini, and Sacchi—as well as the uncomfortable public perception of the castrato's body—all contribute to the tense and unresolved visual depiction articulated in the painting. The figure of Marsyas is a perfect entry into this complex conversation.

Artistic representations of Marsyas often emphasize the flaying of the satyr as the main event of the composition. In Titian's famed *The Flaying of Marsyas* (1576) painting (Fig. 5.6), Marsyas is at the center of the canvas and certainly the center of the narrative. Titian's iconographical choices are clear: the intense emotion inherent in the torture endured by the satyr drive the painting. The hanging and the stretching of Marsyas's arms become common visual gestures allowing for an accurate depiction of tensed muscles, and tension in general. Moreover, the themes of punishment and torture commonly associated

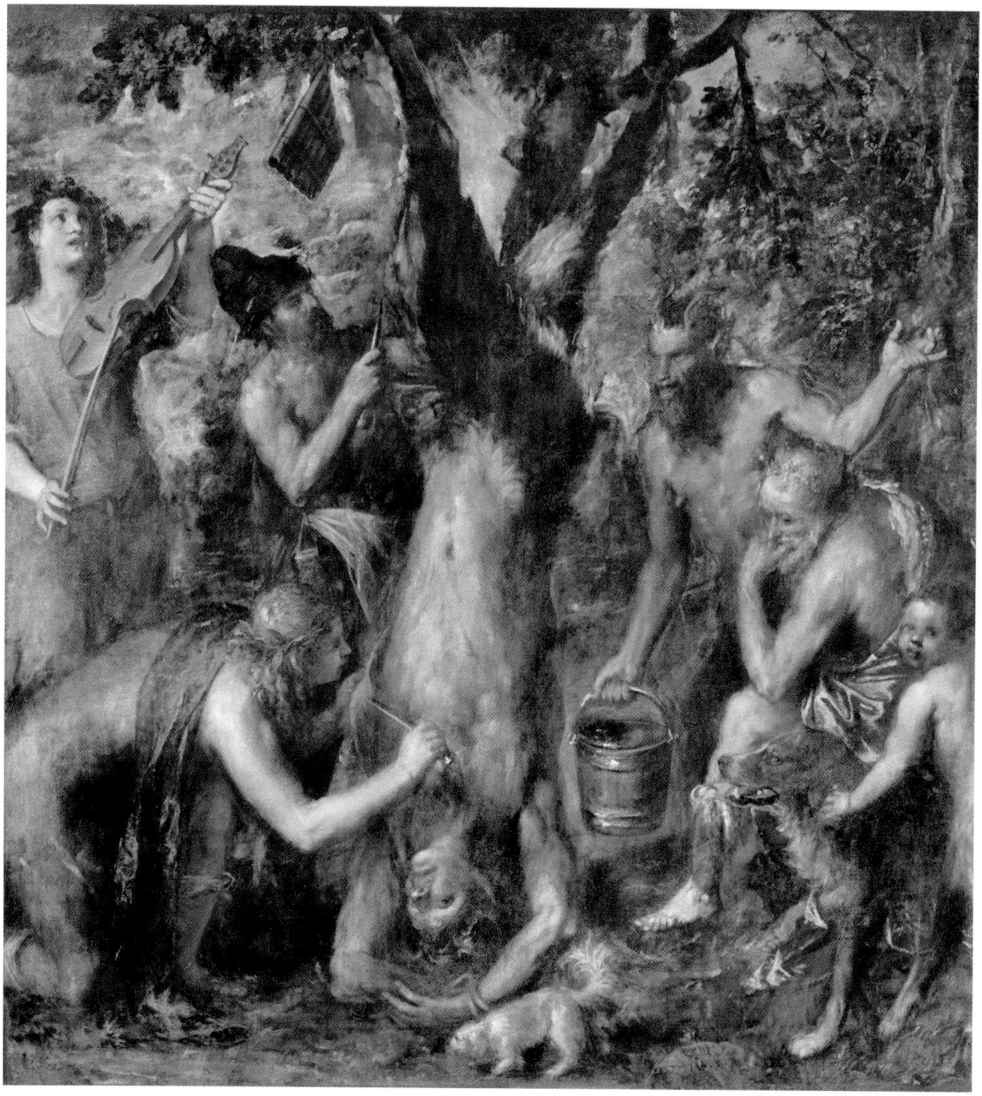

Figure 5.6. Titian, *The Flaying of Marsyas*, 1576, State Museum, Kromeriz. Erich Lessing/Art Resource, New York

with the figure of Marsyas in the Renaissance were reminiscent of dissections. Indeed, Marsyas is also commonly referred to in écorchés figures and myological dissections.[68]

In her persuasive argument regarding the link between Marsyas and dissections, Beth Holman looks at Realdo Colombo's 1559 *De re anatomica*, explaining that the figure of Marsyas provided a perfect pretense for the accurate representation of muscle studies.[69] The illustration for the section on muscles uses the flaying of Marsyas as its heading, just as Andreas Vesalius's second edition of the Fabrica depicts the flaying of Marsyas in one of its first initials.[70] It is therefore difficult to see Marsyas's insertion in Sacchi's painting as a mere mythological reference supporting the narrative of Apollo's, and by proxy, Pasqualini's victory. To begin with, Sacchi's reference to the myth of Apollo and Marsyas was compositionally and visually different from contemporaneous or prototypical depictions of the myth. Sacchi did not emphasize the flaying as a central event; rather he placed Marsyas in the lower background and the instruments used for the imminent flaying are absent. Furthermore, Marsyas is tied to a tree, but his body rests on the ground. Because the physical appearance of Pasqualini does not allow the uninformed viewer to understand his body as that of a castrato, the figure of Marsyas must stand as the signifier of Pasqualini's mutilated body. Cesare Ripa does not mention the need for the figure of Marsyas in an allegory of *poesia*. All that is required is a figure of Apollo with a lyre on his left hand, crowning the subject with a crown of laurel on his right hand.[71] Most examples of crowning by Apollo do not include the figure of Marsyas. A 1641 Claude Mellan engraving of *Apollo Crowning the Poet Virgil* provides a prototype for this basic iconography (Fig. 5.7).

The full-length depiction of both Apollo and Virgil, as well as their physical interactions are seen in Sacchi's composition. If Marsyas's presence is unnecessary to glorify Pasqualini and *poesia*, then the addition of this figure is all the more significant. Whereas the Renaissance favored the story of Apollo and Marsyas, it was not a preferred topic for painters and sculptors after the middle of the sixteenth century; and although the use of Apollo in Sacchi's painting is justifiable because of its iconographical implications, the inclusion of Marsyas is not.[72] In sum, the figure of Marsyas in the middle of the seventeenth century is neither required for the understanding of the allegory of *poesia*, nor a sufficiently popular subject to explain why it appears in Sacchi's painting.

Because of its allusion to mutilation and castration, the figure of Marsyas strikes a chord with the viewer, inserting a strident element of anxiety within the otherwise—or at least on the surface—peaceful narrative of Apollo crowning the artist in glory. This unsettling component of Sacchi's composition summons the equally unresolved tension that exists when the subject of a court portrait is known for his anatomical irregularity. As a visual index for Pasqualini's body, Marsyas's non-human attributes signify the vestige of what turned the man into an audible monster. Furthermore, temporality heightens the anxiety latent in this painting: just as Marsyas is waiting to be flayed, Pasqualini awaits his crown, not yet placed on his head. The glorification of the castrato is, thus far, not fully recognized and in this charged moment, disruptions—in the form of reminders of past mutilations, for instance—may still occur.

The triangle between Sacchi, Pasqualini, and Barberini is critical to establishing a context for the work's production. There are several records in the Barberini *guardarobe* dating payments made to Andrea Sacchi; the first, an entry dated to October 6, 1639, states that Sacchi was paid for the commission he fulfilled.[73] The second entry lists a

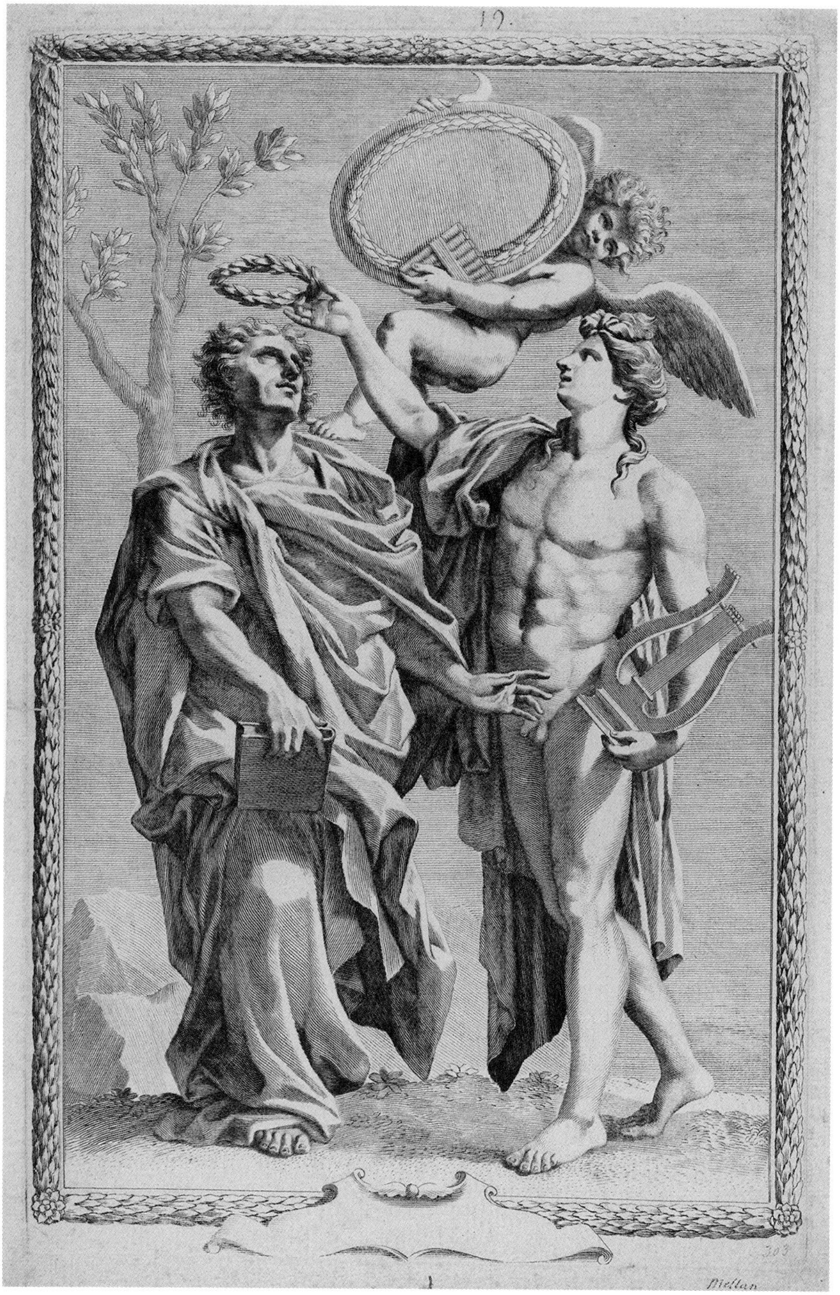

Figure 5.7. Claude Mellan, *Apollo Crowning the Poet Virgil*, 1641, engraving of a drawing by Nicolas Poussin, The Charles M. Lea Collection, 1928–42–2440, Philadelphia Museum of Art, Philadelphia

payment made to Sacchi on November 8, 1641, for the painting representing the feast of *il Gesù*;[74] this seemingly unrelated work is perhaps a key to understanding the composition of Pasqualini's portrait, for Sacchi's preparatory studies for the *Gesù* painting contain studies of Apollo used for the Pasqualini portrait.[75] Though we cannot establish a direct payment connection between the Barberinis and Sacchi, we can find confirmation of the agreement that existed between the cardinal, the painter, and the singer from the incipient preparation of the iconographical program of the portrait to its finalization in 1641. The central question remains as to whether Pasqualini himself had significant input in devising the unusual iconography of this portrait. There is evidence that Marc'Antonio Pasqualini was both literate and schooled in various arts. In addition to his extended musical schooling, Pasqualini himself wrote and copied musical scores, denoting an interest that went beyond mere performance.[76] In 1648, the castrato was also elected *Puntatore*, a high elected office in charge of giving penalty to Vatican choir members who did not fulfill their duties appropriately.[77] This prestigious position was only offered to highly literate individuals, implying therefore that Pasqualini's intellectual abilities were considerable. As commissioner of the painting, Pasqualini was certainly aware of the iconographical message inserted in the composition by his Barberini co-protégé, Andrea Sacchi. Not an exception in this regard, Pasqualini would have been one of many sitters commissioning elaborate allegories imbedded in their own portraits.[78] Various notions point to the fact that Pasqualini may indeed have been active in devising the program of Sacchi's composition, one of which related to the idea of gendered performance associated with castrati in the early modern period.

The period belief that female genitalia were an inversion, and a defective version, of male genitalia determined the way gender related to sexual difference.[79] If, as Thomas Laqueur argues, the Renaissance view was that male and female bodies represented different versions of only one sexual model, then the issue of gender must have been, by default, more closely associated with external signs of difference and less with the appearance of genitals (accordingly, sexual organs may therefore be taken as manifestations of gender, rather than as its determinants). In the case of castrated young boys, the eventual result was an underdeveloped adult penis; though erection was possible, the ability to reach orgasm was (and is) still questioned. Consequently in the Renaissance, based on Aristotelian and humored understandings of sexual difference, castrati fell into the feminine realm, since they could not physiologically produce masculine vital heat.[80] Even though the sensual and hypersexual nature of castrati was never doubted, their virility—also diminished by the fact that they were highly accomplished in the art of music—was seriously questioned.[81] To reiterate, their common denominations as "half-men" or "neither men nor women," as well as their feminine caricaturing, indicate the predicament in which they found themselves as far as asserting their virility.[82] Also, in regard to their sexual relations, accounts differ. While some doubt that castrati could pursue continued sexual relations with men or women, Barbier asserts that castrati had sustained relationships with females, though a generalization in that matter is not possible.[83] Sometime before the Metropolitan Museum of Art acquired Andrea Sacchi's portrait of Marc'Antonio Pasqualini, a different hand had painted a loincloth over the genitals of Marsyas and Apollo.[84] The covering of Apollo's genitals shifted the center of the painting and changed its relative meaning. Indeed, by concealing Apollo's penis, this later hand altered the latent, yet strong, implication of virility present in the compositional juxtaposition of Apollo and Pasqualini. In the original composition, Apollo's posture is shifted so as to make his genitals absolutely central. The presence of Marsyas speaks to the identity of Pasqualini as a castrato while Apollo's genitals become an effective vehicle to assert his constructed virility and counterbalance his status as a feminized male. The crowning gesture reinforces the connection between Apollo and Pasqualini, as Apollo transfers his own victory to the castrato—and by extension his own virility. The figure of Apollo appears to be intended to resolve the intrinsic paradox existing between a castrated male body and its masculinity. The question regarding sexual intimacy between Pasqualini and Barberini may help elucidate the reasons for the insertion of such an obvious affirmation.[85] Though the extent of Barberini's attachment to Pasqualini has not been proven, his deep affection for the castrato was known, and as a present from the castrato to his patron, this portrait could indeed have emphasized a quality dear to the cardinal. The artist may thus have played on other sexual attributes related to the additive insertion of both Marsyas and Apollo. Additionally, as Todd Olson has noted, the homoerotic tenor of the central protagonists is difficult to ignore: "Marsyas alone served as a chaperone to a dangerous homoerotic pairing: not Apollo and Pasqualini, but the cardinal and the favourite castrato."[86]

Aside from the clear anatomical allusions presented by the figure of the satyr about to become an écorché figure, the relation between Marsyas and Apollo also suggests an engagement with the truth. As Apollo will flay Marsyas, he will uncover the reality of his inner body.[87] The conflation between anatomy, myological dissection, and truth is clearly intentional: the glory of Pasqualini is not merely recognized by Apollo—it is *explained* and *revealed* by the god who links Pasqualini's artistic talent to his bodily mutilation, echoed in the body of Marsyas. The violence of the castration procedure and its attached stigma thus find a sympathetic visual articulation that casts the physical attributes of the celebrated singer as a subtle and integral part of the mythological narrative. The myth of Marsyas therefore glorifies the act of castration as an avenue toward *poesia*—it dispels anxiety about the castrato's body precisely by acknowledging its existence. In fact, here we see an apposite link to Fredrika Jacobs's idea that Marsyas is seen as a "metaphor of voluntary sacrificial self-transcendence."[88] Pasqualini shifts from victim to willing partaker in the torture that shaped his identity—through this portrait and through Marsyas, he has now claimed ownership of his artistic prowess.

The figure of Apollo is not the only signifier of masculinity in Sacchi's painting, for the figure of Marsyas may be read on several levels. The violence associated with Marsyas's tortured body may point to the questioned virility of castrati, yet Pasqualini may also have welcomed the allusion to a satyr whose sexuality was seen in explicitly animalistic and virile terms. In combination with the tamed masculinity of Apollo, Marsyas could thus have served as a means to assert Pasqualini's own virility. The combination of the two figures reinforces the castrato's sense of lost masculinity. Through Apollo and his manifest genitals, Pasqualini's virility is established; through Marsyas's strong masculine body and his association with unbridled sexuality, it is reinforced. Satyrs, and Marsyas in particular, came to be associated with crude sexuality and wild behavior during the early modern period. The opposition of two types of music, evoked by Apollo and Marsyas, parallel the two types of masculine sexuality suggested by each mythological figure: whereas Apollo's lyre imparted greatness to the soul, Marsyas's flute induced an immoral effect.[89] In addition, satyrs represented the abundance of nature and, by extension, the sexuality of man.[90] By actively including Marsyas in the painting, Pasqualini, *via* Sacchi's brush, points to his vigorous sexuality; Apollo does not cancel Marsyas's unbridled passions, rather he disciplines them publicly. In the background, the realm of the private, Marsyas's sexuality persists. In fact, merging aural and visual statements, of all the subjects painted by Sacchi in this group portrait, only the voice of Marsyas is heard, accompanied by the keys played by Pasqualini. Additionally, the castrato and the satyr look at the viewer, using us as a direct point of reference that ties them together. Should this painting have an auditory component, it would not be the arias sung by Pasqualini; rather, it would be the deafening scream of Marsyas awaiting torture and death.

The figure of Daphne is the keystone of this arch. Because the laurel—Daphne—and the sun—Apollo—were Barberini emblems, we can see the importance of Pasqualini inserting himself in a narrative that ties him to both. The pain imposed by Apollo is one that Daphne escaped by transforming herself into a laurel tree.[91] Her transformation is, in this composition, occurring as she emerges from Apollo's body: the gold color of the sculpted Daphne mirrors the color of Apollo's hair and the laurel branches that grow from her fingers echo the laurel crown Apollo holds above the head of Pasqualini. The castrato is thus *in the process* of receiving victory, but this fame is one that is tied to pain, torture, and sacrifice—an apt parallel to Pasqualini's life. In fact, Daphne's face is turned away from the castrato, the mythological god, and the viewer, for she is looking at Marsyas, Apollo's other victim. Again, it is not the connection between Apollo and Pasqualini that is strongest, but that between Pasqualini and Marsyas, via Daphne's gaze. Sacchi, in fact, visually asserts the relation between the castrato and the satyr repeatedly. Both Pasqualini's hands are painted touching the keys of the clavicytherium. To their left, another sculpted figure, that of a kneeling and tied Marsyas is part of the instrument's decorative program. Interestingly, Sacchi paints the body of the sculpted satyr and the hands of the castrato with similar brushstrokes, the curves of Marsyas's left thigh almost indistinguishable from Pasqualini's left hand. Marsyas leans into Pasqualini's body, part of his knees merging with the fur worn by the castrato; their wildness becomes one, protected by the shadow the castrato's body offers the sculpted satyr. As the sculpted Marsyas gazes upwards in the direction of Daphne, we follow the narrative toward the nymph once more. But she is looking toward the real, screaming Marsyas. While her body warns Pasqualini of the price one pays for Apollo's love/crowning, her gaze points to the result such a bold glory may bring. Yet, Pasqualini appears calm in receiving this cursed praise; he is impermeable to both Marsyas's scream and Daphne's warning that he, too, may disappear because of Apollo. The castrato's tranquility is disconcerting, but explicable: unlike Daphne, Pasqualini employs his sexuality—in fact both aspects of his masculine sexuality—to welcome Apollo's honor. He is also willingly sacrificing. His controlled virility aurally plays on the strings of the clavicytherium; but this tamed masculinity is not the castrato's sole qualifier since the same hands that reveal musical education are visually coupled to the sculpted body of a hypersexualized satyr. To this rational virility, thus, Pasqualini adds unbridled sexuality, acoustically resounding in the satyr's cries. The castrato—demonstrating that his sexuality holds an additional expression to that of Apollo—therefore dissolves the threat of violence associated with the god's sexual supremacy. Unlike Marsyas, he is fully deserving of the crown Apollo bestows upon him and unlike Daphne he welcomes the god's admiration for it.

The conflicted coexistence of two types of sexuality—and in Pasqualini's representation, both tamed and unbridled—was not uncommon in the early modern treatments of gender dilemmas. Hermaphrodites exemplify an intricate cultural, medical, and juridical case dealing with sexual designation and its consequences; by looking at hermaphrodites and eunuchs, the castrato's legal position becomes more legible. As opposed to the situation castrati faced, hermaphroditism was not the result of a human choice. Although hermaphrodites' sexual difference was often discovered only later in life, the explanation for their condition was either mythical, or medical. The theory of the seven-chambered uterus was used since the Middle Ages to explain hermaphroditism; the concept that three of the purported produced males, three produced females, and the last produced hermaphrodites was a widely acknowledged belief.[92] This view blended in the collective imaginary with the alchemical concept of hermaphrodites as holy beings who restored order on material chaos by trampling over the four elements.[93] However, the treatment of hermaphrodites as monsters, rather than superior creations, prevailed. Jean Riolan in his 1614 *Discours sur les hermaphrodits* argued that hermaphrodites were not wonders since they did not possess full reproductive organs from both genders, but rather a defective version of each.[94] Although Realdo Colombo saw hermaphrodites as curiosities, his pathological approach still placed the hermaphrodite he dissected, and the one he observed, within the realm of the monstrous.[95] The importance of medical discourse in determining the status of hermaphrodites transcended the theoretical, serving to establish their status as full juridical entities. The most famous trial recounting the legal tribulations of a hermaphrodite in the early modern period is undoubtedly that of Marie/Marin le Marcis. In his 1612 *Traité des hermaphrodits*, Jacques Duval devotes twenty chapters to the story of this *fille-homme*.[96] He recounts how he met her, and his subsequent finding of her "membre viril," in spite of opposing opinions from other physicians. The impossibility of reaching a consensus about his/her gendered position eventually led to the release of Marie/Marin and his lover Jeanne. He was, however, forbidden to dress as a man or have any sexual relations until he reached the age of twenty-five.[97] The civic life of hermaphrodites thus appears to have depended almost solely on medical assessment. Paolo Zacchia, in his *Quaestonium medico legalium* (begun in 1621) studied the medico-juridical case of hermaphrodites and eunuchs at length.[98] In book three, Zacchia presents the sixteen questions that pertained to the medico-legal status of eunuchs and hermaphrodites.[99] Interestingly, Zacchia returns to the issues of hermaphrodites in his section on monsters in book seven;[100] juridical personhood for hermaphrodites, eunuchs, and *spadones* boiled down to their ability to reproduce.[101] Zacchia's legal commentaries were inspired by the Pandects—a compendium of civil laws—written by the Emperor Justinian in the 530s, where the seminal powers of a man often determined his legal status. Therefore, if a hermaphrodite or a eunuch (who suffered a partial penectomy rather than a orchiectomy) was able to reproduce, he retained the right to marry, have an heir, and transmit possessions, and thus to possess material goods in his/her name. This juridical determination would thus have kept castrati from marriage, though not from existing as independent beings, at least in state adhering to papal edicts as law. The transmission of name or title would have been a legal intricacy, since bloodlines could not have been directly established for them. However, the case of a seventeenth-century Italian castrato, Bartolomeo Sorlisi, marrying the daughter of a German lawyer demonstrates the complexity of attaching seminal juridical values to men who were born with both X and Y chromosomes and with the capacity for reproduction, but whose choice in the matter was suppressed.[102] This castrato's marriage unraveled many issues inherent in intertwining theological law with juridical assessment of personhood; ultimately, confusion led to a series of complaints gathered in a compendium entitled *Eunuchi conjugium*.[103] In the same vein, an excerpt from an *avviso* dated to November 11, 1662 recalls the predicament of a priest who found himself pregnant after hearing the confessions of a young woman.[104] Though the *avviso* does mention the issue of hermaphroditism, the paradox of such a situation could not have been resolved legally or religiously through the mere application of civil and theological laws based on the reproductive abilities assigned to either hermaphrodites.

Any discussion on juridical personhood and legal rights establishes the liminal position in which Italian castrati found themselves. As successful performers, they had many material possessions and sometimes even occupied positions of courtiers, but they still were legally not granted the permission to marry—which would have allowed them to establish a lineage. This right was granted to those without money, titles, or possessions; however, unable to reproduce, castrati were denied this civil right. Pasqualini's portrait emphasizes the castrato's liminal position. Adored, admired, intellectually sharp, and highly in demand, Pasqualini revels in the poetic glory bestowed upon him by Apollo—yet, in the eyes of God and of civic law, he is a mutilated monster without the possibility of leaving a trace of himself in the form of a subsequent generation. The tension caused by such a social and legal predicament parallels the unresolved tension visible in Sacchi's portrait, a portrait that, ultimately, stands as Pasqualini's strongest material legacy.

The reality of castrati's lives still presents us with numerous unanswered questions. Although their voices will never be heard again, their visual representations contain much evidence that may still be deciphered. The underlying iconological text present in Andrea Sacchi's portrait of Marc'Antonio Pasqualini uncovers many paradoxical realities faced by castrati, while also asserting the prominent place occupied by these artists in the seventeenth and eighteenth centuries. As young boys sacrificed to the altar of musical splendor, castrati may have embraced the glory bestowed upon them, but they were never allowed to forget their deficiency—physically, legally, religiously, or socially. Sacchi's portrait encompasses these intricate and unsettling tensions by juxtaposing two conflicting images: that of a ruling and glorified male god, and that of a defeated and condemned monster. While neither Morgante, nor Antoinette had much agency in their portrayal, Marc'Antonio Pasqualini actually decided on the complex iconographical program of this painting with Andrea Sacchi. In a sense, he constructed his own visual dichotomy by emphasizing the conflict he experienced as a man essentially owned by his patron, but one who exercised considerable influence through the skills given to him by his mutilated body. This active participation of the subject in the creation of a court portrait that ultimately objectifies part of his persona through his body complicates the reading of Sacchi's portrait of Pasqualini. However, this complex script allows this work to participate in the discursive narrative framing the monstrous—as well as its visual articulation through an official representation. Pasqualini's portrait adds to the dialogue started by Bronzino's *Morgante* and Fontana's *Antoinette Gonsalvus* by including the sitter's own voice—in the composition and as a residual memory of his performances—and thus by destabilizing the object/subject balance inherent in depicting an individual whose physical anomaly was the reason for his station in life. The other balance, between *imitare* and *ritrarre*, appears at first to be unmoved in the castrato's portrait. However, the anatomical subtext of the portrait dealing with the physically abnormal body of its subject alters this equilibrium; it is not the body of the castrato that is scrutinized under the *imitare* lens, but rather that of the satyr. And through Daphne's body, Sacchi uses *imitare* to convey Pasqualini's superiority, his idealized sexuality and artistic prevalence. Between *Morgante* and *Antoinette Gonsalvus*, the castrato's portrait holds a more complex composition in which *imitare* seems to surpass *ritrarre*. His latent monstrous body, however, and his subsequent position as a dependent marvel finds resonance in this portrait where *imitare* is in fact not surpassed by *ritrarre*, but slightly veiled. Perhaps this covering resulted from the fact that Pasqualini himself was a full participant in courtly life and his position existed because of civilized taste. Opera and music were central to the civilizing process at court and a complex iconographical program dealing with *poesia* certainly highlighted Pasqualini's intellectual abilities in mastering the social ground on which he walked. And yet, the actuality of his body, undermined his full access to *civiltà* and overwhelmed the visual discourse meant to ennoble the mutilated singer.

Notes

[1] Scholars such as Marie-Hélène Huet have dealt with the complex and extensive relations between monsters, imagination, and procreation. See Marie-Hélène Huet, *Monstrous Imagination* (Cambridge and London: Harvard University Press, 1993). To support his argument, Carlino looks particularly at dissections done by Colombo, most notably the dissection of a hermaphrodite, and discusses monsters as pathological manifestations. Carlino offers a reading that allows for the integration of anatomical inquiries into the investigation of abnormal individuals. See Andrea Carlino, "Strani corpi. Come farsi une ragione dei mostri nel XVI secolo," in *Phantastische Lebensräume, Phantome und Phantasmen*, ed. Hans Konrad Schumtz (Marburg an der Lahn: Basilisken-Press, 1997), 143: "My claim is that Colombo's approach to monstrous subjects through anatomical dissections induced him to conceive their morphological 'difference' as anatomical abnormalities. This approach signifies inscribing monstrosity in pathology; therefore evacuating the merely teratological and superstitious conception, still operating in texts produced by other doctors and anatomists, such as Ambroise Paré."

[2] Patrick Barbier, *The World of the Castrati: The History of an Extraordinary Operatic Phenomenon* (London: Souvenir Press, 1996), 3. Also, for the absence of castrati, see John Rosselli, *Singers of Italian Opera: The History of a Profession* (Cambridge: Cambridge University Press, 1992), 32: "about the castrati there is much we do not and cannot know. We cannot hear their voices; the few recordings made in the infancy of the gramophone only hint at a sound now lost. We cannot interrogate them; this is true of many people studied by historians, but even when there were still castrati living, scholars were too embarrassed to ask them searching questions. We do not really know how they were operated on or what the operation did to human characteristics other than the voice. Nor do we always know who were or were not castrati; so we can make only a rough estimate of how many there were at any time."

[3] These points are further elaborated in this chapter.

[4] Fredrika Jacobs, "(Dis)assembling: Marsyas, Michelangelo, and the Accademia del Disegno," *Art Bulletin* 84, no. 3 (September 2002): 426–48.

[5] Ovid, *Metamorphoses*, book 6, 436–57, as presented in *Ovid: Metamorphoses*, trans. Stanley Lombardo and with an introduction by W.R. Johnson (Indianapolis and Cambridge: Hackett Publishing, 2010), 159–60.

[6] Ovid, *Metamorphoses*, book 1, 470–601, in Lombardo and Johnson, *Ovid*, 18–22.

[7] Sylvie Mamy, *Les castrats* (Paris: Presses Universitaires de France, 1998), 119.

[8] Irina V. Rudakova, *"Uncertain Nature": History of the Castrato Singer in the Early Modern Gender Paradigm*, dissertation (University of Washington, 1999), 86.

[9] I here use the word "mutilation" in accordance with the Oxford English Dictionary's definition: the action of depriving (a person or animal) of a limb or of the use of a limb; the excision or maiming (of a limb or bodily organ); castration.

[10] Rosselli, *Singers*, 34.

[11] Richard Sherr, "Gugliemo Gonzaga and the Castrati," *Renaissance Quarterly* 33, no. 1 (Spring 1980): 33 and James Chater, "Musical Patronage in Rome at the Turn of the Seventeenth Century: The Case of Cardinal Montalto," *Studi Musicali* 16, no. 2 (1987): 180–81.

[12] John Rosselli, "From Princely Service to the Open Market: Singers on Italian Opera and Their Patrons, 1600–1850," *Cambridge Opera Journal* 1, no. 1 (1989): 1.

[13] Rosselli, "From Princely Service," 6.

[14] Ibid.

[15] Barbier, *World of the Castrati*, 126.

[16] In the Clementine Vulgate Bible, elaborated first by Sixtus VI and established by Clement VIII, we find in 1 Corinthians 14:33–35, 37: "As in all the churches of the saints, the women should keep silence in the churches. For they are not permitted to speak, but should be subordinate, as even the law says. If there is anything they desire to know, let them ask their husbands at home. For it is shameful for a woman to speak in church. [...] what I am writing to you is a command of the Lord." Also, for women's ability to perform, Barbier, *World of the Castrati*, 20. Innocent XI banned all women from appearing on stage in 1686, which roughly coincides with the large increase in castrati and in operatic compositions employing them.

[17] Rosselli, *Singers*, 34.

[18] Rodolfo Celletti, *A History of Bel Canto* (Oxford: Clarendon Press, 1991), 108.

[19] Gary Taylor, *Castration: An Abbreviated History of Western Manhood* (New York and London: Routledge, 2002), 39.

[20] Mamy, *Les castrats*, 32.

[21] Lynn Hollen Lees and Paul M. Hohenberg, "Urban Decline and Regional Economies: Brabant, Castile, and Lombardy 1550–1750," *Society for Comparative Study of Society and History* 31, no. 3 (1989): 439–61.

[22] Rosselli, *Singers*, 35.

[23] Rudakova, 92.

[24] Some research has been done on the behavior of castrated rhesus monkeys, but unfortunately it is barely, if not at all, applicable to a human study of castration. Nevertheless, the study concluded that the monkeys developed full sexual behavior when introduced into an environment with non-castrated monkeys. They, however, stopped sexual acts after a short period of time due to their inability to sustain erections. See James Loy, Kent Loy, Geoffrey Keifer, and Clinton Conaway, *The Behavior of Gonadectomized Rhesus Monkeys*, Contributions to Primatology 20 (Basel: Karger, 1984), 3–9. More relevant are studies done in the twentieth century on Skoptzy men and the eunuchs of the Chinese and Ottoman empires. However, because castrating practices on these men were not standardized, their visible and medical expressions varied. See Jean D. Wilson and Claus Roehrborn, "Long-term Consequences of Castration in Men: Lessons from the Skoptzy and the Eunuchs of the Chinese and Ottoman Courts," *The Journal of Clinical Endocrinology and Metabolism* 84, no. 12 (1999): 4324–31. I am indebted to Rolf Nelson for having shared this last reference with me.

[25] Meyer M. Melicow, "Castrati Choir and Opera Singers," *Urology* 3 (1974): 663; and Jacqueline Long, *Claudian's In Eutropium, or, How, When, and Why to Slander a Eunuch* (Chapel Hill: University of North Carolina Press, 1996),108.

[26] Charles d'Ancillon, *Traité des Eunuques* (1707) translated into English under the pseudonym C. d'Ollincan, *Eunuchism Display'd: Describing All the Different Sorts of Eunuchs; ... Written by a Person of Honour* (London: E. Curll, 1718).

[27] Rudakova, 137.

[28] It is interesting to find that up until the mid-twentieth century, such a belief was still prevalent and was still being defended in studies about castration, albeit very biased ones. See M. Riquet, *La Castration* (Paris: P. Lethielleux, Libraire-Éditeur, 1948), 36.

[29] Melicow, "Castrati Choir," 665.

[30] In his 1776 *De diocesana synodo*, Pope Benedict XIV states that "amputation of any part of the human body is never lawful except when the whole body cannot be saved from destruction in any other way."

[31] On a purely medical level, Melicow reproduces and discusses illustrations from a 1559 German medical textbook by Caspar Stromayr, which show the removal of one or two testicles. This reproduction simply serves to assert that the actual procedure of castration was widely known in early modern Europe, though not performed for explicit musical purpose. Melicow, "Castrati Choir," 664.

[32] John Rosselli, "The Castrati as a Professional Group and a Social Phenomenon, 1550–1850," *Acta Musicologica* 60, no. 2 (May–August 1988): 152.

[33] Contract of August 3, 1671 between Salvatore and Olimpia Nannini, represented by Sante Nannini, and the teacher Antonio Masini: "Acciò detto Paolo possa habilitarsi alla musica e mantenere la voce detti signori Salvatore e Olimpia come detto signor Santo promette far castrare il detto Paolo mel mese di settembre prossimo futuro e detto signor Antonio sia tenuto a somministrare a tutte sue spese, le spese che abbisogneranno tanto per l'operatione della castratura, quanto per farlo medicare et d'ogni altra cosa a quest'effeto, e ritenerlo in casa propria con carità paterna." As cited in Rosselli, "Castrati as a Professional Group," 152, footnote 37.

[34] Contract of November 30, 1697 between Giovanni Donato Rizzo, of Castellana, and Niccolò Tricarico of Gallipolli: "[...] havendo un suo figlio legittimo et naturale, d'età al presente di anni otto, nominato Francesco Rizzo, havesse risoluto per maggior profitto d'esso Giovanni Donato, di sua casa, et del detto Francesco di farli imparare perfettamente la professione seu arte di cantar figurato, et in tempo debito farlo castrare per divenir eunuco; et non havendo modo di farli tutti quelli dispendi necessary [...]." As cited in G.A. Pastore, "Un raro documento su l'evirazione dei cantanti nel secolo XVII," *Letture dell'Accademia Salentina di Lettere Scienze e Arti* 1, no. 2 (April 1955).

[35] Orchiectomy—or orchidectomy—is often conflated with castration. However, orchiectomy is a surgical procedure that removed the testicles only, while castration carries cultural connotations of punishment and may include the removal of the penis as well as that of the testicles.

[36] Information gathered and compiled from Celletti, *A History*, 109; Melicow, "Castrati Choir," 665; Rudakova, 18–19; Roger Freitas, *Un Atto d'ingegno: A Castrato in the Seventeenth Century*, unpublished dissertation (Yale University, May 1998), 189; and the *Miller-Keane Medical Dictionary*, 2000.

[37] I am thankful to Dr. Isabelle Kaelin Gambirasio for discussing hormonal effects and their visual expressions on the male body with me.

[38] Piotr O. Scholz, *Eunuchs and Castrati: A Cultural History* (Princeton: Markus Wiener Publishers, 2001), 16. Valeria Finucci discusses at length the nicknames given to castrati and their implications. For instance: *evirati*, *non integri*, *coglioni*, *castratini*, *castratelli*, and *castroni*. See Valeria Finucci, *The Manly Masquerade: Masculinity, Paternity, and Castration in the Italian Renaissance* (Durham and London: Duke University Press, 2003), 239.

[39] Charles Burney, *Men, Music and Manners in France and Italy*, ed. H. Edmund Poole (London: Folio Society, 1969), 128 and 163: the Italians "are so much ashamed at the practice of making [the castrati] that every single city says it is not there, but names some other place."

[40] Though I do agree with Roger Freitas on the labeling of castrati as "others," I do not believe there is a complete absence of familiarity regarding the various socio-economic, theological, or artistic factors that determined their lives. See Freitas, *Un Atto d'ingegno*, 12.

[41] Scholz, *Eunuchs and Castrati*, 22–25. Anthony Milner, "The Sacred Capons," *The Musical Times* 114, no. 1561 (March 1973): 251: "Theologians argued that mutilation was permissible as a punishment for criminals and thus justified the brutal penal codes which increased in severity up to the seventeenth century. The Popes, like other sovereigns, ordered mutilation for criminals in their States, and continued to do so for longer than some."

[42] Melicow, "Castrati Choir," 663 and Joseph Katz, "Testimonia Ritus Italici: Male Genitalia, Solemn Declarations, and a New Latin Sound Law," *Harvard Studies in Classical Philology* 98 (1998): 183–217.

[43] Meyer M. Melicow, "Castration Down the Ages," *New York State Journal of Medicine* 77 (1977): 804–6.

[44] Rosselli, "Castrati as a Professional Group," 143. In his travels through Italy, Jean Jérôme de Lalande also notes that most castrati were made in Naples in the hope that they would participate in operatic compositions, but ended up in the orders when that plan failed. Jean Jérôme de Lalande, *Voyage d'un François en Italie fait dans les années 1765 et 1766. Contenant l'histoire et les anecdotes les plus singulières de l'Italie, et sa description; les moeurs, les usages, le gouvernement, le commerce, la littérature, les arts, l'histoire naturelle, et les antiquités; avec des jugements sur les ouvrages de peinture, sculpture et architecture, et les plans de toutes les grandes villes d'Italie* (Venice and Paris: Desaint, 1769), 6:345–49.

[45] Sacheverell Sitwell, *Baroque and Rococo* (New York: G.P. Putnam's Sons, 1967), 244–45.

[46] John Courtenay, *The Present State of the Manners, Arts, and Politics of France and Italy in a Series of Poetical Epistles from Paris, Rome, and Naples, in 1792 and 1793, Addressed to Robert Jephson, Esq.* (Dublin: Wooan, Byrne, and Jones, 1794), 93–95: "'Twas thus Farinelli delighted all Spain/ When madness he cur'd by his magical strain/ ... / When Ferdinand, insanely grave/ Would neither wash his hands nor shave,/ Nor Olio taste nor jelly;/ His royal confort, sunk in grief,/ When ev'ry faint deny'd relief,/ Thus pray'd to Farineli!/ Sweet Farinelli, swell your throat,/ And pour some soft bewitching note/ ... / Hark! Farinelli squeaks to please her."

[47] In the eighteenth century, up to 4,000 boys were castrated each year. F. Haböck, *Die Kastraten und ihre Gesangkunst* (Stuttgart: Deutsche Verlags-Anstalt, 1927), 238.

[48] For the documents relating to Farinelli's admission to the Order of Calatrava, see Nicolás Soler Quintes, "Nuevas aportaciones a la biografia de Carlo Broschi Farinelli," *Anuario Musical* 3 (1948): 187–204.

[49] For a list of the sitters in this portrait, see the 1783 inventory of Farinelli reprinted in Francesca Boris and Gianmpiero Cammarota, "La collezione di Carlo Broschi, detto Farinello," *Atti e Memorie* (Bologna: Accademia Clementina, 1990), 208: "Un quadro grande bislungo nella sua cornice intagliata e indorata di mano dell'Amiconi, rappresenta Ritratti del Sig.r Testatore, Abbate Metastasio, Teresa Castellini, Giacomo Amiconi stesso, Ussaretto e Cane del Sig.r Testatore. Figure intiere al naturale per il traverso." As for the argument stating that the Hungarian hussar might be Prince Joseph, see Daniel Heartz's argument in Derek Beales, *Joseph II*, vol. 1: *In the Shadow of Maria Teresa, 1741–1780* (Cambridge: Cambridge University Press, 1987), plate I, 172.

[50] Ted Gott and Laurie Benson, *Jacopo Amigoni: Portrait Group: The Singer Farinelli and Friends*, http://bit.ly/QdgZsG, accessed June 26, 2012.

[51] Painted around 1640, this ambitious painting of life-sized figures (243.8 cm x 194.3 cm) has belonged to the Metropolitan Museum of Art since 1981, after it left Lord Spencer's collection, where it had been housed for more than two centuries. First owned by Cardinal Giulio Rospigliosi from 1640 until 1669, the painting then traveled to the palazzo of the Marchese Niccolò Maria Pallavicini where it stayed until approximately 1714. Shortly thereafter, the painting left Italy for England and remained in the collection of Sir Robert Furnese until 1758 when it was sold to the first Earl of Spencer, in conjunction with Guido Reni's "Liberality and Modesty." This information is gathered from: *L'Idea del Bello: Viaggio per Roma nel Seicento con Giovan Pietro Bellori* (Rome: Edizioni De Luca, 2000), 2:449; from Stella Rudolph, *Niccolò Maria Pallavicini: L'ascesa al Tempio della Virtù attraverso il Mecenatismo* (Rome: Ugo Bozzi Editore, 1995), 75; and from the object file related to the Sacchi's portrait of Marc'Antonio Pasqualini and an article in the *Daily Telegraph* dated May 16, 1981 that confirms the dealers and the value of the paintings. Together, these two paintings were sold to Welti Furrer Ltd. of Zurich through the London dealers Wildenstein and Company who first placed a value of 40,000 pounds on the pair.

[52] Nicoletta Guidobaldi, "'Non un semplice ritratto': Marcantonio Pasqualini, Apollo e Marsia in un dipinto di Andrea Sacchi," in *Musica e immagine tra iconografia e mondo dell'opera*, ed. Biancamaria Brumana and Galliano Ciliberti (Florence: Leo S. Olschki, Editore, 1993), 141.

[53] GianPietro Bellori, *The Lives of the Modern Painters, Sculptors and Architects: A New Translation and Critical Edition*, trans. Alice Sedgwick Wohl, notes by Hellmut Wohl, and introduction by Tomaso Montanari (Cambridge: Cambridge University Press, 2005), 390: "This is not a simple portrait, but a most graceful composition, for he represented him in shepherd's costume [...]. His coat, down to the knees, is white, with a fur that crosses from his shoulder."

[54] *Idea del Bello*, 2:450.

[55] This entry is found in an inventory of Cardinal Antonio Barberini's possessions taken in 1636, and included in another 1644 inventory. *Inventoria di Guardaroba di Cardinale Antonio Barberini*, 196v, under the heading *Organi e Cimbali*. The entirety of the seventeenth-century Barberini inventories have been gathered and published by Marylin Aronberg Lavin, *Seventeenth-century Barberini Documents and Inventories of Art* (New York: New York University Press, 1975). For this reference, 156: "un cimbalo in piedi a foggia di arpa con tre figurini in cima, attorno tutto intagliata, e dorato guarnito dinanzi con diverse pietre incastrate, [...] posato su un tavolino di albuccio bianco intagliato con suoi piedi a colonette scallenati [...]."

[56] Letter from Franca Trinchieri Camiz to Keith Christiansen dated to June 28, 1982.

[57] Guidobaldi, "'Non un semplice ritratto,'" 142; *Idea del Bello*, 2:450; and Franca Trinchieri Camiz, "The Castrato Singer: From Informal to Formal Portraiture," *Artibus et Historiae* 18 (1988): 183.

[58] Archivio generale del Vicariato, *Lib. baptiz.* di San Lorenzo e Damaso (1600–1616), 323.

[59] Information gathered from various notes and letters found in Andrea Sacchi's Metropolitan Museum of Art's object file on the portrait of Marc'Antonio Pasqualini.

[60] Freitas, *Un Atto d'ingegno*, 8–9.

[61] Ibid., 9 and Rosselli, "From Princely Service," 5.

[62] The length of a castrato's career does not seem to have been shorter or longer than that of any other performer. Though castrati started their training very early in life, they did not stop singing and performing much earlier than other singers and actors.

[63] Cesare Ripa, *Baroque and Rococo Pictorial Imagery: The 1758–60 Hertel Edition*, ed. Edward A. Maser (New York: Dover Publications, 1971), 183 and Cesare Ripa, *Iconologia* (Rome: Fei, 1603), 408.

[64] Camiz, "The Castrato Singer," 183.

[65] Guidobaldi, "'Non un semplice ritratto,'" 143–49.

[66] Todd Olson, "'Long Live the Knife!': Andrea Sacchi's Portrait of Marc'Antonio Pasqaulini, *Art History* 27, no. 5 (November 2004): 697–722, and 716–17 in particular: "Pasqualini's performance of class, gender and sexuality, seemingly dissociated from a material body, not only effaces women but also regulates male–male sexual, class, and client relations. Castration negotiates the proximate dangers of an erotically charged male body and the spectre of debased carnality, the very risks posed by Caravaggio's paintings. However, the body of Marsyas, constituted as the site of base sexuality and violence, is renounced only to return as the castrato's dematerialized phallic voice, described by contemporaries as forceful, penetrating and ravishing, emitted from the materially violated body of the castrato. [...] Virility and masculinity have been redirected to the artful voice, one deemed entirely independent of both sexuality and commercial pressures. This, I believe, is Pasqualini's achievement: a phallic masculinity is ultimately recuperated by dissociating it from any fixed sexual object, thereby divesting it of heterosexual desire while allaying the fears of both sodomitical relations and, perhaps more importantly, commercial exchange."

[67] Keith Christiansen has stated the likely involvement of Pasqualini in the commissioning of this portrait as a gift for his patron. Keith Christiansen, *A Caravaggio Rediscovered: The Lute Player* (New York: The Metropolitan Museum of Art, 1990), 82, regarding the person who commissioned the portrait: "Any member of the Barberini family may be excluded, since there is no record of a payment for it in their account books and no mention of it in their inventories [...]. The most probable candidate is Pasqualini himself, whose friendship with Sacchi and vain character accord perfectly with the self-adulation implicit in the imagery."

[68] Beth Holman, "Verrocchio's *Marsyas* and Renaissance Anatomy," *Marsyas: Studies in the History of Art* 19 (1977–78): 1–2.

[69] Holman, "Verrocchio's *Marsyas*," 2–4.

[70] Realdo Colombo, *De re anatomica* (Venice: Bevilaqua, 1559) and Andreas Vesalius, *De humani corporis fabrica* (Basel: Oporinus, 1555). Also, see Holman, "Verrocchio's *Marsyas*," 7, footnotes 20 and 21.

[71] Ripa, *Iconologia*, 408, about the iconography of *la Poesia*: "un Apollo ignudo con una corona sulla destra, con la quale faccia sembiante di volere incoronare qualcuno, et ne la sinistra una lira."

[72] Edith Wyss, *The Myth of Apollo and Marsyas in the Art of the Italian Renaissance: An Inquiry into the Meaning of Images* (Delaware: Associated University Presses, 1996), 122.

[73] Biblioteca Vaticana (BV), Archivio Barberini (AB), Computesteria 267, 232: "Andrea Sacchi pittore et architetto di S. Em. Deve dare a di 6 Ott. & cento m.ta buoni a siri pagatigli conforme."

[74] BV, AB, Computesteria 267, 232: "1 cento m.ta. buoni a d[etto] pag[at]i a buon conto della spesa del quadro che rappresenta la fiesta/ del Gesù p[er] il centesimo de P[ad]ri Gesuiti."

[75] Christiansen, *A Caravaggio Rediscovered*, 80.

[76] See Gloria Rose, "Pasqualini as Copyist," *Studien zur italienisch-deutschen Musikgeschichte* 9, no. 4 (1974): 170–75 for Pasqualini's activities as a copyist and collector of musical scores. For

Pasqualini's education and intellectual brush with other famed musical scholars, see A. Cametti, "Musicisti celebri del seicento in Roma: Marc'Antonio Pasqualini," *Musica d'oggi* 3 (1921): 69–71 and 98–99.

[77] Margaret Murata, "Further Remarks on Pasqualini and the Music of *MAP*," *Analecta Musicologica* 19 (1984): 130.

[78] Christiansen, *A Caravaggio Rediscovered*, 82: "Indeed, it now appears that in the seventeenth century musicians emerged not only as outstanding personalities but also as significant patrons: the composer and harpist Marco Marazzoli commissioned an ambitious allegory of Music from Lanfranco that he later gave to Antonio Barberini."

[79] Thomas Laqueur, *Making Sex: Body and Gender from the Greeks to Freud* (Cambridge: Harvard University Press, 1990), 22: the "problematic, unstable female body that is either a version of or wholly different from a generally unproblematic stable male body. [...] The notion, so powerful after the eighteenth century, that there had to be something outside, inside, and throughout the body which defines male as opposed to female and which provides the foundation for an attraction of opposites is entirely absent from classical or Renaissance medicine," and 148: after the eighteenth century, "no longer would those who think about such matters [two distinct and opposite sexes] regard woman as a lesser version of man along a vertical axis of infinite gradations, but rather as an altogether different creature along a horizontal axis whose middle ground was largely empty."

[80] This is a simplified explanation of classical Galenic and Hippocratic beliefs regarding the difference of genders. It is interesting to note an observation about the difference between male and female in regard to the place of eunuchs in that spectrum as stated by Ambroise Paré: "The Nature of Eunuches is to be referred to that of women, as who may seeme to have degenerated into a womanish nature, by deficiency of heate." Cited in Ann Rosalind Jones and Peter Stallybrass, "Fetishizing Gender: Constructing the Hermaphrodite in Renaissance Europe," in *Body Guards: The Cultural Politics of Gender Ambiguity*, ed. Julia Epstein and Kristina Straub (New York: Routledge, 1991), 83.

[81] By hypersexuality, I refer to the idea that castrati were perfect lovers for women. Indeed, their inability to reproduce made sexual intercourse with them extremely safe and therefore attracted many lovers. For the notion of femininity associated with music, see Linda Phyllis Austern, "'Alluring the Auditorie to Effeminacie': Music and the Idea of the Feminine in Early Modern England," *Music and Letters* 74, no. 3 (1993): 347: " music was often perceived by theoretical writers as a vain sensual delight and enemy to masculine rationality."

[82] Rudakova, 191.

[83] Barbier, *World of the Castrati*, 138: "It is also a fact that their exploits with women, which could go as far as marriage, would not have been so numerous if they had been mere pleasant dalliances, even during the century of libertine behaviour. On the other hand one can never generalise in this area, and it seems obvious that sexual appetite among the castrati varied greatly from one man to the next and could be 'voracious' in one case and virtually non-existent in another. This depended in particular on the operation itself, on which organs had been affected, on the circumstances in which it had been performed and at what age."

[84] *Idea del Bello*, 2:449.

[85] Henri Prunières, *L'opéra italien en France avant Lully* (Paris: Champion, 1913), 89 where the author mentions that the Cardinal's passion for the castrato extended beyond his voice.

[86] Olson, "'Long Live the Knife!'" 716.

[87] Wyss, *The Myth of Apollo*, 143.

[88] Jacobs, "(Dis)assembling," 433.

[89] Lynn Frier Kaufmann, *The Noble Savage: Satyrs and Satyr Families in Renaissance Art* (Ann Arbor: UMI Research Press, 1984), 21.

[90] Ibid, 73.

[91] Ovid, *Metamorphoses*, book 1, 470–601, in Lombardo and Johnson, *Ovid*, 18–22.

[92] Michael T. Walton, Robert Fineman, and Phyllis J. Walton, "Of Monsters and Prodigies: The Interpretation of Birth Defects in the Sixteenth Century," *American Journal of Medical Genetics* 47, no. 1 (August 1993): 8.

[93] This view was particularly developed by Paracelsus. See Michael T. Walton, Robert M. Fineman, and Phyllis J. Walton, "Holy Hermaphrodites and Medical Facts: The Depiction of Hermaphrodites in Alchemy and Medicine," *Studies in Hermeticism: Cauda Pavonis* 18, nos. 1–2 (Spring and Fall 1999): 35.

[94] Jean Riolan, *Discours sur les hermaphrodits où il est demonstré contre l'opinion commune, qu'il n'y a point de vrays hermaphrodits* (Paris: Pierre Ramier, 1614), 26 and 67–68.

[95] Colombo, *De re anatomica*, 268: "However, my Boni, or rather good Jacopo, among the many astonishing and rare things which I have observed at different times in the structure of the human body, I consider that nothing is more astonishing , nothing rarer, than what I diligently investigated about a nature neither male nor female." Translation by Moes in Robert J. Moes and C.D. O'Malley, "Realdo Colombo: 'On Those Things Rarely Found in Anatomy,'" *Bulletin of the History of Medicine* 34, no. 6 (November–December 1960): 508–28.

[96] Jacques Duval, *Traité des hermaphrodits: Parties genitals, accouchemens des femmes, etc. Où sont expliquez la figure des laboureurs & verger du genre humain, signes de pucelag, defloration, conception, & la belle industrie don't use Nature en la promotion du concept & plante prolifique*, reimpression of the 1612 Rouen edition (Paris: Isidore Lisieux, 1880). The case of le Marcis is discussed from chapters 60 to 80.

[97] Lorraine Daston and Katharine Park, "Hermaphrodite in Renaissance France," *Critical Matrix* 1, no. 5 (1985): 3. Ten years after his release, Marin was actually living as a man and was employed as a tailor.

[98] Pauli Zacchiae Romani, totius status ecclesiastici proto-medici generalis, *Quaestionum medico-legalium, tomi tres. Editio prima Veneta, Lugdunensi & Noribergensi, quae passim soedis scatebant erroribus multò emendiator: Accedunt Interpolationes, & Auctaria ex novis Inventis & Observationibus Recentiorum Auctorum. Curà Joannis Danielis Horstii, Diversorum S.R.I. Principum Archiatri, & Collegii Medici Moeno-Francofurtani Senioris. Opus omnibus medicinae et juris utriusque peritis, Necnon Tribunalium (Ecclesiastici, Civilis) Assessoribus maximè necessarium* (Venice: Bonifacii Viezzeri, 1737).

[99] Zacchia, Libri Tertii, Titulus I, Quaestio IX: De Hermaphroditis, Spadonibus, & Eunuchis, 223.

[100] Ibid., Libri Septimi, Titulus primus, *De Monstris*, Questio VIII: De Hermaphroditis, 76.

[101] Spadones is the general term for eunuch, though spadones are not always castrated; they simply do not have the ability to reproduce and are usually impotent.

[102] For the story of Bartolomeo Sorlisi's marriage to Dorothea Lichtwer, see Mary E. Frandsen, "Eunichi Conjugium: The Marriage of a Castrato in Early Modern Germany," *Early Music History* 24 (2005): 53–124.

[103] H. Delphinus (pseudonym), ed., *Eunuchi conjugium: Die Capaunen-Heirath, Hoc est Scripta et judicia varia de conjugio inter eunuchum et virginem juvenculam Anno M. DC. LXVI. contracto, T. T. A. quibusdam supremis theologorum collegiis petita, postea hinc inde collecta ab Hieronymo Delphino, C.P.* (Halle, 1718); this represents the third of nine editions; the preface is dated 1685. As cited in Frandsen, "Eunichi Conjugium," 56.

[104] Avviso from Rome of November 11, 1662, Archivio di Stato di Firenze, Mediceo del Principato 4027a, unpaginated folio (ca. f. 386), document no. 19865 in Documentary Sources for the Arts and Humanities listed in the Medici Archive Project. I am very grateful to Sheila Barker for sharing this unpublished document with me: "Dicono affermativamente farsi qui causa di un successo, che un tal prete confessando una giovane si scoprissero esser ambi ermafroditi, restassero vedersi assieme, e doppo vistisi si congiungessero reciprocamente, et in somma il prete restasse pregno."

Epilogue

MICHEL FOUCAULT DEFINED THE NOTION of the "human monster" as one that was essentially juridical. Indeed, for Foucault what defined the monster was the fact that he was, inherently, in violation of societal laws and in violation of natural laws as well.[1] Whereas the rarity of the individuals discussed in this book is not in question, in the portraits produced at court between 1550 and 1650, the violence implied by Foucault though not erased, was not highlighted. Human qualities pervaded their depictions. Mimesis was used to identify the known sitters, and idealization was employed just as it would have been for court portraits of regular human beings. It is precisely this normalizing impulse that was of interest, since it created an unresolved tension within the surface of the canvas. The idealization did not cancel the mimetic emphasis; the two complemented each other while creating a composition whose values lay in the combination of the two. Yet, what was made visible in these portraits was the end result of the civilizing process that tamed the violence of the subversive monster. The portraits served as systems of conventions that integrated dissidence into a regulated frame and were in fact violent in their imposition of a controlled aesthetic for physical dissonance.

Through visual and textual productions, these bodies and their representations became manifestations of political, social, and medical transformations and allowed for alternate epistemologies to occur. Whether difference was used as a wondrous quality aligned with structural power or whether physical anomaly became a projected deformity meant to condemn fallibility, the painted portrait of the bodies studied in this book allow us to elucidate the dialogue between intentions, perceptions, and the intellectual frame that channeled such an exchange. As meanings shifted, the monstrous became porous.

The lack of defined symmetry among the three cases at the center of this book demonstrate the very idea of diversity. In fact, this diversity expands beyond the category of monsters and encompasses the range of cultural histories that compose the Renaissance. It is through portraits of human monsters that we are able to see how heterogeneous the early modern states were and how malleable the concept of truth was—a notion that certainly has relevance today. Far from merely and only reinforcing the norm, the portraits directing this study created an opening that allowed for a glimpse into a world that celebrated difference as a necessary component of life. Without attributing anachronistic qualities to this celebration, the recognition of physical variations as an inherent part of courtly life allows us to approach cultural framing with more nuances.

Neither wondrous objects lying still in a cabinet of curiosities, nor generic anonymous individuals roaming through high social spheres like other courtiers, the beings discussed in this book challenged both structures. Their portraits did not simply mirror their situation at court, they highlighted the liminal position different humans held in both a factual world and its associated collective imaginary. The depiction of anatomically intriguing individuals played with Cinquecento and Seicento discourses on art theory, and ultimately used contemporaneous visual language to convey the dual aspects of these subjects/objects. It also provided agency and voice to those without the direct social ability to establish their own personhood.

The interesting dichotomy present in court portraits of physically anomalous beings in early modern Italy did not vanish with the advent of the Enlightenment and modern scientific standards. Rather, it was explored through different lenses. Court culture lost its dominance; therefore private collections faded in favor of museums and more public venues for objects and individuals of rare interest. The shift from court participant to circus entertainer was certainly one to follow and was pregnant with social significance. Ultimately, however, the fascination with physical difference is one that persists and endures. Achondroplasia has not disappeared, neither has hypertrichosis lanuginosa. Castration for the sake of musical glory does not occur anymore, but gender ambiguity and fluidity plays an active part in social definitions. It is thus not the physical manifestations of non-normative symptoms that are in question; it is the fluctuation of their interpretation that is salient.

Artists such as Agnolo Bronzino, Lavinia Fontana, or Andrea Sacchi actively participated in conventional determinations of court aesthetics through their artistic productions. However, by incorporating marginal subjects into their controlled vocabulary, they expanded what constituted cultural conformity. Ultimately, these portraits speak to the lack of linear cultural hegemony and highlight intellectual exchanges inevitable during a time of self-fashioning and political assertions. The fascination with Morgante's, Antoinette's, and Pasqualini's bodies was articulated through a vocabulary of difference that allowed norms to define themselves against their own limits. The reciprocity between monsters and normative humans grew within a discourse of courtly regulation and scientific discoveries. The subsequent portraits intervened in this discourse as active visual markers of such interactions. Far from being imaginary bodies that suggested a grotesque fascination, the sitters in these portraits confronted the viewers with the reality of their anomalies and with the actuality of their human presence.

Notes

[1] Michel Foucault, *Les anormaux: Cours au Collège de France (1974–1975)*, ed. François Ewald and Alessandro Fontana (Paris: Gallimard Le Seuil, 1999), 51: "Le cadre de reference du monstre humain, bien entendu, est la loi. La notion de monstre est essentiellement un notion juridique—juridique bien sûr, au sens large du terme, puisque ce qui définit le monstre est le fait qu'il est, dans son existence meme et dans sa forme, non seulement en violation des lois de la société, mais violations des lois de la nature."

Bibliography

Adriani, Maurilio. *Arti magiche nel Rinascimento a Firenze*. Florence: Casa Editrice Bonechi, 1980.

Alba, André et al., eds. *Malet et Isaac: L'Histoire Tome 2: L'Age classique: 1497–1789*. Paris: Hachette, 2002.

Alberti, Leon Battista. *On Painting and Sculpture: The Latin Texts of De Pictura and De Statua*. Edited and translated by Cecil Grayson. London: Phaidon, 1972.

Aldini, Tobia. *Exactissima descriptio rariorum quarandarum plantarum quae continentur Romae in Horto Farnesiano*. Rome: Typis Iacobi Mascardi, 1625.

Aldrovandi, Ulisse. *Opera Omnia*. Bologna: Manolesiana, Feronii, Thebaldinum, 1638–1681.

Allegri, Ettore and Alessandro Cecchi. *Palazzo Vecchio e i Medici: Guida storica*. Florence: Studio per edizioni scelte, 1980.

Ariosto, Ludovico. *Orlando furioso*. Edited by Emilio Bigi. Milan: Rusconi, 1982.

Austern, Linda Phyllis. "'Alluring the Auditorie to Effeminacie': Music and the Idea of the Feminine in Early Modern England." *Music and Letters* 74, no. 3 (1993): 343–54.

Avanzati, Elisabetta. "The Unpublished Senesino." *Handel and the Castrati: The Story behind the 18th-century Superstar Singers*. Catalogue of the Handel House Museum, March 2006: 5–9.

Avery, Charles. *Giambologna: The Complete Sculptures*. New York: Moyer Bell, 1987.

Avery, Charles and Anthony Radcliffe. *Giambologna 1529–1608: Sculptor to the Medici*. London and Edinburgh: The Arts Council of Great Britain, the Westerham Press, 1978.

Baccheschi, Edi. *L'Opera completa del Bronzino*. Milan: Rizzoli Editore, 1973.

Bakhtin, Mikhail. *Rabelais and His World*. Bloomington: Indiana University Press, 1984.

Balbiani, Laura. *La Magia Naturalis di Giovan Battista Della Porta: Lingua, cultura e scienza in Europa all'inizio dell'età moderna*. Bern: Peter Lang, 2001.

Banister, John. *The Historie of Man*. Facsimile of the 1578 edition. Amsterdam: Theatrum Orbis Terrarum, 1969.

Barbier, Patrick. *The World of the Castrati: The History of an Extraordinary Operatic Phenomenon*. London: Souvenir Press, 1996.

Barbier, Patrick. *La Maison des Italiens: Les Castrats à Versailles*. Paris: Bernard Grasset, 1998.

Barocchi, Paola, ed. *Scritti d'arte del Cinquecento*. Volume 2. Milan and Naples: Riccardo Ricciardi Editore, 1971.

Barolsky, Paul. *Infinite Jest: Wit and Humor in Italian Renaissance Art*. Columbia and London: University of Missouri Press, 1978.

Baroni Vanucci, Alessandra. *Jan Van Der Straet detto Giovanni Stradano: Flandrus pictor et inventor*. Milan and Rome: Jandi Sapi Editori, 1997.

Barras, Vincent and Michel Porret, eds. *Homo Criminalis: Pratiques et doctrines medico légales (XVIe–XXe siècles)*. Geneva: Association de la revue Equinoxe, 1997.

Barthes, Roland. *S/Z*. Paris: Éditions du Seuil, 1970.

Barzman, Karen-edis. *The Florentine Academy and the Early Modern State: The Discipline of Disegno*. Cambridge: Cambridge University Press, 2000.

Battisti, Eugenio. *L'antirinascimento con una appendice di manoscritti inediti*. Milan: Giangiacomo Feltrinelli Editore, 1962.

Bauer, Günther and Heinz Verfondern. *Barocke Zwergenkarikaturen von Callot bis Chodowiecki*. Salzburg: Reischl-Druck, 1991.

Baumeister, F.A.M. et al. "Ambras Syndrome: Delineation of a Unique Hypertrichosis Universalis Congenital and Association with a Balanced Pericentric Inversion (8)(p11.2;q22)." *Clinical Genetics* 44 (1993): 121–28.

Baxandall, Michael. *Painting and Experience in Fifteenth-century Italy*. Oxford and New York: Oxford University Press, 1988.

Bayer, Andrea. "A Note on Ribera's Drawing of Niccolò Simonelli." *Metropolitan Museum Journal* 30 (1995): 73–80.

Beales, Derek. *Joseph II*, Volume 1: *In the Shadow of Maria Teresa, 1741–1780*. Cambridge: Cambridge University Press, 1987.

Bellori, GianPietro. *The Lives of the Modern Painters, Sculptors and Architects: A New Translation and Critical Edition*. Translated by Alice Sedgwick Wohl, notes by Hellmut Wohl, and introduction by Tomaso Montanari. Cambridge: Cambridge University Press, 2005.

Belozerskaya, Marina. *The Medici Giraffe: And Other Tales of Exotic Animals and Power*. New York, Boston, and London: Little, Brown, and Company, 2006.

Belting, Hans. *Likeness and Presence: A History of the Image before the Era of Art*. Chicago and London: University of Chicago Press, 1994.

Bentini, Jadranka et al. *Il gesto e la memoria: Ritratti a Bologna nella seconda metà del Cinquecento*. Bologna: Editrice Compositori, 2000.

Benveniste, Emile. *Vocabulaire des institutions indo-européennes*. Volumes 1 and 2. Paris: Edition de Minuit, 1969.

Berger, Harry, Jr. "Fictions of the Pose: Facing the Gaze of Early Modern Portraiture." *Representations* 46 (Spring 1994): 87–120.

Berger, Harry, Jr. *Fictions of the Pose: Rembrandt against the Italian Renaissance*. Stanford: Stanford University Press, 2000.

Bernheimer, Richard. *Wild Men in the Middle Ages: A Study in Art, Sentiment, and Demonology*. New York: Octagon Books, 1979.

Bertini, Giuseppe. "Johann Gersmueter's Portrait of a Dwarf of the Farnese Court." *Burlington Magazine* 134, no. 1068 (1992): 179–80.

Blom, Philipp. *To Have and to Hold: An Intimate History of Collectors and Collecting*. Woodstock and New York: The Overlook Press, 2003.

Boaistuau, Pierre. *Histoires prodigieuses*. Paris: Robert le Mangnier, edition of 1566 from the original publication of 1560.

Boiardo, Matteo Maria. *Orlando Innamorato*. Edited by Giuseppe Anceschi. Milan: Aldo Garzanti Editore, 1978.

Bolzoni, Lina. "Parole e immagini per il ritratto di un nuovo Ulisse: L'"invenzione' dell'Aldrovandi per la sua villa di campagna." In *Documentary Culture: Florence and Rome from Grand-Duke Ferdinand I to Pope Alexander VII*, edited by Elizabeth Cropper, Giovanna Perini, and Francesco Solinas. Bologna: Nuova Alfa Editoriale, 1992.

Bonfait, Olivier. "Le collezioni Aldrovandi a Bologna in età moderna." *Il Carrobbio* 13 (1987): 25–50.

Boris, Francesca and Gianmpiero Cammarota. "La collezione di Carlo Broschi, detto Farinello." *Atti e Memorie*. Bologna: Accademia Clementina, 1990.

Brilliant, Richard. *Portraiture*. London: Reaktion Books, 1997.

Brink, Claudia and Andreas Köstler. "The Image of the Individual, ca. 1400–1550." *Kunstchronik* 49, no. 2 (February 1996): 61–64.

Brink, Jean R., Maryanne C. Horowitz, and Allison P. Coudert, eds. *Playing with Gender: A Renaissance Pursuit*. Urbana and Chicago: University of Illinois Press, 1991.

Brock, Maurice. *Bronzino*. Paris: Flammarion, 2002.

Broderius, John R. *The Giant in Germanic Tradition*. Chicago: The University of Chicago Libraries, 1932.

Brooks, Jeanice. "Catherine de Médicis, nouvelle Artémise: Women's Laments and the Virtue of Grief." *Early Music* 27, no. 3 (August 1999): 419–35.

Brown, Beverly Louise. *The Genius of Rome 1592–1623*. London: Royal Academy of Arts, 2001.

Brown, David Alan, ed. *Virtue and Beauty: Leonardo's* Ginevra de'Benci *and Renaissance Portraits of Women*. Princeton and Oxford: Princeton University Press, 2001.

Brown, Katherine T. *The Painter's Reflection: Self-Portraiture in Renaissance Venice 1458–1625*. Milan: Leo S. Olschki, Editore, 2000.

Burckhardt, Jacob. *The Civilisation of the Renaissance in Italy*. Translated by S.G.C. Middlemore. London: George Allen & Unwin, 1921.

Burke, Peter. *Varieties of Cultural History*. New York: Cornell University Press, 1997.

Burney, Charles. *Men, Music and Manners in France and Italy*. Edited by H. Edmund Poole. London: Folio Society, 1969.

Camiz, Franca Trinchieri. "The Castrato Singer: From Informal to Formal Portraiture." *Artibus et Historiae* 18 (1988): 171–86.

Camiz, Franca Trinchieri. "Music and Painting in Cardinal del Monte's Household." *Metropolitan Museum Journal* 26 (1991): 213–26.

Cametti, A. "Musicisti celebri del seicento in Roma: Marc'Antonio Pasqualini." *Musica d'oggi* 3 (1921): 69–71 and 98–99.

Campbell, Lorne. *Renaissance Portraits: European Portrait-Painting in the 14th, 15th, and 16th Centuries*. New Haven and London: Yale University Press, 1990.

Campbell, Mary Baine, ed. *Wonder and Science: Imagining Worlds in Early Modern Europe*. Ithaca and London: Cornell University Press, 1999.

Canguilheim, George. *Le normal et le pathologique*. Paris: Presses Universitaires de France, 1966.

Caprotti, Erminio. *Mostri, draghi e serpenti nelle silografie dell'opera di Ulisse Aldrovandi e dei suoi contemporanei*. Milan: Nuove edizioni Gabriele Mazzotta, 1980.

Carlino, Andrea. "Strani corpi. Come farsi une ragione dei mostri nel XVI secolo." *Phantastische Lebensräume, Phantome und Phantasmen*. Marburg an der Lahn: Basilisken-Press, 1997.

Carlino, Andrea. *Books of the Body: Anatomical Ritual and Renaissance Learning*. Chicago and London: University of Chicago Press, 1999.

Carlino, Andrea. *Paper Bodies: A Catalogue of Anatomical Fugitive Sheets 1538–1687*. London: Wellcome Institute for the History of Medicine, 1999.

Carlino, Andrea. "Fatti contraffatti tra curiosità e scienza: Note su Konrad Gesner e la collezione di fogli volanti di Johann Jacob Wick." *Arte + Architettura in Svizzera* 57, no. 1 (2006): 37–44.

Carlino, Andrea and Michel Jeanneret, eds. *Vulgariser la médecine: Du style médical en France et en Italie*. Geneva: Droz, 2009.

Caroli, Flavio. *Storia della fisiognomica: Arte e psicologia da Leonardo a Freud*. Milan: Arnoldo Mondadori Editore, 1995.

Carolis, Stefano de and Angelo Turchini. *Giovanni Bianchi: Medico Primario di Rimini ed archiatra pontificio*. Verucchio: Pazzini Editore, 1999.

Casciato, Maristella, ed. *Enciclopedismo in Roma Barocca: Athanasius Kircher e il Museo del Collegio Romano tra Wunderkammer e museo scientifico*. Venice: Marsilio Editori, 1986.

Cassani, Silvia. *Luca Giordano 1634–1705*. Naples: Electa Napoli, 2001.

Cazort, Mimi et al., eds. *The Ingenious Machine of Nature: Four Centuries of Art and Anatomy*. Ottawa: National Gallery of Canada, 1996.

Céard, Jean. *Pour une histoire de l'irrationnel: L'imaginaire scientifique au XVIe siècle*. Liège: Section d'histoire, Histoire d'aujourd'hui, 1983.

Céard, Jean. *La nature et les prodiges: L'insolite au XVIe siècle*. Geneva: Librairie Droz, 1996.

Celletti, Rodolfo. *A History of Bel Canto*. Oxford: Clarendon Press, 1991.

Chater, James. "Musical Patronage in Rome at the Turn of the Seventeenth Century: The Case of Cardinal Montalto." *Studi Musicali* 16, no. 2 (1987): 179–227.

Choulant, Ludwig. *History and Bibliography of Anatomic Illustration*. New York and London: Hafner Publishing, 1945.

Christiansen, Keith. *A Caravaggio Rediscovered: The Lute Player*. New York: The Metropolitan Museum of Art, 1990.

Ciardi, Roberto Paolo and Lucia Tongiorgi Tomasi, eds. *Immagini anatomiche e naturalistiche nei disegni degli Uffizi Secc. XVI e XVII*. Florence: Leo S. Olschki, Editore, 1984.

Ciatti, Marco and Diane Kunzelman. *Il* Nano Morgante *di Agnolo Bronzino: Un dipinto "a due dritti" restaurato*. Florence: Edifir, 2012.

Ciociola, Claudio, ed. *"Visibile Parlare": Le scritture esposte nei volgari italiani dal medioevo al rinascimento*. Naples: Edizioni Scientifiche Italiane, 1997.

Clapton, Nicholas. "Machines Made for Singing." *Handel and the Castrati: The Story behind the 18th-century Superstar Singers*. Catalogue of the Handel House Museum, March 2006: 1–4.

Clarke, Paula C. *The Soderini and the Medici: Power and Patronage in Fifteenth-century Florence*. Oxford: Clarendon Press, 1991.

Cochrane, Eric. *Florence in the Forgotten Centuries 1527–1800: A History of Florence and the Florentines in the Age of the Grand Dukes*. Chicago and London: University of Chicago Press, 1973.

Cole, F.J. *History of the Anatomical Museum*. Liverpool and London: The University Press and Constable & Company, 1914.

Coliva, Anna. *Galleria Borghese*. Rome: Progetti Museali Editore, 1994.

Collina, Maria D. *Il carteggio letterario di uno scienzato del settecento (Janus Plancus)*. Florence: Leo S. Olschki, Editore, 1957.
Colombo, Realdo. *De Re Anatomica Libri XV*. Reprint of the 1559 Venice edition. Brussels: Impression Anastaltique, Culture et Civilisation, 1969.
Comelli, G.B. "F.C. & le origini del Museo Civico di Bologna." *Atti e memorie della real deputazione di storia patria per le provincie di Romagna*. 3a serie: 7 (1889): 96–129.
Comment, Bernard. *Le colloque des bustes*. Paris: Christian Bourgeois Éditeur, 2000.
Connell, William J. *Society and Individual in Renaissance Florence*. Berkeley, Los Angeles, and London: University of California Press, 2002.
Conrad, Lawrence, Michael Neve, Vivian Nutton, Roy Porter, and Andrew Wear. *The Western Medical Tradition 800 B.C. to A.D. 1800*. Cambridge: Cambridge University Press, 1995.
Conti, Cosimo. *La prima reggia di Cosimo I de'Medici nel Palazzo già della Signoria di Firenze*. Florence: Giuseppe Pellas, Editore, 1893.
Costa Kauffmann, Thomas da. "Images of Rule: Issues of Interpretation." *Art Journal* 48, no. 2 (1989): 119–22.
Coudert, Allison. *Alchemy: The Philosopher's Stone*. Boulder: Shambhala, 1980.
Courtenay, John. *The Present State of the Manners, Arts, and Politics of France and Italy from Paris, Rome, and Naples in 1792 and 1793; Addressed to Robert Jephson, Esq*. Dublin: Printed for M.F. Wooan, P. Byrne, W. Jones, 1794.
Cox-Rearick, Janet. *Bronzino's Chapel of Eleonora di Toledo in the Palazzo Vecchio*. Berkeley and London: University of California Press, 1993.
Cox-Rearick, Janet. "Art at the Court of Duke Cosimo I de'Medici (1537–74)." In *The Medici, Michelangelo, and the Art of Late Renaissance Florence*. New Haven and London: Yale University Press, 2003.
Cox-Rearick, Janet. "Power-Dressing at the Courts of Cosimo I de'Medici and François I: The 'moda alla spagnola' of Spanish Consorts Eléonore d'Autriche and Eleonora di Toledo." *Artibus et Historiae* 30, no. 60 (2009): 39–70.
Cranston, Jodi. *The Poetics of Portraiture in the Italian Renaissance*. Cambridge: Cambridge University Press, 2000.
Crawford, Katherine. "Catherine de Medicis and the Performance of Political Motherhood." *Sixteenth Century Journal* 31, no. 3 (Autumn 2000): 643–73.
Crimi, Giuseppe and Cristiano Spila, eds. *Nanerie del Rinascimento: "La Nanea" di Michelangelo Serafini e altri versi di corte e d'accademia*. Rome: Vecchiarelli Editore, 2006.
Croizat, Yassana C. "'Living Dolls': François Ier Dresses His Women." *Renaissance Quarterly* 60, no. 1 (Spring 2007): 94–130.
Cropper, Elizabeth. "The Beauty of Woman: Problems of Rhetoric of Renaissance Portraiture." In *Rewriting the Renaissance: The Discourse of Sexual Difference in Early Modern Europe*, edited by Margaret Ferguson, Maureen Quilligan, and Nancy Vickers. Chicago and London: The University of Chicago Press, 1987.
Cropper, Elizabeth. "The Place of Beauty in the High Renaissance and Its Displacement in the History of Art." In *Place and Displacement in the Renaissance*, edited by Alvin Vos. Binghamton: Center for Medieval and Early Renaissance Studies, 1995.
Cunningham, Andrew. *The Anatomical Renaissance: The Resurrection of the Anatomical Projects of the Ancients*. Aldershot: Scolar Press, 1997.

Cunningham, J.D. "The Skeleton of the Irish Giant, Cornelius Magrath." *The Transactions of the Royal Irish Academy* 29, no. 16 (1891): 553–612.

Daniel, Howard. *Devils, Monsters, and Nightmares: An Introduction to the Grotesque and Fantastic in Art*. London, New York, and Toronto: Abelard-Schuman, 1964.

Danti, Vincenzo. *Il primo libro del trattato delle perfette proporzioni*. In *Scritti d'arte del Cinquecento*, volume 1. Edited by Paola Barocchi. Milan and Naples: Riccardo Ricciardi Editore, 1971–77.

Dasen, Véronique. *Dwarfs in Ancient Egypt and Greece*. Oxford: Clarendon Press, 1993.

Daston, Lorraine and Katharine Park. "Hermaphrodites in Renaissance Florence." *Critical Matrix* 1, no. 5 (1985): 1–19.

Daston, Lorraine and Katharine Park. *Wonders and the Order of Nature 1150–1750*. New York: Zone Books, 1998.

Davies, Surekha. *Renaissance Ethnography and the Invention of the Human: New Worlds, Maps, and Monsters*. Cambridge: Cambridge University Press, 2016.

Davis, Natalie Zemon. *Women on the Margins: Three Seventeenth-century Lives*. Cambridge and London: Harvard University Press, 1995.

Debus, Allen G. and Michael T. Walton, eds. *Reading the Book of Nature: The Other Side of the Scientific Revolution*. Kirksville: Thomas Jefferson University Press, 1998.

Delcourt, Marie. *Hermaphrodite: Mythes et rites de la bisexualité dans l'Antiquité classique*. Paris: Presses Universitaires de France, 1958.

Delphinus, H. (pseudonym), ed., *Eunuchi conjugium: Die Capaunen-Heirath, Hoc est Scripta et judicia varia de conjugio inter eunuchum et virginem juvenculam Anno M. DC. LXVI. contracto, T. T. A. quibusdam supremis theologorum collegiis petita, postea hinc inde collecta ab Hieronymo Delphino, C.P.* Halle, 1718.

Diderot and d'Alembert. *L'Encyclopédie: Recueil de planches sur les sciences, les arts libéraux, et les arts méchaniques, avec leur explication: Chirurgie*. Facsimile of the 1776 version. Paris: InterLivres, 2002.

DiFederico, Frank R. *Francesco Trevisani: Eighteenth-century Painter in Rome. A Catalogue Raisonné*. Washington D.C.: Decatur House Press, 1977.

Douthwaite, Julia V. *The Wild Girl, Natural Man, and the Monster: Dangerous Experiments in the Age of Enlightenment*. Chicago and London: University of Chicago Press, 2002.

Dreger, Alice Domurat. *Hermaphrodites and the Medical Invention of Sex*. Cambridge and London: Harvard University Press, 1998.

Duval, Jacques. *Traité des hermaphrodits*. Reprint of the 1612 Rouen edition. Paris: Isidore Liseux, éditeur, 1880.

Eamon, William. *Science and the Secrets of Nature: Books of Secrets in Medieval and Early Modern Culture*. Princeton: Princeton University Press, 1994.

Elias, Norbert. *The Civilizing Process*. Translated by Edmund Jephcott. New York: Urizen Books, 1978.

Elias, Norbert. *The Court Society*. New York: Pantheon Books, 1983.

Emiliani, Andrea. *Il Bronzino*. Busto Arsizio: Bramante Editrice, 1960.

Evans, R.J.W. and Alexander Marr, eds. *Curiosity and Wonder from the Renaissance to the Enlightenment*. Burlington: Ashgate, 2006.

Fabi, Angelo. *Aurelio Bertola e le polemiche su Giovanni Bianchi*. Rimini: Faenza Fratelli Lega, Editori, 1972.

Falciani, Carlo and Antonio Natali, eds. *Bronzino: Artist and Poet at the Court of the Medici*. Florence: Mandragora, 2010.

Farago, Claire J. *Leonardo da Vinci's Paragone: A Critical Interpretation with a New Edition of the Text in the Codex Urbinas*. Leiden and New York: E.J. Brill, 1992.

Farago, Claire, ed. *Leonardo's Writings and Theory of Art*. New York and London: Garland Publishing, 1999.

Felgenhauer, W. "Hypertrichosis Lanuginosa Universalis." *Journal de Génétique Humaine* 17 (1969): 1–44.

Fernández-Armesto, Felipe. *The Canary Islands after the Conquest: The Making of a Colonial Society in the Early Sixteenth Century*. Oxford: Clarendon University Press, 1982.

Ferrari, Giovanna. "Public Anatomy Lessons and the Carnival: The Anatomy Theatre of Bologna." *Past and Present* 117 (1987): 50–106.

ffolliott, Sheila. "Catherine de'Medici as Artemisia: Figuring the Powerful Widow." In *Rewriting the Renaissance: The Discourses of Sexual Difference in Early Modern Europe*, edited by Margaret W. Ferguson, Maureen Quilligan, and Nancy Vickers. Chicago and London: University of Chicago Press, 1986.

ffolliott, Sheila. "Casting a Rival into the Shade: Catherine de'Medici and Diane de Poitiers." *Art Journal* 48, no. 2 (Summer 1989): 138–43.

Fiedler, Leslie. *Freaks: Myths and Images of the Secret Self*. New York: Simon and Schuster, 1978.

Filipczak, Zirka Z. "Poses and Passions: Mona Lisa's 'Closely Folded' Hands." In *Reading the Early Modern Passions: Essays in the Cultural History of Emotions*, edited by Gail Kern Paster, Katherine Rowe, and Mary Floyd-Wilson. Philadelphia: University of Pennsylvania Press, 2004.

Findlen, Paula. *Possessing Nature: Museums, Collecting, and Scientific Culture in Early Modern Italy*. Berkeley, Los Angeles and London: University of California Press, 1994.

Findlen, Paula, Wendy Wassyng Roworth, and Catherine M. Sama, eds. *Italy's Eighteenth Century: Gender and Culture in the Age of the Grand Tour*. Stanford: Stanford University Press, 2009.

Finucci, Valeria. *The Manly Masquerade: Masculinity, Paternity, and Castration in the Italian Renaissance*. Durham and London: Duke University Press, 2003.

Finucci, Valeria and Kevin Brownlee, eds. *Generation and Degeneration: Tropes of Reproduction in Literature and History from Antiquity through Early Modern Europe*. Durham and London: Duke University Press, 2001.

Fischer, Jean-Louis. *Monstres: Histoire du corps et de ses défauts*. Paris: Syros Alternatives, 1991.

Fortunati, Vera. *Lavinia Fontana of Bologna 1552–1614*. Milan: Electa, 1998.

Foucault, Michel. *Herculine Barbin dite Alexina B*. Paris: Editions Gallimard, 1978.

Foucault, Michel. *The History of Sexuality*. New York: Vintage Books, 1990.

Foucault, Michel. *The Order of Things: An Archeology of Human Sciences*. New York: Vintage, 1994.

Foucault, Michel. *The Birth of the Clinic: An Archaeology of Medical Perception*. New York: Vintage, 1994.

Foucault, Michel. *Les anormaux*. Paris: Seuil, 1999.

Fradenburg, Louise and Carla Freccero. *Premodern Sexualities*. New York and London: Routledge, 1996.

Franchini, Dario A. et al. *La scienza a corte: Collezionismo eclettico natura e imagine a Mantova fra Rinascimento e Manierismo*. Rome: Bulzoni, 1979.

Frandsen, Mary E. "Eunichi Conjugium: The Marriage of a Castrato in Early Modern Germany." *Early Music History* 24 (2005): 53–124.

Freedberg, David. *The Power of Images: Studies in the History and Theory of Response.* Chicago and London: University of Chicago Press, 1991.

Freitas, Roger. *"Un Atto d'ingegno": A Castrato in the Seventeenth Century.* PhD Dissertation, Yale University, 1998.

French, Roger. *Dissection and Vivisection in the European Renaissance.* Aldershot, Brookfield, Singapore, and Sydney: Ashgate, 1999.

French, Roger. *Ancients and Moderns in the Medical Sciences: From Hippocrates to Harvey.* Aldershot, Brookfield, Singapore, and Sydney: Ashgate, 2000.

Frey, Karl. *Der literarische Nachglass Giorgio Vasaris.* Munich: Müller, 1923–1930.

Frick, Carole Collier. *Dressing Renaissance Florence: Families, Fortunes, and Fine Clothing.* Baltimore and London: The Johns Hopkins University Press, 2002.

Friedman, John Block. *The Monstrous Races in Medieval Art and Thought.* Cambridge and London: Harvard University Press, 1981.

Fudge, Erica, Ruth Gilbert, and Susan Wiseman. *At the Borders of the Human: Beasts, Bodies and Natural Philosophy in the Early Modern Period.* New York: St Martin's Press, 1999.

Gaffiot, Félix. *Dictionnaire Latin–Français: Le Grand Gaffiot.* Paris: Hachette, 2000.

Galli, Giovanna, "Strano è bello." *Stile Arte* 63 (November 2002).

Garnier, Édouard. *Les nains et les géants.* Paris: Librairie Hachette, 1884.

Garzoni, Tommaso. *La piazza universale de tutte le professioni del mondo.* Edited by Paolo Cherchi and Beatrice Collina. Torino: Einaudi, 1996.

Gentili, Augusto, ed. *Il ritratto e la memoria.* Rome: Bulzoni Editore, 1989.

Geoffroy Saint-Hilaire, Isidore. *Histoire générale et particulière des anomalies de l'organisation chez l'homme et les animaux, ouvrage comprenant des recherches sur les caractères, la classification, l'influence physiologique et pathologique, les rapports généraux, les lois et les causes des monstruosités, des variétés de vices de conformation, ou Traité de tératologie,* 3 vols. Paris: J.-B. Baillière, Libraire de l'Académie Royale de Médecine, 1832.

Gesner, Conrad. *Historiae animalium.* Frankfurt: H. Laurent, 1620.

Gilbert, Ruth. "Seeing and Knowing: Science, Pornography and Early Modern Hermaphrodites." In *At the Borders of the Human: Beasts, Bodies, and Natural Philosophy in the Early Modern Period,* edited by Erica Fudge. New York: St Martin's Press, 1999.

Giustacchini, Enrico. "Leonardo, il ghigno conturbante dell'angelo bisex." *Stile Arte* 51 (September 2001).

Goffen, Rona. "Icon and Vision: Giovanni Bellini's Half-Length Madonnas." *The Art Bulletin* 57, no. 4 (1975): 487–514.

Goguel, Catherine Monbeig. "Sur le chemin de Rome: Le role de Vasari et l'étape florentine." *Bollettino d'arte* 100 (1997): 63–76.

Goldberg, Edward L. *Patterns in Late Medici Art Patronage.* Princeton: Princeton University Press, 1983.

Goldstein, Carl. *Teaching Art: Academies and Schools from Vasari to Albers.* Cambridge: Cambridge University Press, 1996.

Gordon, Archie. *A Wild Flight of Gordons: Odd and Able Members of the Gordon Families.* London: Weidenfeld and Nicolson, 1985.

Grantham Turner, James, ed. *Sexuality and Gender in Early Modern Europe: Institutions, Texts, Images*. Cambridge: Cambridge University Press, 1993.

Grazzini, Antonfrancesco. *Le rime burlesche, edite e inedite, di Antonfrancesco Grazzini, dette Il Lasca*. Edited by Carlo Verzone. Florence: Sansoni, 1882.

Greenham, Peter. *On Velasquez' "Portrait of a Buffoon of Philip IV."* London: Cassell, 1969.

Guerzoni, Guido. "The Italian Renaissance Courts' Demand for the Arts: The Case of d'Este of Ferrara (1471–1560)." In *Art Markets in Europe, 1400–1800*, edited by Michael North and David Ormrod. Aldershot and Brookfield: Ashgate, 1998.

Guerzoni, Guido. "Administrative Knowledge and Renaissance Courts: The Este Case in XVIth Century." Unpublished paper, EBHA Conference, July 2001.

Guevara-Sanguinés, Esther et al. "Congenital Generalized Terminal Hypyertrichosis with Gingival Hyperplasia." *Pediatric Dermatology* 19, no. 2 (2002): 114–18.

Guidobaldi, Nicoletta. "'Non un semplice ritratto': Marcantonio Pasqualini, Apollo e Marsia in un dipinto di Andrea Sacchi." In *Musica e immagine tra iconografia e mondo dell'opera*, edited by Biancamaria Brumana and Galliano Ciliberti. Florence: Leo S. Olschki, Editore, 1993.

Gurrieri, Francesco and Judith Chatfield. *Boboli Gardens*. Florence: Editrice Edam, 1972.

Haböck, F. *Die Kastraten und ihre Gesangkunst*. Stuttgart: Deutsche Verlags-Anstalt, 1927.

Hale, J.R. *Florence and the Medici: The Pattern of Control*. Plymouth: Thames and Hudson, 1977.

Hamby, Wallace B. *Ambroise Paré: Surgeon of the Renaissance*. Saint Louis: Warren H. Green, 1967.

Hammond, Frederick. *Music and Spectacle in Baroque Rome: Barberini Patronage under Urban VIII*. New Haven: Yale University Press, 1994.

Hanafi, Zakiya. *The Monster in the Machine: Magic, Medicine, and the Marvelous in the Time of the Scientific Revolution*. Durham and London: Duke University Press, 2000.

Hanning, Robert W. and David Rosand, eds. *Castiglione: The Ideal and the Real in Renaissance Culture*. New Haven and London: Yale University Press, 1983.

Hansen, Julie V. "Resurrecting Death: Anatomical Art in the Cabinet of Dr. Frederick Ruysch." *Art Bulletin* 78, no. 4 (December 1996): 663–79.

Hansen, Julie V. and Suzanne Porter. *The Physician's Art: Representations of Art and Medicine*. Durham: Duke University Medical Center Library and Duke University Museum of Art, 1999.

Harcourt, Glenn. "Andreas Vesalius and the Anatomy of Antique Sculpture." *Representations* 17 (Winter 1987): 28–61.

Harness, Kelley. *Echoes of Women's Voices: Music, Art, and Female Patronage in Early Modern Florence*. Chicago and London: University of Chicago Press, 2006.

Harris, Constance. *Portraiture in Prints*. Jefferson and London: McFarland & Company, 1987.

Haskell, Francis. *Patrons and Painters: A Study in the Relations Between Italian Art and Society in the Age of the Baroque*. London: Chatto & Windus, 1963.

Haskell, Francis and Nicholas Penny. *Taste and the Antique: The Lure of Classical Sculpture 1500–1900*. New Haven and London: Yale University Press, 1981.

Heikamp, Detlef. "Il Nano Morgante: Tentativo di un ritratto." In *Giambologna: Gli dei, gli eroi*, edited by Beatrice Paolozzi Strozzi and Dimitrios Zikos. Florence and Milan: Giunti, 2006.

Hendler, Sefy. Entry for Bronzino's *Morgante* in *Bronzino: Artist and Poet at the Court of the Medici*, edited by Cristina Acidini, Carlo Falciani, and Antonio Natali. Florence: Mandragora, 2010.

Hendler, Sefy. *La guerre des arts: Le* Paragone *peinture-sculpture en Italie XVe–XVIIe siècle*. Rome: "L'Erma" di Bretschneider, 2013.

Hendler, Sefy. *Gracious and Beautiful Monster: The Literary Universe of Bronzino's Nano Morgante*. Florence: Maschietto Editore, 2016.

Hendrix, Lee. "Of Hirsutes and Insects: Joris Hoefnagel and the Art of the Wondrous." *Word and Image* 11, no. 4 (October–December 1995): 373–90.

Herdt, Gilbert, ed. *Third Sex, Third Gender: Beyond Sexual Dimorphism in Culture and History*. New York: Zone Books, 1994.

Hertel, Christiane. "Hairy Issues: Portraits of Petrus Gonsalus and His Family in Archduke Ferdinand II's *Kunstkammer* and Their Contexts." *Journal of the History of Collections* 13, no. 1 (2001): 1–22.

Heyndels, Ralph and Barbara Woshinsky, eds. *L'autre au XVIIème siècle*. Tübingen: Gunter Narr Verlag, 1999.

Higgs Strickland, Debra. *Saracens, Demons, and Jews: Making Monsters in Medieval Art*. Princeton: Princeton University Press, 2003.

Hochlenert, Dieter. *Das "Tagebuch" des Felix Platter: Die Autobiographie eines Arztes und Humanisten*. Tübingen: Tübingen University, 1996.

Holderbaum, James. "A Bronze by Giovanni Bologna and a Painting by Bronzino." *The Burlington Magazine* 98 (December 1956): 439–45.

Holman, Beth. "Verrocchio's *Marsyas* and Renaissance Anatomy." *Marsyas: Studies in the History of Art* 19 (1977–78): 1–9.

Hopkins, Lisa. *Women Who Would Be Kings: Female Rulers of the Sixteenth Century*. London and New York: Vision Press and St. Martin's Press, 1991.

Howard, Patricia. "Perceptions of the Castrati in Eighteenth-century London." *Handel and the Castrati: The Story behind the 18th-century Superstar Singers*. Catalogue of the Handel House Museum, March 2006: 10–13.

Hsy, Jonathan. "Disability." In *The Cambridge Companion to the Body in Literature*, edited by David Hillman and Ulrika Maude. Cambridge: Cambridge University Press, 2015.

Huber, Katharina. *Felix Platters "Observationes": Studien zum Frühneuzeitlichen Gesundheitswesen in Basel*, Basel Beiträge zur Geschichtswissenschaft 177. Basel: Schwabe, 2003.

Huet, Marie-Hélène. *Monstrous Imagination*. Cambridge and London: Harvard University Press, 1993.

Husband, Timothy. *The Wild Man: Medieval Myth and Symbolism*. New York: The Metropolitan Museum of Art, 1980.

Il teatro della natura di Ulisse Aldrovandi. Bologna: Editrice Compositori, 2001.

Impelluso, Lucia. *Nature and Its Symbols*. Translated by Stephen Sartarelli. Los Angeles: The J. Paul Getty Museum, 2003.

Jacks, Philip, ed. *Vasari's Florence: Artists and Literati at the Medicean Court*. Cambridge: Cambridge University Press, 1998.

Jacobs, Fredrika H. *Defining the Renaissance Virtuosa: Women Artists and the Language of Art History and Criticism*. Cambridge: Cambridge University Press, 1997.

Jacobs, Fredrika. "(Dis)assembling: Marsyas, Michelangelo, and the Accademia del Disegno." *Art Bulletin* 84, no. 3 (September 2002): 426–48.

Jacobs, Fredrika H. *The Living Image in Renaissance Art*. Cambridge: Cambridge University Press, 2005.

Jenkins, Jessica Kerwin. *Encyclopedia of the Exquisite: An Anecdotal History of Elegant Delights* (New York: Doubleday, 2010).

Johnson, Geraldine A. and Sara F. Matthews Grieco. *Picturing Women in Renaissance and Baroque Italy*. Cambridge: Cambridge University Press, 1997.

Jones, Ann Rosalind and Peter Stallybrass. "Fetishizing Gender: Constructing the Hermaphrodite in Renaissance Europe." In *Body Guards: The Cultural Politics of Gender Ambiguity*, edited by Julia Epstein and Kristina Straub. New York: Routledge, 1991.

Jones, Caroline A. and Peter Galison. *Picturing Science, Producing Art*. London and New York: Routledge, 1998.

Jones, Timothy S. and David A. Sprunger, eds. *Marvels, Monsters, and Miracles Studies in the Medieval and Early Modern Imaginations*. Kalamazoo: Board of Medieval Institute, 2000.

Jones-Davies, M.T. *Monstres et prodiges au temps de la Renaissance*. Paris: Diffusion Jean Touzot, 1980.

Judd, Sandra J., ed. *Genetic Disorders Sourcebook*. Detroit: Omnigraphics, 2010.

Kahn-Rossi, Manuela. *Pier Francesco Mola 1612–1666*. Milan: Electa, 1989.

Kane, Eileen. "An Irish Giant." *The GPA Irish Arts Review Yearbook 1990–1991*: 96–98.

Kappler, Claude. *Monstres, démons et merveilles à la fin du Moyen Age*. Paris: Payot, 1980.

Karp, Gerald. *Cell and Molecular Biology: Concepts and Experiments*. New York: John Wiley & Sons, 1996.

Katz, Joseph. "Testimonia Ritus Italici: Male Genitalia, Solemn Declarations, and a New Latin Sound Law." *Harvard Studies in Classical Philology* 98 (1998): 183–217.

Kaufmann, Lynn Frier. *The Noble Savage: Satyrs and Satyr Families in Renaissance Art*. Ann Arbor: UMI Research Press, 1984.

Keller, R. "Hermaphroditism in the Animal Kingdom." *Ciba Symposia* 2, no. 3 (June 1940): 478–85.

Kemp, Martin. *Leonardo da Vinci: The Marvellous Works of Nature and Man*. Cambridge: Harvard University Press, 1981.

Kemp, Martin. "'Wrought by No Artist's Hand': The Natural, the Artificial, the Exotic, and the Scientific in Some Artifacts from the Renaissance." In *Reframing the Renaissance: Visual Culture in Europe and Latin America 1450–1650*, edited by Claire Farago. New Haven and London: Yale University Press, 1995.

Kemp, Martin and Marina Wallace. *Spectacular Bodies: The Art and Science of the Human Body from Leonardo to Now*. Los Angeles: University of California Press, 2000.

Kenseth, Joy, ed. *The Age of the Marvelous*. Hanover: Hood Museum of Art, Dartmouth College, 1991.

Kent, Dale. *The Rise of the Medici Faction in Florence 1426–1434*. Oxford: Oxford University Press, 1978.

Kirke, Sarah B. and Britt Salvesen. *The Incisive Imagination: Jacques Callot and His Contemporaries*. Milwaukee: Milwaukee Art Museum, 2004.

Klapisch-Zuber, Christiane. "Nobles or Pariahs": The Exclusion of Florentine Magnates from the Thirteenth to the Fifteenth Centuries." *Society for Comparative Study of Society and History* 39, no. 2 (1997): 215–30.

Kliemann, Julian. *Il bersaglio dell'arte: "La Caccia di Diana" di Domenichino nella Galleria Borghese*. Rome: Artemide Edizioni, 2001.

Knoppers, Laura Lunger and Joan B. Landes. *Monstrous Bodies/Political Monstrosities in Early Modern Europe*. Ithaca and London: Cornell University Press, 2004.

Konečný, Lubomír. "An Unexpected Source for Jusepe de Ribera." *Source* 13, no. 2 (Winter 1994): 21–24.

Kuczwara, John. *Wonder and Image: Knowledge, Cognition, and Giambattista della Porta*. Unpublished dissertation, University of North Carolina at Chapel Hill, 1998.

Kudlien, Fridolf. "The Seven Cells of the Uterus: The Doctrine and Its Roots." *Bulletin of the History of Medicine* 39, no. 3 (1965): 415–22.

Kudlien, Fridolf. "The Legal Aspect of the Doctrine of the Seven Uterine Cells." *Bulletin of the History of Medicine* 40, no. 3 (1966): 544–46.

Kwakkelstein, Michael W. *Leonardo da Vinci as a Physiognomist: Theory and Drawing Practice*. Leiden: Primavera Pers, 1994.

Lagerkvist, Pär. *The Dwarf*. New York: L.B. Fisher, 1945.

Lalande, Jean Jérôme de. *Voyage d'un François en Italie fait dans les années 1765 et 1766. Contenant l'histoire et les anecdotes les plus singulières de l'Italie, et sa description; les moeurs, les usages, le gouvernement, le commerce, la littérature, les arts, l'histoire naturelle, et les antiquités; avec des jugements sur les ouvrages de peinture, sculpture et architecture, et les plans de toutes les grandes villes d'Italie*. Venice and Paris: Desaint, 1769.

Landini, Roberta Orsi and Mary Westerman Bulgarella. "Costume in Fifteenth-century Florentine Portraits of Women." In *Virtue and Beauty: Leonardo's Ginevra de'Benci and Renaissance Portraits of Women*, edited by David Alan Brown. Princeton and Oxford: Princeton University Press, 2001.

Landucci, Luca. *A Florentine Diary from 1450 to 1516 by Luca Landucci, Continued by an Anonymous Writer till 1542 with Notes by Iodoco Del Badia*. Translated by Alice de Rosen Jervis. New York: E.P. Dutton and Co., 1927.

Langer, Ullrich, ed. *The Cambridge Companion to Montaigne*. Cambridge: Cambridge University Press, 2005.

Laqueur, Thomas. *Making Sex: Body and Gender from the Greeks to Freud*. Cambridge and London: Harvard University Press, 1990.

Lascault, Gilbert. *Le monstre dans l'art occidental: Un problème esthétique*. Paris: Klincksieck, 1973.

Launois, Pierre. "Esquisse iconographique sur quelques nains." *Nouvelle iconographie de la Salpêtrière* 24, no. 1 (1911): 114–21.

Launois, P.-E. and Pierre Roy. *Études biologiques sur les géants*. Paris: Masson et Cie, Éditeurs, 1904.

Laurenza, Domenico. *De figura umana: Fisiognomica, anatomia e arte in Leonardo*. Florence: Leo S. Olschki, 2001.

Lavin, Marylin Aronberg. *Seventeenth-century Barberini Documents and Inventories of Art*. New York: New York University Press, 1975.

Lavin, Marilyn Aronberg. "Art of the Misbegotten: Physicality and the Divine in Renaissance Images." *Artibus et Historiae* 60 (2009): 191–244.

Lecouteux, Claude. *Les nains et les elfes au moyen âge*. Paris: Editions Imago, 1988.

Lees, Lynn Hollen and Paul M. Hohenberg. "Urban Decline and Regional Economies: Brabant, Castile, and Lombardy 1550–1750." *Society for Comparative Study of Society and History* 31, no. 3 (1989): 439–61.

Legati, Lorenzo. *Museo Cospiano: Annesso a quello del famoso Ulisse Aldrovandi E donato alla sua Patria dall'Illustrissimo Signor Ferdinando Cospi Patrizio di Bologna e Senator, ecc.* Bologna, 1677.

Levey, Michael. *Painting at Court*. London: Weidenfeld & Nicolson, 1971.

Levy, Allison, ed. *Sex Acts in Early Modern Italy: Practice, Performance, Perversion, Punishment*. Burlington and Farnham: Ashgate, 2010.

Liceti, Fortunio. *De monstrorum caussis, natura, et differentiis, libri duo*. Padua: Frambotti, 1634.

Liceti, Fortunio. *De la nature, des causes, des differences des monstres*. Translated by François Houssay. Paris: Editions Hippocrate, 1937.

L'Idea del Bello: Viaggio per Roma nel Seicento con Giovan Pietro Bellori. Volumes 1 and 2. Rome: Edizioni De Luca, 2000.

Lomazzo, Giovan Paolo. In *Scritti d'arte del Cinquecento*, Volume 3, edited by Paola Barocchi. Milan and Naples: Riccardo Ricciardi Editore, 1977.

Long, Jacqueline. *Claudian's In Eutropium, or, How, When, and Why to Slander a Eunuch*. Chapel Hill: University of North Carolina Press, 1996.

Loy, James, Kent Loy, Geoffrey Keifer, and Clinton Conaway. *The Behavior of Gonadectomized Rhesus Monkeys*, Contributions to Primatology 20. Basel: Karger, 1984.

Lugli, Adalgisa. "Inquiry as Collection: The Athanasius Kircher Museum in Rome," *RES* 12 (Autumn 1986): 109–24.

Lunsingh Scheurleer, Th.H. "Un amphithéâtre d'anatomie moralisée." In *Leiden University in the Seventeenth Century: An Exchange of Learningi*, edited by Th.H. Lunsingh Scheurleer and G.H.M. Posthumus Meyjes. Leiden: Universitaire pers Leiden / E.J. Brill, 1975.

MacGregor, Arthur. *Curiosity and Enlightenment: Collectors and Collections from the Sixteenth to the Nineteenth Century*. New Haven and London: Yale University Press, 2007.

Maier, Michael. *Symbola auraeae mensae duodecim nationum*. Introduced by Karl R.H. Frick. Graz: Akademische Druck, 1972.

Malacarne, Giancarlo. *Il Palazzo Ducale di Mantova: Immagini da un sogno dinastico*. Mantua: Rossi Edizioni, 1996.

Malvasia, Carlo Cesare. *Le Pitture di Bologna: 1686*. Edited by Andrea Emiliani. Bologna: Edizione ALFA, 1969.

Mamy, Sylvie. *Les castrats*. Paris: Presses Universitaires de France, 1998.

Mandressi, Rafael. *Le regard de l'anatomiste: Dissection et invention du corps en Occident*. Paris: Editions du Seuil, 2003.

Manguel, Alberto. "Lavinia Fontana: The Image as Understanding." In *Reading Pictures: A History of Love and Hate*. New York: Random House, 2000.

Mann, Nicholas and Luke Syson. *The Image of the Individual: Portrait in the Renaissance*. London: British Museum Press, 1998.

Martin, Ernest. *Histoire des monstres depuis l'antiquité jusqu'à nos jours*. Paris: C. Reinwald et Cie, Libraires-Éditeurs, 1880.

Martineau, Anne. *Le nain et le chevalier: Essai sur les nains français du Moyen Âge*. Paris: Presses de l'Université de Paris-Sorbonne, 2003.

Martinotti, Giovanni. "L'Anatomia pubblica a Bologna." *L'Illustrazione medica italiana* 5 (1923): 25–29.

Mauriès, Patrick. *Cabinets of Curiosities*. New York: Thames and Hudson, 2002.

Mazzocut-Mis, Maddalena. *Mostro: L'anomalia e il deforme nella natura e nell'arte*. Milan: Edizioni Angelo Guerini e Associati, 1992.

McComb, Arthur. *Agnolo Bronzino: His Life and Works*. Cambridge: Harvard University Press, 1928.

Melicow, Meyer M. "Castrati Choir and Opera Singers." *Urology* 3 (1974): 663–70.

Melicow, Meyer M. "Castration Down the Ages." *New York State Journal of Medicine* 77 (April 1977): 804–806.

Mendelsohn, Leatrice. *Paragoni: Benedetto Varchi's "Due Lezzioni" and Cinquecento Art Theory*. Ann Arbor: UMI Press, 1982.

Mennell, Stephen and Johan Goudsblom, eds. *Norbert Elias: On Civilization, Power, and Knowledge: Selected Writings*. Chicago and London: University of Chicago Press, 1998.

Meriggi, Marco and Alessandro Pastore, eds. *Le regole dei mestieri e delle professioni Secoli XV–XIX*. Milan: Franco Angeli, 2000.

Methenitis, Marian M. *More than Mirrors: Portraits of Children in Renaissance Italy*. Unpublished dissertation, University of Dallas, 1995.

Mezzetti, Amalia. *Girolamo da Ferrara detto da Carpi: L'Opera Pittorica*. Milan: Silvana Editoriale d'Arte, 1977.

Michler, Andrea Gloria. "Ambiguità e trasmutazione: Discussioni mediche e giuridiche in epoca moderna (secoli XVII e XVIII)." *Memoria: Rivista di storia delle donne* 24, no. 3 (1988): 43–60.

Milner, Anthony. "The Sacred Capons." *The Musical Times* 114, no. 1561 (March 1973): 250–52.

Moes, Robert J. and C.D. O'Malley. "Realdo Colombo: 'On Those Things Rarely Found in Anatomy': An Annotated Translation from the *De Re Anatomica* (1559)." *Bulletin of the History of Medicine* 34 (1960): 508–28.

Monestier, Martin. *Les Nains*. Paris: Jean-Claude Simoën, 1977.

Monestier, Martin. *Les Monstres: Le fabuleux univers des "oubliés de Dieu."* Paris: Tchou Editeur, 1978.

Monestier, Martin. *Human Oddities*. Translated by Robert Campbell. Secaucus: Citadel Press, 1987.

Moreno, Paolo and Chiara Stefani. *Galleria Borghese*. Milan: Touring Editore, 2000.

Morselli, Raffaella, ed. *La celeste Galeria: Le raccolte*. Milan: Electa, 2002.

Mosco, Marilena. *Natura viva in Casa Medici: Dipinti di animali depositi di Palazzo Pitti con esemplari del Museo Zoologico "La Specola."* Florence: Centro Di, 1985.

Muir, Edward and Guido Ruggiero. *Sex and Gender in Historical Perspective*. Baltimore and London: The Johns Hopkins University Press, 1990.

Muller, Sigfrid A. "Hirsutism." *The American Journal of Medicine* 46, no. 5 (May 1969): 803–17.

Murata, Margaret. "Further Remarks on Pasqualini and the Music of MAP." *Analecta Musicologica* 19 (1984): 125–45.

Murphy, Caroline. *Lavinia Fontana: A Painter and Her Patrons in Sixteenth-century Bologna*. New Haven: Yale University Press, 2003.

Musacchio, Jacqueline Marie. *Art, Marriage, and Family in the Florentine Renaissance Palace*. New Haven and London: Yale University Press, 2008.

Museo del Prado. *Alonso Sánchez Coello y el retrato en la corte de Felipe II*. Madrid: Museo del Prado, 1990.

Museo del Prado. *Velázquez, Rubens, Lorrain: Malerei am Hof Philipps IV*. Ostfildern Ruit: Hatje Cantz Verlag, 1999.

Negro, Angela. *Il giardino dipinto del Cardinal Borghese: Paolo Bril e Guido Reni nel Palazzo Rospigliosi Pallavicini Roma*. Rome: Nuova Àrgos, 1996.

Nelson, Jonathan. "Creative Patronage: Luca Martini and the Renaissance Portrait." *Mitteilungen des Kunsthistorisches Institutes in Florenz* 39 (1995): 285–93.

Niccoli, Ottavia. *Prophecy and People in Renaissance Italy*. Translated by Lydia G. Cochrane. Princeton: Princeton University Press, 1990.

Nonni, Giorgio, ed. *Costanzo Felici: Lettere a Ulisse Aldrovandi*. Introduction by Giuseppe Olmi. Urbino: Quattro Venti, 1982.

Norwich, I. "A Consultation between Andreas Vesalius and Ambroise Paré at the Deathbed of Henri II, King of France, 15 July 1559." *SAMJ* 80, no. 5 (1991): 245–47.

O'Bryan, Robin Leigh. *The Dwarf in Italian Renaissance Iconography*. Unpublished thesis, San Diego State University, 1991.

O'Bryan, Robin Leigh. *The Grotesque in Medici Taste and Patronage*. Unpublished dissertation, University of Virginia, 2000.

O'Connor, Eugene. "Panormita's Reply to His Critics: The Hermaphroditus and the Literary Defense." *Renaissance Quarterly* 50, no. 4 (Winter 1997): 985–1010.

Ollincan, C. d'. *Eunuchism Display'd: Describing All the Different Sorts of Eunuchs; ... Written by a Person of Honour*. London: E. Curll, 1718.

Olmi, Giuseppe. *Ulisse Aldrovandi: Scienza e natura nel secondo cinquecento*. Trent: UNIcoop, 1976.

Olmi, Giuseppe. "Il collezionismo scientifico." In *Il teatro della natura di Ulisse Aldrovandi*, edited by Raffaella Simili. Bologna: Editrice Compositori, 2001.

Olmi, Giuseppe and Paolo Prodi. "Art, Science, and Nature in Bologna Circa 1600." In *The Age of Correggio and the Carracci: Emilian Painting of the Sixteenth and Seventeenth Centuries*. Introduction by Giuliano Briganti. Washington, D.C.: National Gallery of Art, 1986.

Olson, Todd P. "'Long Live the Knife': Andrea Sacchi's Portrait of Marcantonio Pasqualini." *Art History* 27, no. 5 (November 2004): 697–722.

Ortiz, Antonio Dominguez, Alfonso E. Pérez Sánchez and Julián Gállego, eds. *Velázquez*. New York: Harry N. Abrams, 1989.

Otto, Beatrice K. *Fools Are Everywhere: The Court Jester around the World*. Chicago and London: University of Chicago Press, 2001.

Ovid. *Metamorphoses*. As presented in *Ovid: Metamorphoses*. Translated by Stanley Lombardo and with an introduction by W.R. Johnson. Indianapolis and Cambridge: Hackett Publishing, 2010.

Pallister, Janis L. *Ambroise Paré: On Monsters and Marvels*. Chicago and London: University of Chicago Press, 1982.

Panormita, Antonio. *Hermaphroditus*. Translated by Eugene O'Connor. Lanham, Boulder, New York and Oxford: Lexington Books, 2001.

Paravicini-Bagliani, Agostino. *The Pope's Body*. Chicago and London: University of Chicago Press, 2000.

Paré, Ambroise. *Vingt cinquième livre traitant des monstres et prodiges*. Paris: G. Buon, 1585.

Paré, Ambroise. *Les Oeuvres d'Ambroise Paré, conseiller et premier chirurgien du roy. Divisées en vingt huict Livres, Avec les figures & portraicts, tant de l'Anatomie, que des instruments de Chirurgie, & de plusieurs Monstres. Revueuës & augmentees par l'Autheur*, 4th edition (Paris: Gabriel Buon, 1585).

Paré, Ambroise. *Des monstres et prodiges*. Translated and annotated by Jean Céard. Geneva: Librairie Droz, 1971.

Park, Katharine. *Doctors and Medicine in Early Renaissance Florence*. Princeton: Princeton University Press, 1985.

Park, Katharine. "The Criminal and the Saintly Body: Autopsy and Dissection in Renaissance Italy." *Renaissance Quarterly* 47, no. 1 (Spring 1994): 1–33.

Park, Katharine. "The Life of the Corpse: Division and Dissection in Late Medieval Europe." *Journal of the History of Medicine and Allied Sciences* 50 (1995): 111–32.

Park, Katharine. *Secrets of Women: Gender, Generation, and the Origins of Human Dissection*. New York: Zone Books, 2006.

Park, Katharine and Lorraine Daston, eds. *The Cambridge History of Science: Early Modern Science*. Volume 3. Cambridge: Cambridge University Press, 2006.

Parker, Deborah. *Bronzino: Renaissance Painter as Poet*. Cambridge: Cambridge University Press, 2000.

Pastore, Alessandro. *Il medico in tribunale: La perizia medica nella procedura penale d'antico regimo (secoli XVI–XVIII)*. Bellinzona: Edizioni Casagrande, 1998.

Pastore, G.A. "Un raro documento su l'evirazione dei cantanti nel secolo XVII." *Letture dell'Accademia Salentina di Lettere Scienze e Arti* 1, no. 2 (April 1955).

Pattanaro, Alessandra. *Girolamo da Carpi: Ritratti*. Padua: Bertoncello Artigrafiche, 2000.

Paulson, Michael G. *Catherine de Medici: Five Portraits*. New York: Peter Lang, 2002.

Pérez Sánchez, Alfonso E. and Nicola Spinosa. *Jusepe de Ribera 1591–1652*. New York: Harry Abrams, 1992.

Piccinelli, Roberta. *Le Collezioni Gonzaga, il carteggio tra Firenze e Mantova (1554–1626)*. Milan: Silvana Editoriale, 2000.

Pierini, Giovanni. *Venefici dalle Quaestiones medico legales di Paolo Zacchia*. Milan: Colonna Mimesis, 2001.

Pinelli, Antonio, ed. *Storia di Roma dall'antichità a oggi*. Rome and Bari: Gius. Laterza & Figli Spa, 2001.

Platt, Peter G., ed. *Wonder, Marvels, and Monsters in Early Modern Culture*. Newark: University of Delaware Press, 1999.

Platter, Felix. *Observationum in Hominis Affectibus plerisa corporie animo, functionum laesione, dolore, aliave molestia et vitio intommodantibus*. Basel: Ludovici König and Conradi Waldkirchii, 1614.

Pliny the Elder. *Natural History*. Translated by H. Rackham. Cambridge: Harvard University Press, 1956–66.

Pomata, Gianna and Nancy G. Siraisi, eds. *Historia: Empiricism and Erudition in Early Modern Europe*. Cambridge and London: The MIT Press, 2005.

Pomian, Krzysztof. *Collectors and Curiosities: Paris and Venice 1500–1800*. Cambridge: Polity Press, 1990.

Pope-Hennessy, John. *The Portrait in the Renaissance*. New York: Bollingen Foundation, 1966.

Porta, Giovan Battista della. *Della fisonomia dell'uomo*. Edited by Mario Cicognani. Parma: Ugo Guanda Editore, 1988.

Pottinger, George. *The Court of the Medici*. London: Croom Helm, 1978.

Privitera, Marta. *Girolamo Macchietti: Un pittore dello Studiolo di Francesco I (Firenze 1535–1592)*. Milan and Rome: Jandi Sapi Editori, 1996.

Provincia di Firenze, Pratolino, Laboratorio di Meraviglie. *L'Appennino del Giambologna-Anatomia e identità del gigante*. Florence: Alinea Editrice, 1990.

Prunières, Henri. *L'opéra italien en France avant Lully*. Paris: Champion, 1913.

Purcell, Rosamond. *Special Cases: Natural Anomalies and Historical Monsters*. San Francisco: Chronicle Books, 1997.

Ragionamenti del Signor Cavaliere Giorgio Vasari pittore e architetto aretino sopra le invenzioni da lui dipinte in Firenze nel Palazzo di loro altezze serenissime con lo illustriss. Ed eccellentiss. Signore D. Francesco Medici allure Principe di Firenze insieme con la invenzione della pittura da lui cominciata nella cupola. Con due tavole, une delle cose più notabili, e l'altra degli Uomini Illustri che sone ritratti, e nominate un quest'opera. Arezzo: Michele Bellotti, 1762.

Ramsden, E.H. *"Come, Take This Lute": A Quest for Identities in Italian Renaissance Portraiture*. Salisbury: Element Books, 1983.

Ravin, James G. and Gerard P. Hodge. "Hypertrichosis Portrayed in Art," *JAMA* 207, no. 3 (1969): 533–35.

Riolan, Jean. *Discours sur les hermaphrodits où il est demonstré contre l'opinion commune, qu'il n'y a point de vrays hermaphrodits*. Paris: Pierre Ramier, 1614.

Ripa, Cesare. *Iconologia*. Rome: Fei, 1603.

Ripa, Cesare. *Baroque and Rococo Pictorial Imagery: The 1758–60 Hertel Edition*. Edited by Edward A. Maser. New York: Dover Publications, 1971.

Riquet, M. *La Castration*. Paris: P. Lethielleux, Libraire-Éditeur, 1948.

Rivosecchi, Valerio. *Esotismo in Roma Barocca*. Rome: Bulzoni Editore, 1982.

Robertson, Clare. *"Il Gran Cardinale": Alessandro Farnese, Patron of the Arts*. New Haven and London: Yale University Press, 1992.

Rocke, Michael. *Forbidden Friendships: Homosexuality and Male Culture in Renaissance Florence*. New York: Oxford University Press, 1996.

Rogers, Mary, ed. *Fashioning Identities in Renaissance Art*. Aldershot and Brookfield: Ashgate, 2000.

Roper, Lyndal. *Oedipus and the Devil: Witchcraft, Sexuality and Religion in Early Modern Europe*. Routledge: London and New York, 1994.

Rose, Gloria. "Pasqualini as Copyist." *Studien zur italienisch-deutschen Musikgeschichte* 9, no. 4 (1974): 170–75.

Roskill, Mark and Craig Harbison. "On the Nature of Holbein's Portraits." *Word and Image* 3, no. 1 (January–March 1987): 1–26.

Rosselli, John. "The Castrati as a Professional Group and a Social Phenomenon, 1550–1850." *Acta Musicologica* 60, no. 2 (May–August 1988): 143–79.

Rosselli, John. "From Princely Service to the Open Market: Singers on Italian Opera and Their Patrons, 1600–1850." *Cambridge Opera Journal* 1, no. 1 (1989): 113–37.

Rosselli, John. *Singers of Italian Opera: The History of a Profession*. Cambridge: Cambridge University Press, 1992.

Rossi, Paolo L. "*Sprezzatura*, Patronage, and Fate: Benvenuto Cellini and the World of Words." In *Vasari's Florence: Artists and Literati at the Medicean Court*, edited by Philip Jacks. Cambridge: Cambridge University Press, 1998.

Rowland, Ingrid D. *The Ecstatic Journey: Athanasius Kircher in Baroque Rome*. Chicago: University of Chicago Libraries, 2000.

Rudakova, Irina V. *"Uncertain Nature": History of the Castrato Singer in the Early Modern Gender Paradigm*. Dissertation, University of Washington, 1999.

Rudolph, Stella. *Niccolò Maria Pallavicini: L'ascesa al Tempio della Virtù attraverso il Mecenatismo*. Rome: Ugo Bozzi Editore, 1995.

Rupp, Jan C.C. "Matters of Life and Death: The Social and Cultural Conditions of the Rise of Anatomical Theatres, with Special Reference to Seventeenth Century Holland." *History of Science* 28 (1990): 263–86.

Rushdie, Salman. *The Enchantress of Florence*. New York: Random House, 2009.

Saslow, James M. *Ganymede in the Renaissance: Homosexuality in Art and Society*. New Haven and London: Yale University Press, 1986.

Saunders, J.B. deC. M. and Charles O'Malley. *The Illustrations from the Works of Andreas Vesalius of Brussels*. New York: Dover Publications, 1950.

Sawday, Jonathan. *The Body Emblazoned: Dissection and the Human Body in Renaissance Culture*. London and New York: Routledge, 1995.

Scappini, Cristiana and Maria Pia Torricelli. *Lo studio Aldrovandi in Palazzo Pubblico (1617 1742)*. Edited by Sandra Tugnoli Pattaro. Bologna: Cooperativa Libraria Universitaria Editrice, 1993.

Scarabelli, Pietro Francesco and Paolo Maria Terzago. *Museo, ò Galleria: Adunata del sapere, e dallo studio del Sig. Canonico Manfredo Settala nobile Milanese decritta in Latin deal Sig. Dott. Fis. Colleg. Paolo Maria Terzago. Et poi in italiano dal Sig. Pietro Francesco Scarabelli Dottor Fisico di Voghera, & dal medemo accresciuta. Et hora ristampata con l'Aggiunta di diverse cose poste nel fine de medemi Capi dell'Opra ed*. Tortona: 1677.

Schaefer, Scott. "The Studiolo of Francesco I de'Medici: A Checklist of the Known Drawings." *Master Drawings* 20, no. 2 (Summer 1982): 125–30.

Scheicher, Elisabeth. *Die Kunst- und Wunderkammern der Habsburger*. Vienna: Molden Edition, 1979.

Schneider, Norbert. *L'art du portrait: Les plus grandes oeuvres européennes 1420–1670*. Cologne: Benedikt Taschen, 1994.

Scheugl, Hans. *Showfreaks and Monsters*. Cologne: Verlag M. DuMont Schauberg, 1975.

Schlosser, Julius von. "Italienische Kuriositätenkammern." In *Dir Kunst- und Wunderkammern der Spätrenaissance*. Leipzig: Klinkhardt & Biermann, 1908.

Schmidt, Olaf. *"Callots fantastisch karikierte Blätter": Intermediale Inszenierungen und romantische Kunsttheorie im Werk E.T.A. Hoffmanns*. Berlin: Erich Schmidt, 2003.

Schneider, Norbert. *L'art du portrait: Les plus grandes oeuvres européennes 1420–1670*. Cologne: Benedikt Taschen, 1994.

Scholz, Piotr O. *Eunuchs and Castrati: A Cultural History*. Princeton: Markus Wiener Publishers, 2001.

Schultz, Bernard. *Art and Anatomy in Renaissance Italy*. Ann Arbor: UMI Research Press, 1985.

Scott, Jonathan. *Salvator Rosa: His Life and Times*. New Haven and London: Yale University Press, 1995.

Secchi Tarugi, Luisa. *Disarmonia brutezza e bizzarria nel Rinascimento*. Florence: Franco Cesati Editore, 1995.

Sherr, Richard. "Gugliemo Gonzaga and the Castrati." *Renaissance Quarterly* 33, no. 1 (Spring 1980): 33–56.

Simon, Robert B. "Bronzino's 'Cosimo I de'Medici as Orpheus.'" *Philadelphia Museum of Art Bulletin* 81, no. 348 (Autumn 1985): 16–27.

Siraisi, Nancy. *Medieval and Early Renaissance Medicine: An Introduction to Knowledge and Practice*. Chicago: University of Chicago Press, 1990.

Sitwell, Sacheverell. *Baroque and Rococo*. New York: G.P. Putnam's Sons, 1967.

Sleptzoff, L.M. *Men or Supermen? The Italian Portrait in the Fifteenth Century*. Jerusalem: The Magnes Press, The Hebrew University, 1978.

Smith, Alistair. *Renaissance Portraits*. London: The National Gallery, 1973.

Smith, D.W. *Recognizable Patterns of Human Malformations*. Philadelphia: W.B. Saunders, 1976.

Smith, Norman R. "Portentous Births and the Monstrous Imagination in Renaissance Culture." In *Marvels, Monsters, and Miracles: Studies in the Medieval and Early Modern Imaginations*, edited by Timothy S. Jones and David A. Sprunger. Kalamazoo: Board of the Medieval Institute, 2002.

Soldini, Francesco Maria. *Il reale giardino di Boboli nella sua pinata e nelle sue statue*. Rome: Multigrafice Editrice, 1976.

Soler Quintes, Nicolás. "Nuevas aportaciones a la biografia de Carlo Broschi Farinelli." *Anuario Musical* 3 (1948): 187–204.

Spilleth, Meg. "The Text in the Jar: Reading the Anatomical *Kunstkammer*." *Eighteenth Century Life* 19 (May 1995): 28–37.

Spinks, Jennifer. *Monstrous Births and Visual Culture in Sixteenth-century Germany*. London: Pickering & Chatto, 2009.

Summers, David. *Michelangelo and the Language of Art*. Princeton: Princeton University Press, 1981.

Summers, David. *The Judgment of Sense: Renaissance Naturalism and the Rise of Aesthetics*. Cambridge: Cambridge University Press, 1987.

Symcox, Geoffrey, Giovanna Rabitti and Peter D. Diehl, eds. *Italian Reports on America 1493–1522: Letters, Dispatches, and Papal Bulls. Repertorium Colombianum X*. Turnhout: Brepols Publishers, 2001.

Taruffi, Cesare. *Storia della teratologia*. Volumes 1 and 4. Bologna: Regia Tipografia, 1881 and 1886.

Taylor, Gary. *Castration: An Abbreviated History of Western Manhood*. New York and London: Routledge, 2002.

Ternois, Daniel. *Jacques Callot: Catalogue complet de son oeuvre dessinée*. Paris: F. de Nobele, 1962.

The Medici, Michelangelo, and the Art of Late Renaissance Florence. New Haven and London: Yale University Press, 2003.

Thijssen, J.M. "Twins as Monsters: Albertus Magnus's Theory of the Generation of Twins and Its Philosophical Context." *Bulletin of the History of Medicine* 61 (1987): 237–46.

Thomson, Rosemarie Garland. *Extraordinary Bodies: Figuring Physical Disability in American Culture and Literature*. New York: Columbia University Press, 1997.

Tietze-Conrat, E., *Dwarfs and Jesters in Art*. New York: Phaidon, 1957.

Torrino, Maurizio. *Giovan Battista Della Porta nell'Europa del suo tempo*. Naples: Guida Editori, 1990.

Toscan, Jean. *Le carnaval du langage: Le lexique érotique des poètes de l'équivoque du Burchiello à Marino (Xve–XVIIe siècles)*. Lille: Presses Universitaires de Lille, 1981.

Trkulja, Silvia Meloni. "Leopolodo de'Medici collezionista." *Paragone* 26 (1975): 1538.

Trkulja, Silvia Meloni. *Al servizio del Granduca*. Florence: Centro Di, 1980.

Tucker, Mark S. "Discoveries Made during the Treatment of Bronzino's Cosimo I de'Medici as Orpheus." *Philadelphia Museum of Art Bulletin* 81, no. 348 (Autumn 1985): 28–32.

Tugnoli, Sandra Pattaro. *La formazione scientifica e il "Discorso naturale" di Ulisse Aldrovandi*. Trent: UNIcoop, 1977.

Tugnoli , Sandra Pattaro. *Metodo e sistema delle scienze nel pensiero di Ulisse Aldrovandi*. Bologna: Clueb, 1981.

Valton, Edmond. *Les monstres dans l'art: Êtres humains et animaux, bas-reliefs, rinceaux, fleurons, etc.* Paris: Ernest Flammarion, 1905.

Vasari, Giorgio. *Lives of the Painters, Sculptors, and Architects*. Translated by Gaston du C. de Vere. Volumes 1 and 2. New York and Toronto: Alfred A. Knopf, 1996.

Veen, Henk Th. van. *Cosimo I de'Medici and His Self-Representation in Florentine Art and Culture*. Translated by Andrew P. McCormick. Cambridge: Cambridge University Press, 2006.

Vesalius, Andreas. *De humani corporis fabrica*. Basel: Oporinus, 1555.

Walker Bynum, Caroline. *Fragmentation and Redemption: Essays on Gender and the Human Body in Medieval Religion*. New York: Zone Books, 2002.

Walton, Michael T., Robert Fineman and Phyllis J. Walton. "Of Monsters and Prodigies: The Interpretation of Birth Defects in the Sixteenth Century." *American Journal of Medical Genetics* 47, no. 1 (August 1993): 7–13.

Walton, Michael T., Robert M. Fineman and Phyllis J. Walton. "Why Can't a Woman Be More Like a Man? A Renaissance Perspective on the Biological Basis for Female Inferiority." *Women and Health* 24, no. 4 (1996): 87–95.

Walton, Michael T., Robert M. Fineman and Phyllis J. Walton. "Holy Hermaphrodites and Medical Facts: The Depiction of Hermaphrodites in Alchemy and Medicine." *Studies in Hermeticism: Cauda Pavonis* 18, nos. 1 and 2 (Spring and Fall 1999): 32–36.

Waquet, Françoise. *Le latin ou l'empire d'un signe: XVIe–XXe siècle*. Paris: Albin Michel, 1998.

Warnke, Martin. *L'artiste et la cour: Aux origines de l'artiste moderne*. Paris: Éditions de la Maison des Sciences de l'Homme, 1989.

Welsford, Enid. *The Fool: His Social and Literary History*. London: Faber and Faber, 1935.

Wendelin, Daniel S., David N. Pope and Susan B. Mallory. "Hypertrichosis." *Journal of the American Academy of Dermatology* 48, no. 2 (February 2003): 161–82.

Wiesner-Hanks, Merry. *The Marvelous Hairy Girls: The Gonzales Sisters and Their Worlds*. New Haven and London: Yale University Press, 2009.

Wiles, Bertha Harris. *The Fountains of Florentine Sculptors and Their Followers from Donatello to Bernini*. Cambridge: Harvard University Press, 1933.

Wilson, Bronwen M.S. *"The Eye of Italy": The Image of Venice and Venetians in Sixteenth-century Prints*. Dissertation, Northwestern University, 1999.

Wilson, Jean D. and Claus Roehrborn. "Long-term Consequences of Castration in Men: Lessons from the Skoptzy and the Eunuchs of the Chinese and Ottoman Courts." *The Journal of Clinical Endocrinology and Metabolism* 84, no. 12 (1999): 4324–31.

Wind, Barry. *"A Foul and Pestilent Congregation": Images of "Freaks" in Baroque Art*. Brookfield: Ashgate, 1998.

Wittkower, Rudolf. "Marvels of the East: A Study in the History of Monsters." *Journal of the Warburg and Courtauld Institutes* 5 (1942): 159–97.

Wohl, Helmut. *The Aesthetics of Italian Renaissance Art: A Reconsideration of Style*. Cambridge: Cambridge University Press, 1999.

Woodall, Joanna, ed. *Portraiture: Facing the Subject*. Manchester and New York: Manchester University Press, 1997.

Woods-Marsden, Joanna. *Renaissance Self-Portraiture: The Visual Construction of Identity and the Social Status of the Artist*. New Haven and London: Yale University Press, 1998.

Wynne-Davies, R., C.M. Hall and A.G. Apley. *Atlas of Skeletal Dysplasias*. Edinburgh: Churchill Livingstone, 1985.

Wyss, Edith. *The Myth of Apollo and Marsyas in the Art of the Italian Renaissance: An Inquiry into the Meaning of Images*. Newark and London: University of Delaware Press and Associated University Presses, 1996.

Zacchiae Romani, Pauli, totius status ecclesiastici proto-medici generalis. *Quaestionum medico-legalium, tomi tres. Editio prima Veneta, Lugdunensi & Noribergensi, quae passim soedis scatebant erroribus multò emendiator: Accedunt Interpolationes, & Auctaria ex novis Inventis & Observationibus Recentiorum Auctorum. Curà Joannis Danielis Horstii, Diversorum S.R.I. Principum Archiatri, & Collegii Medici Moeno-Francofurtani Senioris. Opus omnibus medicinae et juris utriusque peritis, Necnon Tribunalium (Ecclesiastici, Civilis) Assessoribus maximè necessarium* (Venice: Bonifacii Viezzeri, Superiorum Permissu, 1737).

Zanca, Attilio. "Mostri nelle leggende popolare." In *I naifs e l'arte popolare* (Rome, 1975)

Zanrè, Domenico. *Cultural Non-Conformity in Early Modern Florence*. Burlington: Ashgate, 2004.

Zapperi, Roberto. "Arrigo le Velu, Pietro le Fou, Amon le Nain et autres bêtes: Autour d'un tableau d'Agostino Carrache." *Annales: Économies – Sociétés – Civilisations* 40, no. 2 (March–April 1985): 307–27.

Zapperi, Roberto. *Un buffone e un nano fra due cardinali: Aspetti della comicità a Roma nell'ultimo Cinquencento*. Rome: Fondazione Camillo Caetani, 1995.

Zapperi, Roberto. *Il selvaggio gentiluomo: L'incredibile storia di Pedro Gonzalez e dei suoi figli*. Rome: Donzelli, 2005.

Zorach, Rebecca. *The Virtual Tourist in Renaissance Rome: Printing, Collecting, and the Speculum Romanae Magnificentiae*. Chicago: University of Chicago Press, 2008.

Index